Third World Challenge
to Psychiatry

Third World Challenge to Psychiatry

Culture Accommodation and Mental Health Care

HOWARD N. HIGGINBOTHAM

An East-West Center Book
from the Institute of Culture and Communication

Published for the East-West Center
by the University of Hawaii Press

Library of Congress Cataloging in Publication Data

Higginbotham, Howard N., 1949–
  Third World challenge to psychiatry.

  "An East-West Center book from the East-West Culture
Learning Institute."
  Bibliography: p.
  Includes index.
  1. Mental health services—Asia, Southeastern.
2. Mental health services—Taiwan. 3. Mental health
services—Philippines. 4. Mental health services—
Thailand. 5. Psychiatry, Transcultural. I. East-West
Center. Culture Learning Institute. II. Title. [DNLM:
1. Culture. 2. Developing countries. 3. Ethnopsychology.
4. Mental health services—Asia, Southeastern. 5. Mental
health services—Taiwan. 6. Psychiatry. WM 30 H635t]
RA790.7.A785H54   1984   362.2'0959   83-24259
ISBN 0-8248-0894-0 (pbk.)

With abundant thanks
Alena Shelburne
Anthony J. Marsella

Contents

Illustrations

Tables

Preface

The student of social science who traverses the interface of two disciplines will encounter a wellspring of captivating research questions. In 1976, I was fortuitously assigned the task of preparing a critique of Juris Draguns and Raymond Prince's contributions to the encyclopedic *Handbook of Cross-Cultural Psychology*. Through that rare vantage I gained an overview of culture and psychopathology studies in juxtaposition with the literature describing culture and psychotherapy. It became obvious that theoretical and applied research were disconnected. Health planners and service innovators were in no way guided by the thinking and research on the relationship between culture and psychopathology, its causes and its treatment.

From that moment my course was clear. I would commit my energies toward bridging this hiatus by addressing three questions: First, in what ways does culture impinge upon the delivery of formal psychological care? Second, in what fashion should a system of mental health services adapt or accommodate itself to gain a closer fit with the community's distinct culture pattern? Third, will a closer fit maximize acceptance, use, and satisfaction with a service as well as minimize its iatrogenic effects and diminish pressure for disruptive cultural transformation?

Armed with these questions, I scanned the literature and eventually undertook a field study to identify authentic dimensions of culture accommodation which would serve the interests of both community and planner in the development of clinical care systems. Of course, there will be those who insist that these two domains should never be brought together. They feel that studies of culture and mental health can contribute to our theoretical understanding of social processes involved in disorder and its remediation, but that our research should not enter the political marketplace of treatment service development. These voices further argue that the separation of cultural research from psychiatric practice is necessary to prevent social scientists from serving narrow professional interests and aiding the mental health industry to consolidate its power over already scarce community resources. While I sympathize with the view that psychiatric resources are often misdirected, I would argue that it is for this very reason that social scientists must focus on psychiatric service delivery. Through our efforts, clinical problems can be reconceptualized in sociocultural terms, and alienated clinical systems can be transformed into care-giving resources congruent with community-sanctioned modes of healing.

Interestingly, the genesis of my investigation coincided with medical anthropology's expansion into the domain of ethnopsychiatry, crystallized in Arthur Kleinman's new journal, *Culture, Medicine, and Psychiatry.* However, the preparation and execution of my fieldwork in Southeast Asia was undertaken without the benefit of knowing the ethnographic methodologies and theory building of Kleinman, Fabrega, the Goods, Leslie, and the other ethnomedical specialists. My orientation was shaped more by the survey research traditions of cross-cultural psychology, as practiced by my mentor, Tony Marsella, at the University of Hawaii and promulgated through Richard Brislin's projects at the East-West Center Culture Learning Institute. Also, my frame of reference was colored by the concerns of clinical psychologists manning American community mental health centers and the critique of their labors proffered by prevention-oriented community psychologists. Therefore, my approach to understanding culture accommodation was structured by a clinical-experimental reality of verifiable evidence—i.e., ask standardized interview questions, gather responses to attitude scales, and synthesize personal observations of institutional behavior into case study descriptions from which inferences may be drawn.

Initially, the strategy I envisaged for answering the culture accommodation question required a community study in a setting where clinical services are offered to non-Western clients. First, I would describe the model underpinning the provision of extant mental health care by formal organizations. Second, cultural patterns regarding mental health care would be determined through probing client and family expectations of effective treatment modes and descriptions of indigenous healing practices. Authentic dimensions of culture accommodation could thereby be distilled through pinpointing the links between popular expectations and actual institutional practices in response to cultural forms. This strategy defines culture accommodation as the process of representation in the design of agency operations, selected community beliefs, cognitive styles, and patterns of health and healing that enhance user acceptance and diminish disruption of existing folk care practices.

Starting in June, 1977, I sought to implement this general strategy through a seven-month study tour of Southeast Asia sponsored by the Culture Learning Institute. Unfortunately, I had to abandon the original plan of a detailed community study because of turmoil within the institution hosting my proposed investigation. Instead, the opportunity available was to document the status of psychiatric resources throughout Southeast Asia and to assess treatment ideology through the eyes of indigenous professionals. I could also tap conceptions of culture accommodation shared by agency personnel and their judgements of viable accommodation practices. To map community expectations of healing, I had to rely on staff opinions also, as well as ethnographic accounts of the settings visited.

This monograph is a distillation of what I learned through scores of interviews with mental health practitioners and planners as well as observations of the psychiatric facilities they operate. With few exceptions, these findings from three of the Asian countries visited are generalizable to other developing nations in Southeast Asia, and quite probably to most Third World countries around the globe. Chapter 1 provides the reader with a background of how historical and contemporary forces have shaped the evolution of psychiatry in the region. Chapter 2 raises two fundamental challenges to modern psychiatry as a standard for mental health care in the Third World: Is the Western model feasible within the context of developing countries? and, Does psychiatry manifest cultural sensitivity or harbor forces for social transformation?

Chapters 3 through 6 present the results of comprehensive case studies of the mental health systems of Taiwan, the Philippines, and Thailand. I describe for each nation how Western biomedical psychiatry has been transmitted, the formidable barriers preventing achievement of what psychiatrists consider to be a "modern standard of care," and the failure of institutional psychiatry to gain community acceptability, integration, and continuity with prevailing health beliefs. I argue, in conclusion, that the Western model, suitable for some industrialized settings, cannot be lauded as even remotely feasible as a standard for nationwide service delivery in the Third World, and that institutional sites are generally insensitive and isolated in relation to healing customs prescribed in the popular health sector.

The final chapter offers the authors' vision of how psychiatric care can be initially transformed through culture assessment methods and eventually reformulated altogether. The radical reformulation perspective draws upon the ideology of strengthening culture-specific alternatives to institutional intervention. It recasts psychiatric resources into a form that is simultaneously immediate and accessible, community controlled, and an invisible part of community life.

Deep appreciation goes to individuals from Japan, Taiwan, the Philippines, Thailand, Malaysia, Singapore, Indonesia, and Australia who gave their time and resources to help this undertaking. To those dozens of extremely busy professionals who welcomed the traveling investigator with warm Asian hospitality and unselfishly served as key contacts and informants, I offer my most sincere gratitude. A partial list of these generous individuals would include: Dr. E. K. Yeh, Dr. K. K. Hwang, Dr. C. C. Chen, and Ms. Agnes Wu in Taiwan; Philippine professionals Dr. Eleanor Elequin, Ms. Estrella Aragon, Dr. Jaime Castañeda, and the entire staff of the Philippine Mental Health Association; and Dr. Sangun Suwanlert, Mrs. Somsong Suwanlert, Professor Phon Sangsingkeo, Dr. Narongsak Chunnual, and Dr. Chamlong Disayavanish in Thailand.

Professor Anthony J. Marsella was a central force in the genesis of this project. For more than a decade he has devotedly provided the stimulus for my scholarship as well as wise personal counsel, for which I am ever grateful. The East-West Center Culture Learning Institute (now the Institute of Culture and Communication) generously funded the field project and my studies at the University of Hawaii. Greatly appreciated were the untiring support and assistance of Dr. Richard Brislin, Ms. Lyn Anzai, and Mrs. Judy Rantella. Furthermore, I am indebted to the new generation of leadership at the Culture Learning Institute, especially Dr. Geoff White and Mr. Greg Trifonovitch, who have come forward again to support the publication of this manuscript. I thank Professor Marc Pilisuk and the Department of Applied Behavioral Science, University of California at Davis, for allowing me the resources to rework this manuscript into publishable form. Appreciation goes to Marjorie Muecke, Richard Lieban, Arthur Kleinman, and Juris Draguns for their substantive comments on an earlier draft of this manuscript. I also thank Michael Macmillan for performing his eloquent editorial magic on the final draft.

Finally, I am pleased to acknowledge the significant contribution of my coauthor and partner, Dr. Linda H. Connor. She assisted with writing the first and final chapters and offered incisive critical comment on several others. Linda's willingness to join the revision process broke the ice and brought the final report to fruition. My warmest Aloha to them all.

Abbreviations

CGC   Child Guidance Center of Bangkok

CU   University of Chiangmai Department of Psychiatry

DOH   Philippines Department of Health

DMH   Division of Mental Health, Thailand Ministry of Public Health

DMS   Department of Medical Services, Thailand

ECT   Electroconvulsive Therapy

MC   Medical City Hospital, Rizal, Philippines

MHD   Mental Hygiene Division, Philippines Department of Health

MOPH   Ministry of Public Health, Thailand

NACMHC   Northern Area Community Mental Health Center, Taipei

NEDA   National Economic and Development Authority, Philippines

NHA   National Health Administration, Taiwan

NMH   National Mental Hospital, Mandaluyang, Philippines

NTUH   National Taiwan University Hospital, Department of Psychiatry, Taipei

OT   Occupational Therapy

PGH   University of the Philippines General Hospital, Department of Psychiatry, Manila

PHD   Provincial Health Department, Taiwan

PM   Prasri Mahaphodi Regional Mental Hospital, Ubol Province, Thailand

PMHA	Philippine Mental Health Association
PN	Prasart Neurological Hospital, Bangkok
PYO	Pan Ya On Mental Retardation Hospital, Bangkok
RH	Ramathibodi Hospital, Mahidol University, Bangkok
SCP	Somdej Chaopraya Hospital, Bangkok
SH	Srithunya Hospital, Bangkok
SP	Suan Prung Hospital, Chiangmai, Thailand
TCCMHP	Taipei City Community Mental Health Project
TCMHC	Taipei Children's Mental Health Center
TCPC	Taipei City Psychiatric Center
THD	Taipei City Health Department
TSP	Tri-Service Hospital Department of Psychiatry, Taipei
UERM	University of the East, Ramon Magsaysay Hospital, Quezon City
UNESCO	United Nations Educational, Scientific, and Cultural Organization
UST	University of Santo Tomas Hospital, Manila
VL	Victoria Luna Medical Center, Quezon City
VMH	Veterans Memorial Hospital, Quezon City
WFMH	World Federation of Mental Health
WHO	World Health Organization

chapter 1

The Influence of
Western Psychiatry
in Southeast Asia

(WITH THE ASSISTANCE OF
LINDA H. CONNOR)

"Modern" psychiatry has a firm foothold in the developing nations of
Southeast Asia. Western visitors are often surprised to find psychiatry
practiced and taught in capital cities throughout this region. The surprise
stems from an assumption that traditional societies have less stress and,
hence, fewer psychological problems. It also comes from the incongruity
that modern psychiatry could be readily exported to the nonindustrialized world.

An examination of the historical and contemporary conditions underlying the development of psychiatry in Southeast Asia illuminates the
critical forces that have shaped the Western-derived treatment systems
found in this region and the forces that continue to influence efforts to
plan and to expand these services.

HISTORICAL FACTORS

The fifteenth-century voyages of Portuguese traders into Southeast Asia
were harbingers of European colonialism, and this form of domination
did not end until well after World War II in some countries. Beginning in
1619, the Dutch exerted control over large areas of what is now Indonesia, while the Spanish, based in nearby Manila, were transforming the
economy, political structure, and religion of the northern Philippines.
The British were late arrivals, establishing colonies at Penang in 1786 and
Singapore in 1819 at the expense of their Dutch rivals. English involvement in this region was initiated to secure the eastern flank of the Indian
Empire and to protect the shipping routes to China. Only Thailand
escaped the yoke of direct colonization, although it was influenced by
European powers in other ways.

Following the Napoleonic Wars, and spurred on by the Industrial Revolution, Europeans launched a political and commercial offensive in

Southeast Asia which brought most of the territory under their formal control by 1870. As the mercantile powers extended their influence from the coastal harbor towns into the hinterlands, traditional states were annihilated or their rulers became the instruments of indirect rule. In fertile and accessible areas, plantation agriculture often replaced peasants' subsistence cultivation, thereby transforming the conditions of existence of rural populations. Through these offensives grew new sociopolitical structures and apparatuses for public administration as well as an increased dependence of indigenous populations on the vicissitudes of world markets.

Although colonial powers transformed the political and economic life of indigenous populations, their influence in other areas, especially social welfare, is more uneven. Members of local elites, who mediated colonial rule to the masses, often had access to Western-style education, bureaucratic jobs, and medical assistance. The vast majority of the colonized populations remained peripheral to these advantages.

Health care for the most part remained confined to elite urban populations and took the form of individualized medical treatment (see Gunaratne 1981). Very few clinics or hospitals were to be found in rural areas, and peasant populations sought most medical assistance from traditional, village-based practitioners. Limited programs of public vaccinations made some inroads in the war against infectious diseases, primarily smallpox, in the late nineteenth century and the early twentieth century. The Dutch record in Java and Bali, for example, is particularly creditable in this regard. However, for the most part the vast majority of government health resources were directed towards a very small elite population, and it has taken many decades for this imbalance to be remedied in even a small way.

European concepts about mind and body, illness and health, do not always articulate well with indigenous conceptions, and this is never truer than in the case of the ideas about mental illness and its treatment that the newcomers brought to their colonies (Marsella and White 1982). In the earlier years of colonization, the British, Portuguese, Dutch, and others incarcerated disturbed individuals along with common criminals. Secular definitions of madness had already overtaken medieval religious notions, but had yet to be tempered with a disease-oriented approach to the phenomenon. It is fair to say that in the early nineteenth century Westerners had somewhat less sophisticated therapeutics than native healers in the region who practiced many forms of community-based psychotherapy.

Institutional and custodial care began in Southeast Asia and the United States at approximately the same time. Colonial powers were not averse to confining political dissidents as well as deviants in these institu-

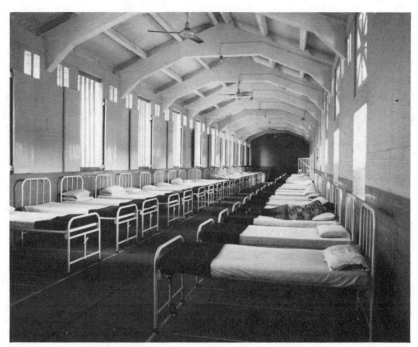

Enormous, rambling dormitories housing dozens of patients in a single space are hallmarks of British-designed facilities, such as this one in Singapore.

tions (see, for example, Van der Kraan 1980). The earliest mental hospitals in this region preceded by a decade the opening of city mental hospitals in New York and Boston as well as Dorothea Dix's quest to hospitalize every "insane" individual, ending "moral" treatment in the United States. In 1829 Penang had a "lunatic asylum" populated by Chinese, Portuguese, and Indians (Tan and Wagner 1971). H. B. M. Murphy's (1971) search of records in Singapore yielded an 1841 decree to "lose no time in commencing the erection of an Insane Hospital" (p. 14). Twenty years after it opened, this hospital, accommodating 100 patients for a colony of 82,000, was providing Singapore with a higher psychiatric bed ratio than that of the United States.

By the close of the nineteenth century, colonial architects and health administrators had created rambling custodial enclaves—all remarkably alike—stretching from India to Southeast Asia (Haq 1975; Setyonegoro 1976; Tan and Wagner 1971). Even the Royal Thai Government had in 1912 engaged British architects and administrators to create a mental health system in that country. These facilities were isolated and alien to the culture of their surrounding populations, and for this reason alone it is not surprising that they were regarded as a last resort. Often built in rural zones remote from areas of dense population, these institutions aimed only at custodial care of inmates to protect the community at large. Largely untrained staffs functioned more as jailers than as care-takers or therapists. Of course, for most referrals the mental hospital was the end of the road (Harding 1975), and the ominous images associated with such an institution still shapes the perceptions of surrounding popu-lations. The names of towns where large mental hospitals were founded are now synonymous with "madness." Their historical administrators are sometimes household names, who are jokingly threatened to be sent for when someone behaves oddly.

Such psychiatric facilities, increasingly cut off from the mainstream of medical and psychological theory in the Western cultures that spawned them, and oblivious to the more global, spiritual, and humanistic notions of health and illness amongst the populations they supposedly served, did not disappear in the years of national independence after World War II. Indigenous elites, just as cut off from local rural cultures as their colonial mentors had been, had no resources with which to bridge the immense gulf between indigenous ideas and practices and these imported institutions. The fortunate few who could afford it were offered individ-ual psychotherapy by privately practicing psychiatrists in affluent urban locales; the majority of sufferers continued to arrive at the mental hospi-tals only when more accessible and comprehensible community-based forms of care had been exhausted. Colonialism had not offered the newly independent countries any realistic or innovative means with which to come to terms with their problems as developing countries, in health care as in many other spheres.

CONTEMPORARY FACTORS

National independence did not end the pattern of colonial psychiatry in Southeast Asia, nor did it herald the resurgence of indigenous healing forms as a serious component of government social welfare policy. In-stead, several factors have combined to insure the continued importation and expansion of Western therapeutics to the exclusion of locally availa-ble alternatives. These include governmental requests based on national development needs; the unsettling effects of rapid "modernization" on mental health; the rationale that psychiatric medicine is transcultural and disorders are uniformly identifiable; and the standards of international consultation and training, which offer no alternatives to this form of mental health planning. The following sections examine these factors in relation to establishing a need, rationale, and means for psychiatric care.

ESTABLISHING A NEED FOR PSYCHIATRIC CARE

Governmental Request Based on National Development Needs

The quest for economic and industrial development is the principal organizer of national priorities in Southeast Asia. Nationalist leaders are ushering in "modernization" with breathtaking intensity to offset their countries' dependency on the world's more advanced states (Butwell 1975). Modernization is also expected to bring a higher standard of living and a fuller life for the people through expanded educational and job opportunities and improved health conditions. To the extent that social welfare services and management of the psychologically distressed can contribute to these development goals, such services are given governmental attention.

Several writers have sought to link psychiatry with national development. Among them, Kiev (1972, 1976) and Benyoussef, Collomb, Diop, and Zollner (1975) have made the strongest case for including mental health as a national priority. They use a cost-benefit logic to argue that mental *ill* health is detrimental to socioeconomic development. Mental illness is depicted as a national burden because disordered individuals have a smaller chance of participating in the full range of employment roles and attaining job productivity. Kiev (1972) further points out the critical need for human resources and the unaffordable loss arising from mental problems among college students, technical specialists, and government leaders. In a struggling economy, there is also a disproportionately greater impact of such problems on absenteeism, poor motivation, and crime and drug addiction, as well as the economic strain of long-term patients. Kiev (1976) asserts that psychiatry is a valuable tool for development when its techniques can be employed to motivate and commit people to the development process and prepare individual initiative towards modernization.

The struggle to modernize and the need to prepare citizens for new social and economic roles has moved some governments to request psychiatry's participation in the process. In this respect, psychiatry has two functions: to set up a "modern" social institution supporting the philosophy of development and to alleviate its negative human consequences. Modernization is a two-edged sword, a topic considered next.

Stress from Socioeconomic Change

Irrespective of present priorities, there is consensus among indigenous professionals, international consultants, and researchers throughout developing countries that psychological problems are on the upswing and that socioeconomic transformation is clearly to blame (Burton-Bradley

1973; Cawte 1972; Kiernan 1976; Lin 1981; Marsella 1978; Murphy 1955; Sangsingkeo 1966; Santoso 1959). This belief has become a second prompt for health leaders to request and plan for a Western system of care. It is assumed to be the modern solution for meeting the increasing casualties of sociocultural change.

Epidemiological evidence for rising incidence rates in Southeast Asia is sketchy and difficult to document (Hartog 1972a; Kapur 1975). The World Health Organization (WHO 1975a) reports an estimate of 40 million untreated cases of mental illness in world developing regions; perhaps 200 million suffer from less-severe disorders. Trends do show increasing survival rates for brain-damaged children and disorders of the aged as a consequence of public health measures (WHO 1980).

In Indonesia, Widjono (1975) reports an increase in drug abuse, a finding that he attributes to newly found affluence among the youth. This concern has been recently echoed in Singapore, Malaysia, and Thailand with initiation of programs and public education campaigns (e.g., Ratanakorn 1975). In Taiwan, Ko (1975) tried to establish rising rates for depression among urban dwellers, while Lin, Rin, Yeh, Hsu, and Chu (1969) carried out a fifteen-year longitudinal study revealing significant increases in the prevalence of all disorders, particularly among in-migrants there. Kiernan (1976) suggests that Thailand shares with other countries in Southeast Asia a rising prevalence rate due to continued incidence of traditional forms of illness and the appearance of newer patterns related to stress, overindulgence, growing numbers of old people, and iatrogenesis.

In harmony with this, adjustment problems of adolescents at a mental health clinic in the Philippines were attributed to the new technological demands of society (Aragon 1977).

Concern for the mental health effects of industrialization and rapid social transformation among health professionals (e.g., Ignacio 1976; Ko 1975; Prasetyo 1977; Sangsingkeo 1966; Sanvictores 1976) has been stimulated by extensive literature on this topic by Western writers. In particular, researchers have shown an interest in social change (Guthrie 1971; Lindemann 1969; Marsella 1978; Shore and Mannino 1975). Singled out for study are those instances where the fabric of a society cannot endure the pace of change; increased social pathology presumably follows.

Leighton and his colleagues began in the early 1950s to lay a theoretical foundation linking community disorganization with individual impairment (Leighton 1959). They found data suggesting that when the sociocultural setting no longer met essential individual needs, and in fact disrupted patterns of personal striving for security, love, status, and so forth, rates of disorder increased (D. Leighton 1963, 1971).

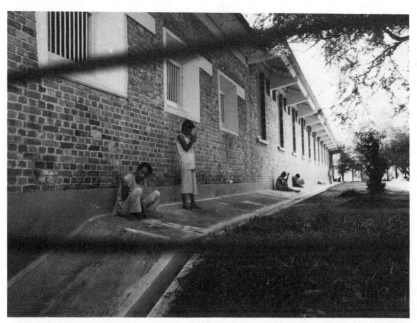

Women patients in an activity yard at a Singapore hospital find solitary space along a wall.

Wittkower is a second influential psychiatrist explaining the tie between culture and disorder (Wittkower and Dubreuil 1973; Wittkower and Termansen 1968). He identifies three pathogenic dimensions of culture: *cultural content,* including taboos, antagonistic values, and role deprivation; stressful *social organization* characterized by anomie or social rigidity; and *social change,* which becomes noxious with the accumulation of value diversity, role deprivation, and heightened anomie.

Undergirding all of these writings is an assumption about the functioning of cultures and societies. Namely, that cultures represent systems with mutually dependent parts. Kluckhohn and Leighton (1946) evolved this conception from their studies of Navajos undergoing acculturation stress. They found that, "instead of a patterned mosaic, Navajo culture is becoming an ugly patchwork of meaningless and totally unrelated pieces . . . [with] personal and social chaos as the byproducts" (p. 237).

Specifically, the complex systems of belief that people share in a society are core elements that hold people together and make enduring social relationships possible. When the belief systems are threatened, the society is in danger of becoming disorganized (Kunitz 1970). This theme, promulgated by influential international psychiatrists, has become the explanatory framework used by mental health professionals for examining the rates of disorder in their rapidly acculturating and developing countries.

Echoing the culture disorganization theme, social observers in Southeast Asia lament and fear the passing of traditional cultural forms and institutions (Kiev 1976). This change was initially restricted to the capital cities when Europeans began it two centuries ago. Now, however, it is spreading beyond its former enclaves to the 80 to 90 percent of the people living in the countryside (Butwell 1975). With the current widespread effects, Kamal (1975) notes the abandonment of the stable, traditional ways of life that gave people security, identity, and perhaps some immunity from mental breakdown. He asks if it is possible to preserve spiritual elements of traditional life—community and family ties, religious convictions—without affecting the desired national "progress."

Other writers have commented on the specific dangers of modernization and abandonment of old ways. Thailand's Professor Phon Sangsingkeo, an enlightened leader of psychiatry in his homeland, points to the effects of technological changes on interpersonal relationships. The extended family is dissolved as machinery makes farming less labor-intensive and young people move toward urban centers. No one remains in the village to care for the old (Sangsingkeo 1966).

Indonesian psychiatrists are concerned that the tremendous speed of change will significantly affect marital patterns and the household authority structure and bind the family with conflicting values as children are socialized to old loyalties that have little meaning for them (Indries 1971; Santoso 1959). Widjono (1975) believes that the youth gangs springing up in Jakarta are a result of the breakdown in the family's ability to maintain the loyal ties of its younger members.

Urbanization has other consequences. Recent migrants are at high risk of disorder as they seek to adjust, usually without a firm economic base, to conditions of overcrowding, poor housing, status loss, sex role changes, depersonalization, crime, and drug addiction (Ignacio 1976; Kiev 1972, 1976; Widjono 1975). The break in cultural continuity—from rural to urban, from traditional to modern—especially affects child-rearing patterns. The family network and value structure are thrown into confusion (Prasetyo 1977; WHO 1981a). Moreover, emergence of the nuclear family under the pressure of urban living further reduces the family's capacity to care for its ill and psychologically distressed (Kiernan 1976). Each member is now required to find work outside the home.

Along with sociocultural disorganization, a second factor, the revolution of rising expectations, has been identified as a determinant of disorder rates. Parker and Kleiner (1966), working with samples of American

Blacks, and Marsella, Escudero, and Gordon (1972), studying urban Filipinos, provide a theoretical understanding of how an individual's aspira-
tions, compared to what is actually achieved, lead to stress and psychiatric symptoms. As suggested by Sangsingkeo (1966) in Thailand and
Sanvictores (1976) in the Philippines, widespread frustration accrues
when people view the goods, services, and life styles of developed countries, yet lack the economic means to secure them.

Pressure on the poor intensifies as they perceive wider horizons
through the mass media, only to find the fruits of national development
reserved for the elite. Poor people, without the resources of a close-knit
family, employment, or a philosophy of life to mediate the frustration,
experience a rise in mental distress (Marsella et al. 1972). As the gap
remains unbridged between what is desired and what is obtained, the
incidence of disorder theoretically increases along with pressure on the
government to provide psychiatric assistance.

Some authors dispute the scenario just depicted. Murphy (1961) points
out that mental health may be either worsened or bettered in some situations of change. Inkeles and Smith (1970), in their six-culture study of
modernization and personal adjustment, found that individual stress is
not an inherent accompaniment of industrialization and urbanization.
These authors concur with Lambo (1978) that village life can be just as
stressful as the urban center. Some young migrants rushing from the
countryside into towns are in fact escaping from an oppressive psychological environment—one with limited roles and individual opportunities.

Irrespective of whether or not modernization per se is related to increases in adjustment problems, mental health workers in the region
believe this to be the case. This perception has led to the request for assistance from WHO and other international consultants for manpower
training and expanded services (Hassler 1971; WHO 1977a, 1981a).

ESTABLISHING A RATIONALE FOR PSYCHIATRIC CARE

A third reason for the continuing exportation of psychiatry is the strong
conviction that Western physicians have in the cross-cultural suitability
of their methods. Practitioners, socialized in biomedical theory, assume
the uniformity of mental illness worldwide (Draguns 1980). Some physi-
cian-investigators admit to cultural coloring of symptoms, especially for
nonpsychotic dysfunctions, yet they believe that the basic disease process
is not culturally determined (Fabrega 1982).

The epidemiological approach for measuring and comparing disorder
rates is predicated on this assumption. A methodological drawback to

using this approach in the past was the lack of agreement among professionals on a worldwide classification scheme and standard procedures for case finding. In the early 1960s, the Scientific Group of Mental Health Research of WHO (1964) made epidemiological research top priority and stimulated the development of the mental illness glossary for the International Classification of Disease (ICD) to alleviate this problem.

A major issue in culture and mental health research has been to demonstrate the universal invariance of disorder manifestations (Draguns and Phillips 1972; Marsella 1982). This impetus has indirectly built support for cross-cultural application of psychiatry. Several studies are often cited as supporting this hypothesis (see Draguns 1980). Casual observation in Thai hospitals led Bowman (1959) to conclude that disorders in Thailand closely resemble those in the United States. Using the same method in Tahiti, Berne (1960) reported that cultural factors are of negligible significance at the hospital level. More systematic in their method of inquiry, Murphy, Wittkower, and Chance (1970) found "primary" or universal symptoms of depression in their thirty-nation survey of practitioners. Comparing Yoruban and Nova Scotian taxonomies of psychological disturbance, A. Leighton, Lambo, Hughes, D. Leighton, Murphy, and Macklin (1963) found convergence on several criteria that these societies use for deciding disorder. This finding was later extended to an Eskimo group by Jane Murphy (1972). She reported that the same disorders were located in all three groups and were recognized as such by culture members and psychiatrists alike.

Summarizing this body of research, and drawing upon anthropological findings from other cultures, Murphy (1976) concluded that patterns, rates, and causes of mental illness are more similar than different for all human groups. She thus rejects the notion that each culture independently shapes psychopathology. The scope of this generalization can be challenged, however, given that her argument rests on cases representing the most severe, chronic, and deteriorated forms of "schizophrenic reaction" (see Fabrega 1982: 54).

The most ambitious project to address this issue, and one which has had a direct impact on international psychiatry, has been the International Pilot Study of Schizophrenia undertaken in nine countries by WHO (1973). This study yielded an impressive demonstration of similarity across facilities in terms of: (1) rank ordering of schizophrenic symptoms as measured by the Present State Exam (Wing et al. 1967); (2) symptom clustering; and (3) the emergence of a core (concordant) group of schizophrenics with identical profiles of dysfunction. Ironically, a two-year follow-up of these schizophrenic patients found very marked

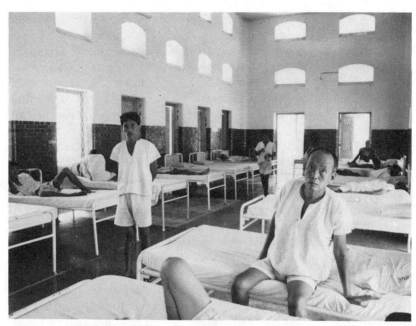

Chinese, Malay, and Indian patients share a large sleeping area in this West Malaysian hospital. Colonial architects adjusted their design to the tropical climate through the use of high, vaulted ceilings and window ventilation.

variability in their prognosis based on cultural setting. Patients in developing countries have more favorable course and outcome than their counterparts in developed countries (Sartorius, Jablensky, and Shapiro 1978). This discovery sparked WHO researchers to take a keen interest in cultural factors and prepare collaborative projects to identify community and family system (as well as biological) variables favoring non-Western schizophrenic patients (WHO 1978b).

Nevertheless, this monumental effort yielded two messages. First, international diagnostic instruments can be developed and interviewers trained to reliably code selected individuals. Secondly, the "disease" of schizophrenia is the same in Denmark and the United States as it is in India, Nigeria, and Colombia, even though its prognosis may vary across cultures. Aside from criticisms of methodology and validity that could be levelled against the results of this project (see Marsella 1982: 372) and other epidemiological and hospital record investigations (e.g., Margetts 1965; Murphy, Wittkower, and Chance 1963), the message for developing countries is quite clear. Namely, that the same mental illness exists everywhere and, by medical analogy, the same disease deserves the same therapeutic interventions.

The studies just reviewed permit another assertion contributing to the exportation of psychiatry: treatment successful in one culture should be successful in another (German 1972; Kamel, Bishry, and Okasha 1975; Kiev 1972; Murphy, Wittkower, and Chance 1970). Giel and Harding (1976) echo the sentiments of a growing number of psychiatrists around the world that an expansion of psychiatric services is overdue, that such services offer viable care, and when provided, will be readily acceptable.

Spearheading the dissemination of mental health technology are psychopharmaceuticals. Psychotropic drugs are touted as an immediate solution to handling the heavy backlog of chronic cases and are seized upon by overburdened physicians (Giel and Harding 1976). Kiev (1972) places high faith in this intervention mode. He urges that an active program based on drugs should be established at the earliest possible moment in developing countries. Among the benefits of drug treatment, according to Kiev, are: elimination of long hospital stays; dramatic effects that change family attitudes toward the patient; establishment of community programs based around drug care; and removal of the patient's symptoms from his or her responsibility, relieving guilt and anxiety and creating faith in treatment.

Other intervention modes have been tried in Southeast Asia as well. Lubis (1975, 1977) has worked steadily to introduce dynamic psychotherapy to Indonesia. In his doctoral dissertation he found that highly educated clients with neurotic problems could benefit with this modality without modifications. The urbanized, educated Indonesian, a tiny minority of the population, is seemingly more suited to psychotherapy than folk therapies (Lubis 1975). Moreover, Indonesia does not have time for trial and error methods in developing its mental health system, so psychotherapy is perceived as a scientific, responsible, and economical choice (Lubis 1975).

Psychiatrists in this region are also trying other interventions. For example, Chen and Yang at the National Taiwan University Hospital have adopted group therapy and behavior modification programs for adults and brain-damaged children. Deva created a day care and industrial rehabilitation program at the University Hospital in Kuala Lumpur. In Bangkok, Suwanlert operates a similar center to promote behavioral adjustment among preschoolers. In the Philippines, token economy wards were begun at the Philippine General Hospital and the Veterans' Administration Hospital. Drug abuse units are springing up within established psychiatric facilities throughout the region. In short, Western therapeutics, whether drugs, psychotherapy, special units, or behavior modification, are perceived as valuable tools for dealing with the mental health problems of Southeast Asia as defined by indigenous professionals.

ESTABLISHING A MEANS FOR PSYCHIATRIC CARE

Once the need for intervention is established, and a rationale offered for the suitability of psychiatry, the next concern becomes the means by which psychiatric technology is transferred and the form it assumes. Several mechanisms have evolved to insure the transference of Western technology in the mental health domain. First, influential health leaders in Southeast Asia received most or all of their professional training in Europe or the United States. Second, international agencies like WHO provide ongoing consultation, coordination, and technical assistance to nations in this region. Through these mechanisms, models have been suggested and tried for assessing mental health needs and designing programs intended to meet those needs. This section details the consultation practices, service delivery models, and needs assessment found in these countries.

Western Training

International psychiatry is the comparative study of problems that arise in teaching, hospital administration, and treatment due to resource shortages in certain settings (Wittkower and Termansen 1968). One solution to problems of this sort is to send trainees to resource-intensive centers in Britain or the United States, for example, to receive specialized instruction. Historically, WHO (1963) and the World Federation for Mental Health (WFMH 1961) endorsed this practice, as did degree-granting facilities in the United States (e.g., Lin 1971; McDermott et al. 1974), the Agency for International Development, and various governments (e.g., Australia Development Assistance Bureau 1977).

The impact of this approach is considerable. The majority of national decision makers in medicine and psychiatry were educated under Western auspices. Supporting this point, Tan (1971) revealed that psychiatry started in Malaysia when the first psychiatrist returned from England. A WHO fellowship provided the first foreign certification for an Indonesian psychiatrist in 1956 when Professor Salan made his way to the Netherlands (Salan 1968). Among the eighty key professionals I interviewed in thirty-four psychiatric agencies in the region, 50 percent received graduate diplomas abroad. Surprisingly, the trend of sending physicians overseas for advanced instruction has not abated (Lin 1981), although early returnees have built specialized courses within home universities and hospitals (e.g., Philippines, Indonesia). Administrators maintain that without complementary programs for disciplinary research, knowledge and practice brought back quickly grow stale, necessitating further trips abroad to update information.

Influence of the World Health Organization

The WHO is a significant influence in Southeast Asia as well as in other developing world regions. At its first meeting thirty years ago, the World Health Assembly approved in principle a set of recommendations from the World Federation for Mental Health (WFMH). These recommendations set in motion WHO's involvement in mental health, which has grown steadily in recent years. Today the WHO Mental Health Division enjoys the status of a "major program," involving interlocking projects, research centers, and collaboration on a truly global level.

The WFMH's guidelines proved enduring as a series of Expert Committees convened to steer the activities of the Mental Health Division and make technical recommendations for programs of research, professional training, standardization of nomenclature, consultation, service delivery alternatives, and regional coordination. The organizing principle, as laid down in the 1949 Expert Committee meeting, has been to work toward the incorporation into public health work of the responsibility for promoting the mental as well as the physical health of the community (Hassler 1971).

A watershed year for the Mental Health Division was 1964. Work initiated by an Expert Committee a few years earlier, devoted to assessing the application of epidemiological methods to developing mental health programs, laid the foundation for a Scientific Group recommendation that a full-scale epidemiological research program be undertaken with the highest priority (Lin 1967). This was to be the first major involvement in research and gave the Mental Health Division the visibility, direction, and energy it needed to establish parity with other programs within WHO. The long-term plan on epidemiology began in 1965 with a four-component research operation (Sartorius 1971): standardization of psychiatric diagnosis; comparative research on specific diseases; epidemiological studies of diseases in geographically defined populations; and training in epidemiology and social psychiatry. Out of this undertaking came the well-known studies comparing diagnostic differences among American and British psychiatrists (Cooper et al. 1972) and the International Pilot Study of Schizophrenia (WHO 1973, 1975d).

Mental health achieved higher prominence when the 1974 and 1975 World Health Assemblies urged the promotion of mental health within the general and public health services. The Assemblies further urged

WHO member states to promote the development of new low-cost treatments, bolster local research potential and information systems, train multiple categories of health workers to manage the mentally ill, and standardize the classification system in mental health (WHO 1978a: 23). The director general was requested to organize multidisciplinary projects examining the influence of "psychosocial" factors (i.e., those involving individual psychology and the functioning of groups) on health, mental health, and health service delivery (WHO 1981b: 65–66). Mental health received the designation "major program" in 1977, further enhancing its status, with budgetary levels proposed—at up to $5 million per year—that would provide the basis for a further evolution of its work (WHO 1977a, 1977e). By 1980 the mental health program had attained both peak visibility within international health circles and strong endorsement by WHO member states (WHO 1978c: 358–364). This was facilitated by articulate and persuasive presentations delivered by WHO leadership describing the program's rationale and new integrated role within WHO (Lambo 1977; Sartorius 1977, 1978).

The newfound prominence of mental health, long considered low man on the medical totem pole, can be linked to a shifting focus in the content and philosophy of the Mental Health Division's activities and to a pioneering effort in formulating its program's organizational structure. In the former case, the new image of mental health eschews dependence upon the medical model of education, psychiatry as a specialized profession, and mental illness per se as its sole defining characteristics. Instead, stress is on the public health and social-psychological aspects of mental health and the "whole team" approach, embracing other social services, the local community, and pertinent social sectors such as education, social welfare, law, labor, and so forth. The multidisciplinary framework gives new roles to anthropology, psychology, and social work, with problems defined as psychosocial in character. Core objectives include the adoption of mental health considerations in overall socioeconomic plans, integration of the former with existing health networks, and movement of psychiatric services and training into the community arena through reliance upon the primary health worker.

Complementing the new image in content is an innovative structure for defining and carrying it out—the Coordinating Group. Structurally there are coordinating groups at the national, regional, and global levels, linked to each other as mechanisms to insure coherence, social relevance, and coordination of all mental health activities (WHO 1977a). This approach is aimed at establishing the highest level of involvement from member states, as well as collaborating institutions, nongovernmental organizations, and the social sciences, and fostering technical cooperation among the developing nations themselves. Coordinating these views and resources is thought to be the key to program effectiveness and relevance to the needs of developing countries.

The first meeting of the Coordinating Group in 1976 yielded the "Medium-Term Program in Mental Health" (WHO 1976). Underpinning the new program is the desire to confront priority problems in developing countries with strategies that are simple, realistic, and culminating in fast results. The four main areas of activity include two new endeavors, psychosocial aspects of human environments and program coordination at all levels, plus two historical foci: development of services and manpower and research to improve, prevent, and treat specific forms of mental disorder.

The action arm of the Mental Health Program involves several mechanisms. First, in response to requests from member states, experts are sent for periods of from one month to four years (Hassler 1971). Consultants sent to Southeast Asia have made a lasting impression with their advice and evaluations (e.g., Kiernan 1976; Lin 1964b; Stoller 1959, 1963). These experts draw upon the latest thinking of WHO and their own countries to recommend policies, projects, and education schemes. An excellent example is E. C. Dax, who in 1962 and 1969 filed assignment reports regarding the proposed expansion of psychiatric programs in Malaysia. His recommendations were modelled after the service that he had established for the State of Victoria in Australia, where he was director of the Mental Health Authority (Tan 1971).

Interestingly, Alan Stoller, who followed Dax as director for the Victoria Authority, was on assignment for WHO and gave a comprehensive set of recommendations for further planning and elaboration of mental health care in Thailand in 1959 and Indonesia in 1963. T. Y. Lin, father of Taiwanese psychiatry, visited Thailand a year after Stoller and established the framework for manpower development and teaching psychiatry to medical students there (Lin 1964b).

Secondly, WHO regional seminars and workshops are devices for implementing program goals. By 1975, five seminars on the teaching of psychiatry in the South-East Asia Region (SEAR) had been successfully held (WHO 1975c, 1977d, 1978a). Output from these events included specific recommendations and technical advice: for example, teaching methods and curriculum for providing personnel with skills for doing community mental health work. Surveys followed-up the recommendations to appraise progress made by member states in meeting the guidelines and noted the barriers that prevent attainment.

Improved coordination among national, regional, and global levels of mental health action is the third mechanism. Following the leadership of the Coordinating Group, SEAR held its first intercountry group meeting in December, 1977, to set up its own regional advisory and coordinating body. An important outcome of this meeting was the decision that each country should have a medium-term program plus an advisory group on mental health. This national group would be vested with the authority to establish priorities, reallocate resources, evaluate and implement projects, and provide continuous input into the national health and social policy-making apparatus (WHO 1978a). By 1981 some twenty countries had established national mental health coordinating groups with members representing health, education, welfare, labor, and other sectors (WHO 1981a: 34).

This second recommendation underscores WHO's present movement to build clout at the national level in its member states and to bring into governmental awareness the new directions and opportunities offered by the Medium-Term Program (WHO 1977a). To insure this, a new project, "Mental Health in National Health Policy Formulation," is proposed to make sure that WHO plays an active role in national policy formulation and cooperates with each country's health authority in the inclusion of mental health within the overall health planning. If WHO's mental health activities are not felt in the drafting of national policy, then their intended effect has been lost.

Fourthly, more than forty WHO collaborating and resource centers are operating in as many countries. Resource centers support the national coordinating groups with their technical advice. While some centers are broadly based to concentrate on the diverse problems of developing countries, others operate more narrowly with specialized research and training on such topics as psychotropic medication effects, drug dependency, mental health benefits of family life, and mental health planning using national-level demographic and social indicators (WHO 1978b: 124–126). They are intended to evolve appropriate technology for prevention and treatment schemes, insure that psychosocial input is felt in social action programs, and carry out WHO research as well as initiate local studies. Both collaborating and resource centers provide needed leadership for formulating and implementing policies and offering health education training models (WHO 1977a).

Lastly, WHO trainee fellowships and collaborative research projects form channels for implementing Mental Health Division objectives. Indonesia, Thailand, and Malaysia cooperated in a project testing an epidemiological case-reporting instrument for gathering data on drug users in contact with treatment facilities (WHO 1978a). The Philippines collaborated with six other developing countries to test the feasibility of assigning primary health workers in local clinics the task of detecting and managing priority mental disorders. Interim results have been used to argue that psychiatric disorders are commonplace among clients using community health posts (from 10.5 to 17.7 percent of adults seen) and that only limited additional resources enable these workers to acquire and use basic mental techniques and safely dispense selected psychoactive drugs.

Five years after the inauguration of this "new image" program, WHO Mental Health Division staff and their consultants sought further philosophical changes and evolution in the program's development. This group produced a far-reaching position paper calling for the "radical rethinking" of mental health principles and activities in harmony with a fundamental value position they offered (WHO 1981a). Their position is that the quality of people's mental life—the capacity to "think, feel, aspire, strive and achieve, and to be social—is what makes people's life valuable" (WHO 1981a: 5). Thus health promotion involves equal attention to: (a) the preservation of human biology and (b) the enhancement of mental life in tandem with preventing disability.

Corollary assumptions and guidelines filling out the program's new framework follow on from this core value. Prominent among these assumptions is, first of all, the assertion that mental health knowledge must become a vital tool for preventing the harmful psychosocial consequences of rapid socioeconomic change and mass migration. Fully discussed are the health promotive effects of maintaining family cohesion, especially in the face of community development, and how mental health principles could guide formulation of legislation and legal procedures. Second, mental health technology integrated into the general health system can improve the health sector's ability to gain community participation and acceptance and offer a psychosocial critique of the all-too-common dehumanizing practices found in medical facilities. Furthermore, the program's architects contend that neuropsychological dysfunctions are indeed preventable and treatable via the application of simple, effective measures. This technology can be effectively delivered to those who have previously found it inaccessible through a system whereby primary health workers are trained to incorporate psychiatric care into local clinic functions. The mental health specialist's role thereby shifts from provider for the selected few to that of an advocate of urgent preventive measures, trainer and supporter of community health workers, as well as researcher developing appropriate knowledge of the roots of psychosocial problems affecting community members.

WHO now enjoys a greatly enhanced capacity to weave the fabric of mental health programming, especially in developing nations. In so doing, it exemplifies the dynamic process of psychiatric technology's ascendence in these settings and raises the unexamined issue of its sociocultural consequences for non-Western peoples—two central foci of this monograph. WHO activities also typify the paradoxes arising when planners, operating within a medical or even "medicosocial" paradigm of disorder, seek to extend service delivery to "unreached" people and places. For example, WHO strives to operate as a facilitator, enabling developing countries to work together sharing their own technical resources and self-developed methods for handling mental health needs as they are understood locally. Yet, the medium-term program's success is apparently predicated on a deepening penetration of its guidelines for assessing mental health legislation, research, and new technology into national decision making.

WHO's expressed philosophy embraces active community participation in setting program priorities arising from self-assessed needs and even providing care for its own members. But the mechanisms that assure local program resource control and allow people to share responsibility for planning their own health systems are not given prominent attention. It may well be that the involvement of primary health workers in this arena will strengthen the grip of centralized health administrators on local healing practices at the expense of traditional sources of self-help and further remove the practitioner's accountability to local interests. Moreover, the WHO position that neuropsychiatric syndromes are by and large expressed identically in different cultures detracts from the importance of attending to the subtle sociocultural context of health and healing. Proponents argue that a safe, simple, and effective set of standard procedures (emphasizing psychotropic medication) can be taught to health workers for handling identified cases. We may well ask, given this accounting, if WHO planners can envision the development of care-giving systems in response to unmet needs which (a) do not further centralize health care at national and international levels and into the hands of an elite circle of health leaders and (b) do not promote the homogenization of treatment ideology into some blend of biomedical psychiatry to the exclusion of alternatives already existing in the form of traditional healing systems?

Service Delivery Models

Mental health technology is skillfully being transmitted into Southeast Asian settings through WHO seminars, consultants, regional meetings, collaborative research, resource centers, and so forth. Yet what form does this technology assume when it reaches a non-Western context? What models of service delivery have been suggested or tried, and what data are amassed in planning for psychiatric systems? Characteristic approaches to needs assessment and treatment delivery are described below.

Needs assessment. Ideally, needs assessment is a systematic procedure for sampling problem domains within a population and deciding priorities for intervention. The process is problematic, however, because it must first be determined who decides what the problems are, the form of assistance necessary for their alleviation, and the type of information required to make these decisions. Potential participants in mental health planning include patients, their families, interested community members, professionals, outside consultants, politicians, and government administrators. The trend in the United States, and that used by WHO (1975a) to make services acceptable in the community, is toward an increasing degree of citizen involvement, either through surveys, interviews, forums, or citizen advisory groups (MacMurray 1976; Rossi and Freeman 1982).

Services now available in the region did not originate through such rational planning or surveys of user needs. Rather, they were derived from vicissitudes of the colonial era, the orientation of visiting advisors, and the type of foreign education received by indigenous professionals. These factors, in combination with economic and political realities of developing nations, are the actual determinants of the scope and role of clinical psychiatry.

Given these constraints, there nevertheless have been needs assessments undertaken to guide some phase of planning, or at least to record the existence of problems. The most frequently used methods of case finding have been epidemiological surveys and descriptions of patients in contact with agencies (e.g., Jayasundera 1969).

The epidemiological approach, where the incidence of new cases and prevalence of existing cases are estimated for a given population, was used successfully by Lin in the late 1940s to argue for the creation of psychiatric care and training in Taiwan (Lin 1961). An important use of this method is to document the extent of untreated disability, or "residual deviance," and thus provide ammunition for lobbying to secure more funds, manpower, and facilities. It may also give impetus to a "seeking mode" of therapy—going out to find clients where they live and work (Rappaport and Chinsky 1974).

The recent plan of action for Filipino mental health workers (Aragon 1977) is predicated on a 1965 epidemiological survey that found a prevalence of thirty-six cases per 1,000 and a hospitalization estimate of 1.26 per 1,000. WHO efforts in SEAR take into account a population survey carried out in South India in 1972 (WHO 1978a). Carstairs and Kapur found that 8 percent of the adult population there were experiencing two or more mental symptoms that were sufficiently distressing to cause them to consult one or another of the local sources of healing. Rates of this sort are also used to assess the impact of a program, identify high-risk groups, and link sociocultural conditions with magnitude of disorder (cf. Cooper and Morgan 1973).

The second method of uncovering mental health needs is to tabulate detailed information on those people who find their way into the treatment system. Demographic data were found useful in Malaysia for learning which sex, age, income, and ethnic groups use facilities and from which part of the country they are drawn (Hartog 1972b; Teoh, Kinzie, and Tan 1972). Data for presenting problems and differential diagnoses are instructive to the extent that such indicators reflect the need for different types of staff, intervention techniques, specialized units, and programs. A variation of this method is the case register, a standard, precoded questionnaire administered to all new admissions or outpatients. Indonesia has pioneered in the case register approach at the national level. Computer assistance enables data collected from the General Purpose Questionnaire, administered to more than 5,000 yearly admissions to Indonesia's thirty-five inpatient facilities, to be summarized and cross-tabulated (Salan 1975; Setyonegoro 1976; Tenny 1971). Kiev (1972) and Tenny (1971) point out that monitoring such as this has direct implications for national budgeting, program development, and manpower deployment.

Although epidemiological and hospital case-counting approaches appear useful to planners, they have been strongly criticized on methodological and conceptual grounds (Dohrenwend and Dohrenwend 1965; Draguns 1973, 1980; Giel 1975; Kapur 1975; Mintz and Schwartz 1964).

Treatment models. Programs and facilities to handle psychiatric needs are the intended products of needs-assessment research. Reviewing the reports of consultants and indigenous professionals, however, reveals an overall lack of clarity in program objectives and intervention strategies. These reports fail to conceptualize how systematic criteria (theoretical or empirical) are to be used to structure services and evaluate outcome (Higginbotham 1976). WHO recently sought to deal with this confusion through the publication of guidelines taken from social psychiatry (WHO 1975a, 1975b). Nevertheless, there remains an absence of systematic procedures for designing therapeutic programs appropriate to community problems. Reviewing the existing programs in the region, two basic models for service design do emerge. These are "traditional" psychiatry and the public/community health approaches.[1]

The first model represents the extension of traditional North American or European psychiatry, unmodified, to non-Western settings. Typically, inpatient or outpatient facilities are added to existing hospitals, or present treatment centers are given consultation on "modern methods" (Dax 1962; Lin 1961; Murthy 1977). Emphasis is placed on the development of institutional settings where the patients are removed from general populations (Baasher 1975; Thong 1976). The drawback is that expensive custodial care ties up personnel and resources; it perpetuates chronicity through lack of inpatient or follow-up care and long-term confinement

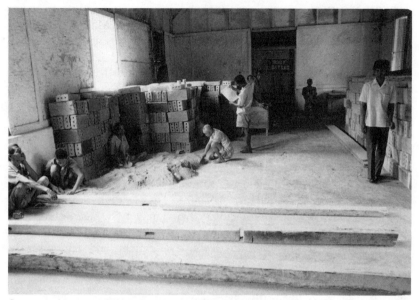

Some patients provide labor for hospital manufacturing activities, as in this brickmaking unit in Indonesia, and may receive a small payment for their efforts.

of cases thought too violent, unmanageable, or incompetent to release (Benyoussef et al. 1975). This approach carries the legacy of colonial times. It is currently deemed an anachronistic and inapplicable element of modern psychiatry (Harding and Curran 1978; Kiev 1972; WHO 1981a).

Treatment within these settings ranges from custodial management only to active programs of work "therapy": farming, woodshop, sewing, and daily chores around the hospital for lifelong residents. For those newly admitted, or residing in "acute" wards, treatment often follows classic psychiatric formulae of psychotropic drugs—chlorpromazine, reserpine, lithium carbonate—and physical therapies like electroconvulsive shock (ECT) (Hartog 1972a; Kinzie and Bolton 1973). One-to-one psychotherapy is less commonly reported as a treatment modality. It is a luxury absent from the training of practitioners (Santoso 1959), or else they reserve it for a more profitable private practice. Recently, psychotherapy has become popular among those able to afford private sessions, as shown by Lubis's (1977) work in Indonesia. Seemingly more fruitful have been extensions from two contemporary psychiatric notions, group therapy and the therapeutic community (Chen 1974; Lubis 1975; Visuthikosol and Suwanlert 1976).

Within this model, there are examples of accommodation to local social conditions and customs. Chen (1972), doing inpatient group psychotherapy in Taiwan, uses occupational and recreational activities to facilitate desired patient interaction. Kinzie and Bolton (1973) describe a program where hospitalized Malaysian aborigines are accompanied by relatives who encourage them to carry on normal daily activities. Also, long-acting phenothiazines are administered to discharged patients in their West Malaysian jungle homes.

A second approach to the design of therapeutic systems, the public/community health model, is rapidly replacing "traditional" psychiatry as treatment of choice among workers in developing countries (e.g., Argandona and Kiev 1972; Kiev 1971; Harper, Shapiro, and Zusman 1975; Sartorius 1977). Community mental health programs in the United States are fundamentally derived from the public health model (Rappaport 1977). Principles of community and social psychiatry evolved from community settings serving multiethnic populations with diverse problems. These principles are thus considered applicable across cultural boundaries. A key article by Mehryar and Khajavi (1974) delineates the features of this approach which are common to programs recently begun in Southeast Asia (e.g., Hsu and Lin 1969; Kinzie, Teoh, and Tan 1974): (1) emphasis on primary prevention; (2) training of paraprofessionals; (3) extension of professional resources through consultation and education activities; and (4) mobilization of community resources to maintain the patient outside the hospital.

To this list can be added WHO's new thrust to incorporate psychosocial factors in health delivery and training and its concern with the prevention of disorder among high-risk participants in settings of social change, urbanization, and economic development (WHO 1977a). Moreover, WHO planners have historically given strong encouragement to the integration of psychiatric with general health delivery (WHO 1950). The full scope of this approach involves multiple levels of specialization and referral. A primary health worker at the village level would be trained to screen psychological disorders for referral to a nearby rural health clinic. There, the client would be attended by a nurse or paraprofessional with some psychiatric training under the supervision of a physician from the psychiatric unit of the district hospital. If the problem were unmanageable at the primary level, the client would be referred again, this time to the district hospital.

At the secondary level, psychiatrist and staff operate a small inpatient unit along with a weekly outpatient clinic and consultation visits to rural health clinics. The regional mental hospital, the tertiary and final level, is reached only after efforts to manage the problem closer to home have been exhausted. This system was tested with favorable results in rural and semirural settings of seven developing countries, including the Philippines (Climent et al. 1980). In Sarawak, Schmidt (1967) pioneered in the creation of such a referral network to avoid hospitalizing his Chinese, Malay, Dyak, and Murato clients.

ESTABLISHING A STANDARD OF MENTAL HEALTH INTERVENTION

The introduction of a public/community health delivery system includes set criteria for its structure and characteristics. These criteria represent standards of mental health care desirable for the adequate coverage of a community. Standards for WHO member states are set forth in the publication, *Organization of Mental Health Services for Developing Countries* (WHO 1975a). If these standards are adopted by member states, and the priority of mental health services reversed, WHO personnel like Harding (1975) believe that effective care can be brought to the 90 percent who are without it.

According to the public/community health model of intervention, four components are essential to complete the system. First, the service should be *comprehensive,* with a diversity of treatments and units. Among them are emergency, outpatient, partial hospitalization, inpatient, rehabilitation, domiciliary, and after-care. Second, a *preventive* focus should guide the service activities. Primary duties are consultation with social agencies, other community services, and the public education system. Prevention includes the training of and collaboration with general health-care workers. The third component of the model is *continuity* of care. Patients should be handled by a team of multidisciplinary staff —psychiatrist, psychologist, nurse, social worker, occupational therapist—who share continuous contact with their charge while hospitalized and during transition back into the community. This principle implies setting up an integrated referral network among different service agencies responsible for the client's welfare. Finally, the model mental health system should be *accessible* to the potential users. Accessibility can be defined in several ways. It can mean ease of referral, immediate attention without an appointment or long wait, manpower availability, or no educational sophistication required to use the system successfully (Quah 1977b). Sometimes it is viewed as a ratio of hospital beds per population, as in the 1953 WHO recommendation of one bed per 10,000 severely disturbed. More recently, accessibility has been defined as the extent to which mental health programs are integrated with primary health care (WHO 1975a). Concern is with how best to intermingle mental with general health delivery, either through retraining health personnel or sharing their facilities. This effort is aimed at reaching more of the 10 to 15 percent of the population who presently receive basic health care in developing countries.

These four standards, along with the recognition that the programs must somehow be acceptable to the community (WHO 1975a), are lifted up as the attributes of a modern service. They are also criteria employed by the National Institute of Mental Health and the Accreditation Council for Psychiatric Facilities to evaluate the network of community mental health centers in the United States (Errion 1979; Windle, Bass, and Taube 1974). International agencies, consultants, indigenous professionals, and visitors evaluate existing systems of delivery according to these standards. They are the foundation for recommendations about future development, allocation of resources, manpower training, national legislation, international collaboration, and research. Because of their profound significance, these criteria should be carefully analyzed and the full extent of their implications and suitability for these Asian countries brought to light.

NOTE

1. Lin (1981) offers a more elaborate discussion of service delivery systems, analyzing the mental health models adopted by Third World pioneers into five forms: (1) hospital based; (2) medical school based; (3) community based; (4) voluntary organizations; and (5) primary health care. Lin sees the fifth development model as holding great promise for the future for reasons similar to those expressed in WHO's medium-term program.

chapter 2

Psychiatry as a Standard for Mental Health Care in Southeast Asia

Chapter 1 described how Western psychiatry became firmly established in Southeast Asia. An enterprise of this magnitude and scope has far-reaching implications. It is essential, therefore, to inquire both as to the feasibility of following the Western model and as to its responsiveness to non-Western cultures. Are there socioeconomic barriers that limit the feasibility of psychiatry's full development? Are Western therapeutics sufficiently sensitive to Asian cultures? The investment of resources required and the potentially disruptive impact of Western psychiatry make it imperative to examine the current status of treatment delivery with regard to (1) the socioeconomic capability of developing countries to attain the essential standards of modern care, (2) community acceptability of psychiatric facilities, and (3) efforts to accommodate cultural needs and customs.

THE FEASIBILITY OF THE WESTERN MODEL IN THE CONTEXT OF DEVELOPING NATIONS

Observers and practitioners in Southeast Asia recognize the immense difficulty of creating and implementing any therapeutic system. Failure to provide access to clinical psychiatry for the millions who are without it is part of a much wider failure to provide basic health services to the populations of developing countries (Giel and Harding 1976). For reasons discussed below, developing nations today are unable to meet the four standards of modern psychiatry—comprehensive, preventive, accessible, and continuous care. Nationwide systems of modern psychiatry do not now exist in Southeast Asia, and for many Asian settings such systems will remain unobtainable in the decades ahead. From this we infer that patterns of treatment delivery followed by Western industrialized countries are inappropriate templates for regional needs.

A number of forces operating at the national level limit the attainment of Western standards of clinical intervention. The most critical of these is the low priority assigned social and medical welfare services in general, and psychiatric care in particular (Indris 1971; Sartorius 1977; Tan 1971; WHO 1975a). Meeting in New Delhi, prominent planners of the World Health Organization South-East Asia Region (WHO-SEAR) termed this problem the "lack of national will" to elevate mental health concerns (WHO 1978a). Only programs for dental care receive less attention during national budgeting for health items.

Projects for industrialization, rural development, and food production—not to mention defense—have top priority in settings where at present 70 to 90 percent of the citizens reside in rural areas (Gunaratne 1981; Neki 1973a). Crises in population growth, nutrition, internal migration, infectious disease, water purification, and education press intensely upon the perceptions of national leaders (Harding 1975; WHO 1975a). Nevertheless, Neki (1973a) found that in 1970, public health funding was only .6 percent of national expenditure for Indonesia, 2.7 percent for Thailand, and 7 percent for the states of India. Mental health was the lowest allocation within these expenditures. The money available went toward maintaining large custodial hospitals with their backlog of "incurables."

The political aspect of establishing mental health care is a study in and of itself. Politicians are moved to address this issue primarily in relation to political gain: as publicity during election time, when a mental patient commits a sensational crime, or when a scandal erupts at the national mental hospital (Sartorius 1977; Tan and Wagner 1971). With intense competition for scarce resources, general health providers, already entrenched in government circles, lobby against psychiatry as premature for areas where infectious disease remains unchecked (Harding 1975).

Such competition fosters an unwillingness to coordinate with other agencies, leading to interdepartmental conflict and political turmoil that stalls mental health legislation (Dasnanjali 1971; Kiev 1972). National legislation, outlining precise mental health goals and policies for institutions, is clearly lacking (Curran and Harding 1977; Harding 1975; Widjono 1975). A permanent government coordinating body, situated at the directorate level, is recommended by WHO advisors for giving mental health political clout (Kiernan 1976; Tan 1971; WHO 1976). Directorates of mental health, such as the one in Indonesia, can be responsible for coordination and evaluation of services, planning, policy making, and manpower development. They can also serve as the focal point for collaboration with international agencies and research.

Insufficient organizational development, characteristic of emerging nations, also affects health care. From the perspective of Western social welfare administration, an efficient government bureaucracy with ample revenues for planning and executing health policy simply doesn't exist.

Butwell (1975), a political scientist, bolsters this point by suggesting that governments in Southeast Asia have generally coalesced under the authority of powerful individual leaders. Political, economic, and health programs fall with the figures that proposed them when long-term governing structures (i.e., incipient bureaucracy) fail to develop.

For example, in some medical schools, there is no teaching department of psychiatry; psychiatrists are subsumed under other medical departments. This is lamented as a barrier to the recruitment of able specialists and a contributor to the paucity of leadership (WHO 1978a), although ironically it augers well for the recent argument to diffuse psychiatry throughout the general health system. Benyoussef et al. (1975) complain of resource mismanagement by incompetent administrators within fledgling institutions. Poor managerial skills prevent effective service utilization as drugs and equipment are stolen or lost. Professional time is dissipated also through poor coordination, overlap, or involvement in nonclinical functions.

From an anthropological vantage, Foster (1977) posits that the culture of bureaucracies, and the psychology of the specialists operating within them, determines the shape of medical service delivery. Forces that determine how a professional actually acts within the system include his status and training, salary, personality, and convenience. As Carstairs (1973) notes, no one wants to work within the village. Therefore, 75 to 90 percent of the mental health resources serve 10 to 20 percent of the population—the urban dwellers (Kiernan 1976; Kraph and Moser 1966). On these occasions, Foster (1977) concludes, professional and client culture fail to overlap.

INTENSIVE TECHNICAL AND ECONOMIC DEMANDS OF THE WESTERN MODEL

Actualizing the standards of modern care delivery requires an intensive investment of resources (Murthy 1977). A delivery system that is structured to provide comprehensive, preventive, accessible, and continuous treatment demands manpower, training programs, integrated facilities, and supportive research (Harper, Shapiro, and Zusman 1975). Southeast Asia, and developing nations in general, are characterized by their acute lack of these resources (Kraph and Moser 1966; Neki 1973a; WHO 1975a). The magnitude and implications of these shortages are described below.

Manpower and Training

The shortage of manpower across all helping professions, especially at the supervisory level, is the most lamented scarcity (Benyoussef et al.

1975; Carstairs 1973; Chaudhry 1975; Kline 1963; Sartorius 1977; WHO 1975a, 1976; Widjono 1975; Wig 1975). Compounding the thinness of manpower is the uneven distribution of personnel (Kraph and Moser 1966; WHO 1976). Most are ensconced in a few urban inpatient facilities since general practitioners and specialists alike prefer to work and live in cities.

This condition evolved from lobbying by biomedical model proponents for professional care-giving, a system only affordable by industrialized economies. Professionalism artificially circumscribes the pool of indigenous helpers available to a people by defining certain human conditions as requiring professional solutions (Sarason and Lorentz 1979). The official sanction for healing is thereby limited to those few capable of earning elite credentials. Consequently, governmentally mandated facilities, operating without sufficient manpower, impose a rigid stamp upon the nature of client care. Psychiatrists feel their treatment options constricted when they face dismal manpower-to-client ratios. Sartorius (1977) estimates that there are approximately 700 psychiatrists for 800 million people in the South-East Asia Region. Based on 1970 records, Neki (1973a) found ratios of .08, .05, and .34 psychiatrists per 100,000 population for India, Indonesia, and Thailand respectively. These figures are in sharp contrast with the *First Report* of the World Health Organization Expert Committee On Mental Health calling for one psychiatrist per 20,000 in order to provide satisfactory treatment (WHO 1950). It is not surprising that patient management consists almost entirely of drug therapy and other brief somatotherapeutic modes applied chiefly to acute cases (Leon 1972).

The source of manpower shortage lies in the absence of Western-style training facilities and university departments to prepare careers in the helping professions (Chaudry 1975; Hartog 1972b; Kiernan 1976; WHO 1978a; Wig 1975). Settings that have initiated psychiatrist education may completely lack training opportunities for supporting professionals— social workers, psychiatric nurses, and psychologists. Psychology within these countries remains largely an academic discipline, unmotivated and unqualified to produce service providers (WHO 1976).

Some governments, like Singapore, deny the need to train professionals in this field, although they could afford to do so. Their rationale is that society should progress through the hard work of its members without such crutches. The Singapore government's policy may also be influenced by the presence of a well-organized network of Chinese folk medicine practitioners catering to a full spectrum of presenting problems, including "psychosomatic" complaints (see Quah 1977a).

Prejudice within academic medicine and traditions of nonspecialization in some countries are also curtailing influences (Carstairs 1975;

Maguigad 1964). In a survey of thirty-three countries, Kraph and Moser (1966) found psychiatric specialization unattractive to medical students because of poor-quality courses, unattractive working conditions, low status, and low salary. Tan (1971) confirms this image, recalling that doctors assigned to work in mental hospitals by the Malaysian Division of Health reacted as if they were being disciplined or outcast. The following actual conversation about one Malaysian psychiatrist communicates the attitudes of some physicians toward psychiatric hospitals (Wagner and Tan 1968: 28–29):

> FIRST PHYSICIAN: "Have you heard that Eng-Seong is now in Tanjong Rambutan (the large psychiatric hospital of 4,500 beds 150 miles north of Kuala Lumpur)?"
> SECOND PHYSICIAN: "Gosh, what happened to him?"
> FIRST PHYSICIAN: "Oh no, he is there as a doctor, not as a patient."
> SECOND PHYSICIAN: "My God, that's even worse!"

This fear may not be unfounded. Besides the low financial and bureaucratic reward of being assigned to the two Malaysian hospitals is the awareness that patients' relatives may threaten the lives of the medical staff when they are upset (Hartog 1972). The prejudice and lack of support in general make it difficult to get either treatment or training materials. Up-to-date journals, books, and reprints are as unavailable as newer drug therapeutics (Giel and Harding 1976; Wig 1975).

Specializing in psychiatry is just as difficult in Indonesia. To survive economically, psychiatrists employed by the government must do private practice in the evenings. Since most patients cannot afford the high fees of talk therapy, drugs are extensively relied upon. Frequently, the therapist finds it more economically rewarding to simultaneously carry on a general medical practice (Lubis 1975).

Lubis laments that the introduction of newer modes, like psychotherapy, are hindered in Indonesia by traditional Kraepelinean teaching curricula and emphasis on drug management. Since the government supports medical training, it is only concerned with those problems that can be solved in large numbers. The restricted scope of individual psychotherapy is considered to be a poor dividend.

Training Abroad

The consequences of having few training opportunities at home is that those interested must seek advanced degrees abroad. Several problems are associated with this practice. Recently, sentiment has turned against offering overseas fellowships. Regional experts agree (WHO 1977a) that it is more useful to invite experts to their countries and train nationals in subjects identified as high priority by the government. Another preference is to send trainees to centers in nearby countries where psychiatric needs are relatively similar (Wig 1975).

In the past, fellows have returned from highly developed countries with expertise inapplicable to the needs and resources of their home settings (Neki 1973b; Lin 1981). Such "overtrained" professionals, with interests in esoteric therapies like psychoanalysis or Gestalt therapy, face colleague resentment and may grow frustrated in their inability to incorporate new approaches (Kiev 1972). Moreover, training in the West in a foreign tongue may inhibit communication with clients seeking care from the local community. Regional leaders are insisting that psychiatrists be trained within the cultural setting where the work is applied and in the language of the people served (Neki 1973b).

Another problem is that foreign training frequently leads to a loss of manpower when trainees remain overseas. Their host country attracts them with higher-paying positions than they would receive back home (Quah 1977b; UNESCO 1975). Elite applicants, trained at home, often graduate only to slip away to jobs in more-industrialized countries where their labor is also more appreciated (Mejia, Pizurki, and Royston 1979). The former chairman of psychiatry and neurology at National Taiwan University, Dr. Hsin Rin, remarked that the mental health system in his country would be quite different if the numerous graduates trained in the last twenty years had remained at home (Rin, personal communication).

Approximately one-third of the psychiatrists, and many other medical specialists, have left Malaysia since 1976. Government policies of discrimination, politics at the national university, and the mood of the country, coupled with Australia's loosened immigration restrictions, are the key reasons for this "brain drain."

Facilities

A number of deficits characterize available facilities. Inpatient beds are particularly scarce (Benyoussef et al. 1975). Industrialized societies make available anywhere from one to six beds per 1,000 population; for example, Japan has 1.8 and Finland, 4.5 (Kiernan 1976). In 1959, WHO consultant Alan Stoller estimated that Thailand needed an additional 70,000 beds (Stoller 1959). Twenty years later, follow-up consultant Kiernan (1976) estimated that a fourfold increase in beds was needed to bring the .2 beds per 1,000 up to acceptable standards. With referrals feeding into these limited residential facilities from police, courts, general medicine, and families, overcrowding reaches 50 to 250 percent (Neki 1973a).

There is an acutely felt shortage of comprehensive and specialty care (Kiernan 1976; Kraph and Moser 1966; WHO 1975a; Widjono 1975). The "essential" units for a standard comprehensive care system advo-

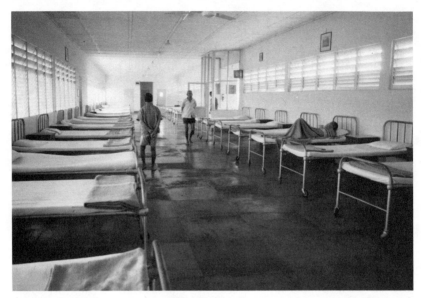

With few activities to structure their time, patients pace the corridors of a hospital in Sarawak, East Malaysia.

cated by planners include inpatient, outpatient, partial hospitalization, emergency, rehabilitation, and specialized services for forensic, retardation, geriatric, child, and substance abuse cases (Kiev 1972; Tjahana 1976; WHO 1975a). These are extremely rare and do not exist at all in rural zones. It is a common sight to see masses of patients, some having travelled quite far, waiting long hours for outpatient consultation which lasts a few brief minutes (Carstairs 1973). Under these conditions, it is not surprising that psychiatry is used as a last resort.

Pressure on these facilities will only increase as public health measures enable brain-damaged and senile populations to survive longer (WHO 1971, 1978b). Will native healers also experience difficulty shouldering the burden of care as modernization and official disapproval curtail their maneuverability and new trainees become scarce (Foster 1977)? Adding to this, WHO (1975a) foresees no prospect in the next ten to twenty years of providing enough specialized workers to meet even the basic needs. For example, Wig (1975) notes that if India were to double the number of psychiatrists in the next ten years, there would then be one psychiatrist for every one million population.

Two additional problems plague existing facilities. First, despite efforts of WHO, mental health services remain isolated from the general/ public health network. The absence of referral pathways linking the primary health worker with psychiatric units contributes to the lack of integration between the two systems. This fosters a related problem of wasted and misused resources: up to 18 percent of adults and 29 percent of children visiting outpatient medical units are potential psychiatric cases (Climent et al. 1980). WHO consultants fear that insufficiently trained health workers misdiagnose and mismanage these clients. This places an extra burden on the system and negates more appropriate treatment (Giel and Harding 1976; Kiernan 1976; WHO 1975a).

Needs Assessment

The last component international advisors consider essential to the complete treatment system is evaluation research. It provides four functions: assessing community needs, deciding program priorities, monitoring program implementation, and determining program effectiveness (Rossi and Freeman 1982). Although WHO now considers the design of national information systems a key priority (Rosen, Goldsmith, and Redick 1979; WHO 1978c: 125–126), current delivery systems operate in an information vacuum. They lack data regarding mental health problems and intervention outcome (Murthy 1977; Widjono 1975; WHO 1976). Knowledge relevant to community needs, essential for rational priority structuring, is rarely sought through epidemiological surveys—they are quite expensive and technically demanding (Giel 1982; Kiev 1972). Moreover, epidemiological data alone are useless for setting priorities and making other planning decisions. These data cannot provide a clear statement by the government of what constitutes proper mental health care and how this can be achieved (Giel 1975).

Mental health priorities are ultimately value judgments superimposed on the survey process by observers with a particular orientation (Giel and Harding 1976). These observers may also take into account evidence of community concern, perceived seriousness of problems, susceptibility to management, and their own therapy preferences as guidelines for priority setting (Morely 1973). Giel and Harding (1976) undermine the fallacy that prevalence or incidence rates alone determine priorities. They show that the disorder with the lowest prevalence rate, functional psychosis, makes up two-thirds to three-fourths of those in mental hospitals and consumes the greatest proportion of health resources.

Outcome research for evaluating treatments may be slightly less expensive than full-scale epidemiological assessment. However, the methodological sophistication essential to carry out valid systems evaluations is perhaps more demanding. Fine-tuning of mental health programs using experimental designs that employ rigorous controls (e.g., Cook and Campbell 1979) is clearly beyond the present means of developing countries.

Indeed, it has only recently emerged as an important aspect of funding for health care in the United States (Schulberg and Baker 1979). It can be argued that evaluation is more important for settings where misdirected and ineffective programs are less tolerable economically. Even so, with social science disciplines struggling for recognition vis-à-vis the more heavily funded applied sciences, there is no one qualified to set up projects for systems analysis. Throughout all of Southeast Asia there are fewer than a handful of Ph.D. psychologists. Those having anything to do with mental health have difficulty gaining access to patients, even for personality and mental testing. The study of administrative decision making, policy implementation, and the impact of medical staff and facility operations on patient change is unthinkable for both practical and political reasons.

In summary, it appears that the developing nation context affords little support at present for actualizing the comprehensive mental health model. Its feasibility for these settings is hindered by forces at the national level, including socioeconomic barriers, patterns of political power, and limited institutional development. Furthermore, the psychiatric model makes demands for manpower, training, expertise, facilities, and research that at this time and for the foreseeable future are too intensive to meet even partially. We must conclude, therefore, that standards endorsed by the industrialized West are inapplicable to Third World societies which do not maintain a heritage of richly endowed public health bureaucracies capable of building and feeding the elaborate superstructure of professional class and culture.

CULTURAL SENSITIVITY AND THE WESTERN MODEL OF HEALTH DELIVERY

Even if it were feasible to fully develop a modern mental health system in Southeast Asia, is it legitimate, ethical, or even desirable to do so? What are the implications for Asian societies? These are questions of cultural sensitivity and continuity. It is imperative to appraise the cultural sensitivity of any intervention system. If the system lacks sensitivity, the community is unlikely to accept and use the services, except in limited circumstances. Also, discontinuity between services and culture has far-reaching implications for social change, some of which may be undesirable. Some calculation must determine whether the assets of innovation outweigh their potential liabilities.

COMMUNITY ACCEPTANCE OF SERVICES

Acceptance of services by the community in Southeast Asia has been a problem historically. The negative evaluation of psychiatric care can be traced to a number of factors bearing on the relationship between the cultural traditions of the communities and the facilities placed in their midst.

Mental hospitals have not transcended their historical stigma (Darmabrata 1971; Carstairs 1973; Tjahana 1976). Organizationally they have remained a closed system to the larger community. Alien and isolated, their inhabitants—staff and patients—are cut off from the surrounding pattern of social life (Baasher 1975). The perception of the mental hospital as a prison, a holdover from the colonial days (Tjahana 1976), is coupled with the social stigma of seeking outside help. In Malaysia, some consider going to others for help with psychological problems as an admission of failure or irresponsibility and an invitation to family disgrace (Teoh, Kinzie, and Tan 1972). Rural people are especially remote from psychiatric clinics or hospitals. Yet for the above reasons, it is doubtful whether many would seek such help even if access were available (Connor 1982a; Giel and Harding 1976).

A vicious circle operates to keep these mental hospitals isolated. Existing prejudice forces families to wait a long time before admitting the patient (Darmabrata 1971; Draguns and Phillips 1972; Quah 1977b; Neki 1973a; Wolff 1965). Typically, after family remedies are tried, initial consultations are made with nearby religious healers and folk health specialists (see Kleinman 1980). Should these front-line providers fail to effect a satisfying change, and the family continue to judge the individual unmanageable given the resources present in their setting, then hospitalization is finally sought.

When it becomes apparent that there is little hope for recovery, the family loses contact and abandons the patient. This is especially true if the person was violent or severely upset his family and community. Thus, the prophecy is fulfilled: the hospital becomes the institution of last resort, reserved for conditions of extreme disturbance for which rehabilitation back into the community is improbable. It remains an isolated entity, unacceptable except as a place of abandonment.

Another cultural factor influencing acceptance of psychiatry is the community's perception of deviance and behavioral disorder. Centuries-old beliefs about the causes of disorders involve, along with less-alarming interpretations, notions of punishment for sin, violation of taboo, malevolent spirits, and witchcraft (Asuni 1975; Baasher 1975; Connor 1982b; Marsella and White 1982; Murthy 1977). The "traditional" family reaction is to seek a definitive explanation. They fear that the person may have sinned or neglected ritual obligations, or that someone else in the village is using sorcery to bring illness to their kinsmen (Lieban 1967).

Being labelled "mad," *orang gila,* in Malaysia and Indonesia is a shameful and humiliating experience for the person and his family. It is

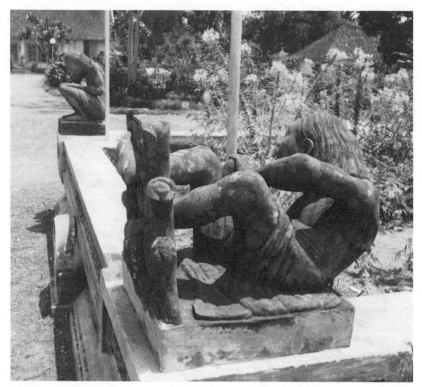

The legacy of harsh confinement measures has contributed to the stigma associated with psychiatry in Southeast Asia. These stone statues, commissioned by a doctor, depict the historical use of stocks and were carved by Balinese patients at Bangli Hospital, Indonesia.

second only to having leprosy (Darmabrata 1971; Hartog 1972). Taking the patient to a psychiatric facility only reinforces this stigma. Moreover, such services have little to offer. They ignore the real wellspring of suffering (Asuni 1975; Neki 1973b; Torrey 1972). Indigenous healers are called upon to propitiate the malevolent spirit or cast off the malicious spell, returning the patient to his normal self without the stigma of institutionalization (Connor 1982a).

   The attitudes of other health workers toward psychiatry also determine its acceptance (Baasher 1975). A number of sources report strong negative bias against mental health among other professionals (Baasher 1975; Neki 1973b; Tan 1971; WHO 1975a, 1976). For example, Carstairs (1975) sampled the attitudes of senior medical faculty in eight Southeast Asian countries. He found a high degree of prejudice and ignorance among professors of medicine, surgery, anatomy, and physiology. These medical leaders still maintained "outdated ideas about psychiatry, regarding it as exclusively concerned with the treatment of insane in mad houses" (Carstairs 1975, 109).

WHO (1975a) regards negative attitudes held by health personnel, planners, and politicians as a major obstacle to the development of rational mental health care. Entrenched conservatism, with personnel favoring institutional treatment and resisting introduction of new, community-based methods, is also seen by WHO as perpetuating the negative, archaic image of psychiatry. Lastly, a new breed of indigenous professionals is beginning to challenge the blind borrowing of Western patterns of training and intervention without testing their relevance to local conditions (Wig 1975). Such challenges may play a larger role in the future acceptance of new psychiatric technology.

DISCONTINUITY OF SERVICES WITH CULTURE

The second characteristic of a mental health service relevant to cultural sensitivity is the continuity of its goals and operations with the pattern of indigenous culture. Led by the writings of medical historian Michel Foucault (1971), there is a growing awareness that the purely secular discourse about madness expounded by psychiatry forces a kind of "epistemological break" with traditional formulations embodied in many non-Western cosmologies and in European thought prior to the eighteenth century. The language of madness in some of these societies retains the potential of divine intervention and even suggests exalted access to another reality transcending the everyday world (Connor 1982a). In contrast, psychiatry's "logical-positivism," with its "monologue of reason about madness" (Foucault 1971:10), manifests a deep incongruity with understandings inspired by religious belief. Secular psychiatry thus becomes an impetus for culture change. However, the use of psychiatry as a force of innovation raises serious ethical questions when community members have no influence over the direction of that change (Neki 1973b).

Visiting consultants and their in-country counterparts share a common education. Undergirding it are philosophical assumptions about the nature of humanity that are specific to the cultures of Europe and America. These assumptions shape the course of psychiatric discourse and action. Definitions of disorder, the curing process, and the ideal outcome of therapy are all determined by culture-specific values, just as they are in traditional societies of Africa and Asia (Collomb 1973; Neki 1973b). Many writers have commented on the cultural bias of modern psychiatry and psychotherapy as social institutions seeking to meet the deficits in the Western way of life (e.g., Gains 1982; Meadow 1964; Pande 1968; Yap 1968). Sampson (1977), for example, presents a fine illustration of how psychotherapy evolved in the United States as a peculiarly American medium for securing socially prescribed values of "self-actualization," autonomy, and mastery.

In broad terms, psychotherapy serves culture as a process of resocializing the person to expected norms (Draguns 1975). To the extent that cultures differ, the goal and modality of resocialization differ as well. Draguns (1975) offers the following typology of culture and therapy: societies with internal locus of control practice insight-oriented, reconstructive, and open-ended psychotherapy; cultures preferring external control of members employ authoritarian, directive techniques with focused outcomes. When indigenous professionals trained abroad in psychotherapy return home, with whom are their interventions appropriate? Kiev (1972) suggests that these returnees may have to unlearn newly acquired methods and seek out other approaches more congruent with the needs encountered.

Since each system of curing is geared to fulfilling the sociocultural needs of its society, each system becomes culture-specific and cannot be transferred intact to another society (Asuni 1975). With the transference well under way, though, something must be happening. Is the curing system being modified? Or are elements in the host society changing to accept a better fit?

Disease Notions

A review of ethnographic and transcultural psychiatric literature suggests that prevailing notions about disease in a culture may be replaced when new health technology is introduced (Clement 1982; Kiev 1972; Neki 1973b). Wolff (1965) underscores this point in viewing medicine as a potent agent of culture change on the Malay Peninsula: "For really good medical services to be established, it is necessary to acquaint the people with not only more modern tools, more efficient techniques, but with a new and acceptable way of thinking about disease, about causation of disease, about treatment of disease" (pp. 344–345).

The Western classification of diseases is intended to replace indigenous conceptions, including notions of behavior disorder. Making psychological evaluations from the standpoint of Western culture, Neki (1973a) argues, means holding Western criteria as normal and assuming any departures from its prevalent pattern as deviant. This tendency runs counter to the assertion by ethnographers that diagnostic labels developed and employed in industrialized countries are not applicable in divergent societies (Marsella 1982; Wittkower and Termansen 1968).

Attitudes and Values

Secondly, cultural values and attitudes may come under attack. Ari Kiev warns against "psychiatric imperialism." Yet, at the same time, he advocates psychiatry stepping into the political arena. Psychiatrists, armed with social science knowledge, should involve themselves in leadership selection, educational planning, and suppression of tribal customs impeding the development of "psychological autonomy" among the young. Such customs, Kiev reasons, hinder modernization (Kiev 1976: 147–148).

Comments such as these reveal elements of blatant ethnocentrism and the fallacious reasoning underlying the "evolutionist" model of culture "progress" (Shweder and Bourne 1982: 101–102). These same elements, in more subtle form, compose the common theme in international psychiatry that the professional should assume the role of community educator and modifier of "archaic" and "harmful" attitudes. Baasher (1975) sees the need to study communities intensively to identify incorrect attitudes, particularly the stigma of treatment, that need to be changed. WHO planners expect mental health technology to play a vital role in enabling workers to change community perceptions of health and medical programs, thereby mobilizing community participation in the activities of general health providers (WHO 1981: 17–18). These same authorities advocate social planning measures to strengthen the "normal psychosocial functioning of the family" and to protect the vulnerable or "incomplete" family (WHO 1981: 15). The family at risk of experiencing behavioral problems is defined as one with either one parent missing or no children present to gratify the "basic psychosocial needs of adults."

Upon reflection, this attempt to enshrine the nuclear family as the ideal building block for psychosocial health in the world is empirically dubious and fails to consider the fact that nurturing, caring, and enduring relationships can assume myriad forms, including homosexual couples, childless heterosexual pairs, communal ties, single-parent families, and other alternatives (Pilisuk and Parks, in press). In essence, psychiatry is value-laden (London 1965), employs a single standard to establish deviance and normality (Neki 1973b; Rappaport 1977), and advocates altering individuals' values and life styles. Thus, there is an ethical and human rights obligation to gain community approval before it is introduced. Practitioners should clarify psychiatry's value system to community leaders and take great pains to insure that those affected have the freedom to offer or withdraw their informed consent to receive tratment.

Social Relationships

Social relationships are a third cultural element at risk of being altered. An established psychiatric service places explicit role demands on those involved. The medical system is hierarchical and prescribes role relationships among levels of staff, as well as among staff and patients, their families, and other involved community agents. In taking on the responsibility of caring for patients, the medical system competes with, and undermines, an intricate pattern of interpersonal relationships (Lewis 1955).

Interpersonal contact with the identified client may be quite complex. The social matrix may include his immediate family, other kinsmen, village elders, religious leaders, teachers, local authorities, folk doctors, and so forth (e.g., Hartog 1972b). Foster observes that changes in health behavior "almost always produce, or require, major restructuring of traditional and valued social relationships. When the 'social' costs of this restructuring [or any innovation] are seen as outweighing the potential advantage, the decision will be against change" (Foster 1977: 530; see also Fairweather 1972; Lewis 1955; Rappaport 1977).

In particular, the family/patient relationship is most likely to be affected. The authority of the family, with its responsibility for making health decisions and overseeing the member's recovery (Kleinman and Sung 1976), is often sacrificed for the sake of medical expediency (Clark 1959; Prasetyo 1977). This is especially tragic as maintenance of family contact—and involvement with the patient during admission—is an important determinant of early discharge.

Existing Power Structure and Local Control

Fourthly, the introduction of mental health services has implications for strengthening or weakening prevailing patterns of power within a society (Lewis 1955; Lieban 1973). Some Western writers characterize psychiatry as a device for political and social control. They argue that as an institution, its goals are to maintain the status quo or to discredit and silence opponents of those in power (e.g., Laing 1967; Szasz 1978).

In Southeast Asia, the introduction of modern institutions has served to stratify communities into small Westernized elites—those in leadership positions—and the vast majority of traditional farmers and peasants (Neki 1973a). The former group is a separate class: a body of nationals different from the majority as a result of their economic position and acculturation. In many instances, they are the remnants of elites co-opted during colonization. The domain of this class is government service, big business, education, the professions, communication, and the military. They have travelled abroad, have gone to college, and speak English (Butwell 1975). For the latter group, the village is their world and the focus of their identification and loyalty.

Historically, family ties and the welfare of the family business in the village were placed above that of the nation (Butwell 1975). However, for convenience in administering public health, educational, and other social programs, villages are in the process of being rearranged. Although well-intentioned, newly introduced programs of village welfare represent an unprecedented assault on the ways of village life (Steinberg 1971). Older rulers had exploited, but seldom intruded into, village affairs. Contemporary governments have done so in drawing the peasants into new administrative frameworks (Steinberg 1971). Administrative rearrangement of village units serves the needs of psychiatric delivery as well.

While the introduction of psychiatry adds to the rationale for political changes in these areas, authorities control how the treatment system will be introduced and used. This insures that, at minimum, it will not prove disruptive to the desired status configuration. Kiev (1972) warns international consultants that those in power may not be willing to help disadvantaged groups through the distribution of services. He encourages consultants to be watchful that authorities don't manipulate them into becoming a tool of their own political ends. In a similar warning, Westmeyer and Hausman (1974) add that authorities may try to limit direct consultant contact with clients and engage in other paternalistic practices. These can only be overcome by devising administrative machinery guaranteeing community control of both the form and substance of local mental health resources (cf. Denner and Price 1973; Thursz and Vigilante 1978).

Indigenous Healing

The final cultural element to suffer as a consequence of imported psychiatry is the system of indigenous healing (Draguns and Phillips 1972; Kleinman and Sung 1976; Torrey 1972). The net result of introducing a modern, formal system for psychological problems may be less help for those in need. This situation arose for poor people in the United States with the development of comprehensive community mental health centers (Kelly 1966). Rappaport (1977) explains that services to the poor were actually reduced when other agencies stopped treating them. Instead, these clients were referred to the new community mental health centers which also had little to offer.

Creating an ineffective new institution—like the alienated residential facilities described earlier—results in less support for the community. This occurs when legislation, official disapproval, and referral patterns combine to undermine the existing healing network. Leslie (1976), Kleinman (1980), and Hartog (1972) found that traditional healers are extensively relied upon by all layers of Asian society. Native institutions are curative, serve important social functions, and assist in mediating the stress of rapid social change. Yet, folk healers, shamans, spiritualists, and other practitioners seldom receive official sanction and in some places are dying out (Foster 1977; Hartog 1972; Weinberg 1970). The formal programs intended to replace them are scarce, not well accepted, and suffer from the other deficiencies outlined earlier.

CULTURAL CONTINUITY OF INDIGENOUS HEALING

The critical feature of folk healing that Western methods lack is continuity with the language, values, and customs of the local cultural setting. This points to the major deficit of modern psychiatry—cultural discontinuity. The repercussions of discontinuity involve disruption of the integrated set of cultural elements governing perception and response to mental health problems. What are the specific ways in which indigenous treatment provides cultural continuity and modern medicine does not?

Kleinman's (1980) analysis of the cultural mechanisms governing the health care system suggests a means for understanding the cultural continuity of folk healing. He sees a radical discontinuity between contemporary care and traditional forms of healing. While healing takes into account the control of sickness and provision of meaning for the individual's experience of sickness, modern health care attends solely to the former. While modern medicine is only interested in disease—the malfunctioning of psychological and biological processes—healers are interested in the patient and his family's psychosocial reaction to the disease. Kleinman states his theoretical position as follows:

> Healing is not so much a result of the healer's efforts as a condition of experiencing illness and care within the cultural context of the health care system. Healing is a necessary activity that occurs to the patient, and his family and social nexus, regardless of whether the patient's disorder is affected or not. The health care system provides psychosocial and cultural treatment (and efficacy) for the illness by naming and ordering the experience of illness, providing meaning for that experience, and treating the personal, family, and social problems which comprise the illness, and thus it heals, even if it is unable to effectively treat the disease (Kleinman and Sung 1976: 55–56).

To the extent that folk practitioners provide culturally legitimate treatment of illness, they *must* heal. To the extent that professional clinicians focus exclusively on disease, they must *fail* to heal.

The cultural continuity of traditional medicine begins with the folk healer. In a significant way, the healer is a medium for transmitting subcultural ideology. Her ceremonial activities integrate clients with traditional religious philosophy and ideals of human relationship in the face of socioeconomic transformation affecting agrarian life styles (Connor 1982c). Folk specialists maneuver with full knowledge of their patient's and audience's expectations of therapy. The personal manner, ritual

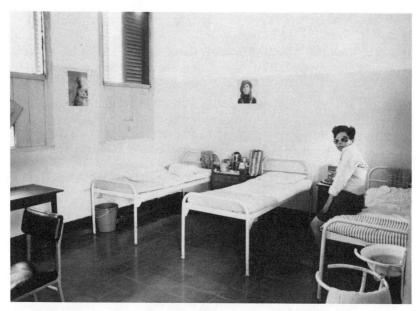

A woman patient in Indonesia has added pictures to her bedroom walls, a personal gesture rarely seen in the largely depersonalized institutions of Southeast Asia.

drama, symptom interpretation, even style of dress selected by the healer synthesize to instill within the onlooker hope, faith, and expectancy of success (Higginbotham 1977).

Unlike the generally individualistic and rationally oriented therapies of the West, folk doctors employ purposefully dramatic healing ceremonies where patient and audience are actively engaged. These are public events (Lebra 1982; Lieban 1967); activities assaulting the sensory systems of patient and onlookers are intended to intensely captivate the patient or induce altered conscious states. The shaman, often with a supernatural connection and aura of wonder about him, creates a ritual structure that powerfully transmits the message of healing and change to the participants (Connor 1982a; Kennedy 1973).

In summary, the concept of cultural continuity is critical for understanding the disruptive potential and failure of Western psychiatry in Southeast Asia. When modern medicine is imported to traditional societies in this region, it fails to provide ritual and philosophic bases considered necessary by members of these societies (Chen 1975). Villagers view Western treatment as depersonalizing, mechanistic, and fragmented. Scientific doctors seem aloof and uncaring of family and friends (Chen 1975; Wolff 1965). In short, scientific medical systems fail to satisfy both basic health requirements and the social and metaphysical needs related to them (Foster 1977; Kleinman and Sung 1976; Lambo 1978). Lambo, speaking from the African perspective, but equally applicable to Asia, makes a statement ideal for summarizing the cultural continuity theme:

> The character and effectiveness of medicine for the mind and body always and everywhere depend on the culture in which the medicine is practiced. In the West, healing is often considered to be a private matter between patient and therapist. In Africa, healing is an integral part of society and religion, a matter in which the whole community is involved. To understand African psychotherapy one must understand African thought and its social roots (Lambo 1978: 32).

CULTURAL ACCOMMODATION OF PSYCHIATRY

Recently, ethnopsychiatry has sought to come to terms with the cultural barriers inhibiting the introduction of "modern" services and, in the process, modify psychiatry to make it more acceptable (e.g., Benyoussef et al. 1975; Draguns 1975; Lebra 1976; Leighton 1969; Prasetyo et al. 1977). Experimentation with various strategies and recommendations has occurred worldwide. The village system of Nigeria and Senegal encourages psychiatric patients to live with a relative in a traditional community especially provided to handle them close to the mental clinic (Collomb 1972; Lambo 1966; Osborne 1969). Treatment progresses through the natural therapeutic elements of village life, use of native healers, drugs, and group psychotherapy. Wig (1975) feels that community needs found in Asia call for a new type of psychiatrist: one who serves as a community planner, organizer, and supervisor of nonprofessionals and is trained within the home country.

Other authorities recommend that services achieve greater acceptability when: they are planned in strict collaboration with local leaders (Asuni 1975; Bhaskaran 1975; Hassler 1975); users have easy access to care in terms of location, reduced waiting, and affordable fees (Foster 1977); and personnel share a common background and language with the clients (Schmidt 1965). Finally, the literature of ethnopsychiatry notes favorable outcomes when new services are integrated with existing helping networks (Higginbotham 1976). This may take the form of collaboration with agencies in a positive relationship with the public, relying on traditional healers (Kapur 1975; Prince and Wittkower 1964; Wittkower and Warnes 1974), or choosing the family home as the site for care. In this regard, culture-specific concepts of illness and classification of disorder are treated with sensitivity and respect (Fabrega 1971; Torrey 1972).

What these strategies and recommendations have in common is an intention to modify the system of mental health delivery to make it more continuous with elements of community life style and client expectations. Culture accommodation efforts presumably engender a closer fit between the treatment system and the culture system which determines health behavior. An accommodating program seeks not to replace existing patterns of helping, but rather to support and build upon them. New service elements should be introduced only where none exists and the community recognizes the value of innovation.

Very little has been written about the process of culture accommodation in Southeast Asia and the planning necessary to insure it in the design of new services for the region's diverse ethnic and income groups. This topic demands research attention because it is an important consideration in designing services in any community, including those for ethnic minorities in the United States (e.g., Manson 1982; Padilla, Ruiz, and Alvarez 1975; Sue 1977). It would be valuable to have descriptions of the accommodation practices and dimensions of accommodation that Asian facilities have evolved in responding to the unique cultural demands placed upon them.

A SURVEY OF MENTAL HEALTH SERVICES
IN SOUTHEAST ASIA

Two major points can be distilled from this discussion of international psychiatry. First, there is clear doubt as to the feasibility of following the Western model of mental health care in Southeast Asia. Second, it is critically important for any helping program to accommodate itself to the surrounding cultural milieu in order to gain community acceptability and avoid cultural discontinuity. At this point, however, the methods and dimensions of accommodation remain speculative.

At present, there is little systematic information on the suitability of Western psychiatry from the perspectives of feasibility and cultural sensitivity. Gaining these perspectives was sought through a survey of services operating in Southeast Asia during 1977. The purpose of this survey was to describe the status of mental health programs in terms of (1) their ability to attain the criteria of comprehensive mental health care as delineated by the modern psychiatric model and (2) the practices of culture accommodation within these facilities aimed at enhancing community acceptability.

These two perspectives on psychiatry's suitability in Southeast Asia were approached through intensive interviews with personnel assigned to mental health agencies and through the collection of written materials, including ethnographic information, pertinent to agency operations. The research strategy was conceptualized as a case study approach integrating these various information sources.

During the field work, the case study data were viewed as belonging to three domains of agency functioning. First, to obtain an overview of the services each agency provided, an interview was constructed tailored to the administrator's knowledge. Questionnaire 1 covered sources of funding, staffing, capacity, clients, staff training, referral paths, discharge rates, primary prevention efforts, therapies, family involvement, and community participation in agency policy formulation. (The questionnaires used and a discussion of the survey procedure are included in the Appendix.) Hospital annual reports, statistical yearbooks, and public relations brochures were reviewed to obtain additional documentation of service components. Additional inquiries regarding "global" or national variables affecting the mental health institutions' capacity to function as an integrated system were posed to knowledgeable people in universities, government, and international agencies. These included questions about the availability of national health insurance, communication and cooperation among institutions, mental health legislation, and regional health planning. Consultant reports and evaluations by WHO experts assigned to the region were particularly valuable for grasping an overview of the psychiatric system. Some of these documents were the blueprints for establishing the current systems of care and training.

Second, the survey pinpointed characteristic problems encountered by agencies as perceived by treatment staff. Questionnaire 2 elicited the viewpoints of doctors, psychologists, social workers, nurses, and their co-workers regarding problems with funding, staffing, professional support, treatment outcome, community acceptability, and other resource difficulties.

The third domain of agency functioning involved considerations of culture accommodation found in agency policies, practices, and personnel activities. Items from Questionnaire 2 tapped staff judgments related to patient and family concepts of disorder and treatment expectations, cultural barriers in using the agency, therapy goals, staff accommodation to patients' conceptions of disorder, adjusting inpatient services to culture, accessibility of services, and involving community helpers. A brief (sixteen-item) attitude scale measuring the degree to which the professionals agreed with practices of culture accommodation was distributed to as many personnel as possible within each facility.

To complement the structured interviews with staff, open-ended discussions were held with selected administrators, therapists, representatives from national health ministries, and authorities from academic institutions—anthropologists, psychologists, and ethnopsychiatrists.

Discussion notes were taken regarding: (1) culturally unique aspects of mental health problems and psychiatric care; (2) considerations given to gathering culture-specific information during treatment; (3) the degree of integration of this knowledge into services; (4) the perceived value of culture accommodation processes; and (5) barriers to this approach.

Last, in order to discover how pertinent and comprehensive culture-accommodation practices actually were in relation to local life styles, an intensive search was made for ethnographic documentation of folk conceptions of behavioral disorder and traditional healing. The juxtaposition of these rich anthropological descriptions of healing systems with our case studies of formal psychiatric care offers a dramatic image both of how accommodation could proceed and of the sharp discontinuities between the "traditional" and "modern" care-giving modes.

To compose a case study from these diverse sources, it was necessary to synthesize the information into a set of variables (table 2.1). They form a framework for integrating data from questionnaires, open-ended interviews, actuarial and published reports, and consultant evaluations. The case studies presented in the following three chapters are uniformly organized according to this set of variables.

The extent to which the survey covered the inpatient facilities in each of the three countries is shown in table 2.2. The facilities chosen for observation account for the majority of the psychiatric beds in the Philippines and Thailand, but not in Taiwan. The highest percentage of beds

TABLE 2.1 Variables for Analyzing Case Study Data

Resource potential variables
1. Comprehensive services
2. Preventive orientation
3. Continuity of care within the facility: Manpower
4. Continuity of care: Interinstitutional
5. Continuity with community care-giving
6. Accessibility of facilities
7. Staff evaluation of resource strength

Community integration and acceptability variables
8. Community involvement in treatment
9. Community integration via review and consultation
10. Staff evaluation of acceptability

Cultural accommodation and continuity variables
11. Institutional Practices: Selected Examples
12. Staff attitudes toward accommodation

TABLE 2.2 Extent of Inpatient Facility Sampling by Country
          and City

Country and city	Total number of mental hospitals and inpatient beds available	Total number of mental hospitals and inpatient beds visited
Taiwan	±12 "active" treatment facilities ±3,000 beds	4 facilities visited 323 beds (11% sampled)
Taipei	6 treatment facilities 774 beds	4 facilities visited 323 beds (40% sampled)
Philippines	23 treatment facilities 6,500 official beds	8 facilities visited 3,801 beds (58% sampled)
Manila	9 treatment facilities 3,831 official beds	7 facilities visited 3,781 beds (99% sampled)
Thailand	14 treatment facilities 7,865 beds	7 facilities visited 4,885 beds (62% sampled)
Bangkok	6 treatment facilities 4,290 beds	5 facilities visited 3,990 beds (95% sampled)
Chiangmai	2 treatment facilities 865 beds	2 facilities visited 865 beds (100% sampled)

visited, 62 percent, was in Thailand; only 11 percent were sampled in Taiwan. Nearly 100 percent of the beds in Manila, Bangkok, and Chiangmai are located in the sampled institutions. Clinics accounting for 40 percent of Taipei's beds were studied. The data are believed to be highly representative of urban psychiatry and moderately exhaustive of the nations' inpatient resources in general.

In twenty-two facilities in the three countries, an administrator filled out the intensive overview questionnaire (six in Taiwan and eight each in Thailand and the Philippines). The number and diversity of staff answering Questionnaire 2 is especially important (table 2.3). It is the principal tool for gathering multidisciplinary perspectives on agency operations, problems, and community accommodation. Fifty staff members from twenty-two agencies were interviewed with this instrument. The strength of the results lies in the large number of psychiatrists—directors, supervisors, and line staff—who were sampled. Psychologists, social workers, and occupational therapists interviewed were fewer, but were in proportion to their numbers.

While we may be confident that the data reflect the perspectives of psychiatrist-administrators, there is less certainty regarding the represen-

TABLE 2.3 Occupation of Respondents for Questionnaire 2: Staff Perceptions of Agency

Country	Psy-chiatrist	Psy-chologist	Social worker/ occupational therapist	Nurse	Total
Taiwan	6 (4)*	1 (1)	2 (2)	2 (2)	11
Philippines	12 (8)	5 (4)	2 (2)	3 (3)	22
Thailand	11 (6)	5 (4)	1 (1)	0	17
Total	29 (18)	11 (9)	5 (5)	5 (5)	50 (22)

*First number indicates the number of respondents; the number in parentheses is the number of facilities from which they were sampled.

tation of psychologists, social workers, and occupational therapists, even though nonmedical staff are numerically weak in these institutions. Furthermore, there is little confidence that the data represent the perspective of nurses, only five of whom were interviewed, even though they are the largest portion of trained staff and bear the burden of day-to-day care for inpatients.

Of the fifty staff completing Questionnaire 2, most were from large government hospitals with more than 500 beds or from small government hospitals with fewer than 200 beds (table 2.4). These two types of institutions, along with university psychiatric units, account for the majority of mental health manpower in the region.

The prevalence of foreign-educated professionals in the sample is noteworthy. Forty-two percent of the fifty respondents had specialty education abroad, eighteen (36 percent) in the United States and three (6 percent) in the British system, either in England or in Australia. Thailand alone accounted for 57 percent of those educated overseas. The remaining twenty-nine (58 percent) were trained in their home countries.

Nearly all of the hospital directors and supervisors had overseas experience, but so did several senior psychologists and social workers. This points to the lack of training facilities in the allied disciplines in earlier years.

Far more workers in all categories—especially the allied professions—were able to complete the sixteen-item attitude scale on culture accommodation (table 2.5). Thus there is more confidence that differences found in comparing attitudes across disciplines reflect variations in the perspectives of these workers. With a total of ninety-two respondents from twenty-four agencies, there is also greater confidence that the atti-

TABLE 2.4 Number of Personnel Completing Questionnaire 2 within Each Facility Type

Type of facility	Number of respondents
Unit in university department	9
Community mental health center outpatient department	4
Large government hospital: > 500 beds	17
Medium government hospital: 201–500 beds	2
Small government hospital: < 200 beds	14
Private mental hospital	2
Unit in private general hospital	2
Total	50

TABLE 2.5 Occupation of Respondents for Questionnaire 3: Attitudes Toward Culture Accommodation

Country	Psy-chiatrist	Psy-chologist	Social worker/occupational therapist	Nurse	Total
Taiwan	7 (3)*	5 (3)	5 (1)	3 (2)	20
Philippines	22 (8)	10 (4)	10 (3)	7 (5)	49
Thailand	10 (6)	9 (5)	3 (2)	1 (1)	23
Total	39 (17)	24 (12)	18 (6)	11 (8)	92 (24)

*First number indicates the number of respondents; number in parentheses is the number of facilities from which they were sampled.

tudes expressed accurately represent the perceptions of Taiwanese, Filipino, and Thai mental health workers toward the value of accommodating programs to meet cultural needs.

It is wise to keep in mind the bias and limitations of the data. First, the case studies are restricted to the perspective of mental health professionals and administrators employed in various government and private institutions. The interviews and the supplementary information collected represent as thorough an analysis as possible of what they *say* they are doing. Staff responses are influenced by their attitudes, prejudices, world views, and the desire to look good. These aspects are part and parcel of the professional perspective under investigation.

From an anthropological perspective, it is just as legitimate to study the "culture" of the mental health provider and his or her setting as it is to do field work among the intended recipients of psychiatric services. It would have been ideal to do both. The community perspective enters the case studies through the anthropological and ethnopsychiatric writings used and therapists' statements regarding client expectations and beliefs encountered in clinics.

Second, it would be naive to accept the statements of these professionals at face value. Unquestionably, the desire for "impression management" motivates workers describing their facility to an outsider. Also, they are constrained to present an optimistic or "official view" of what they do and what the agency's capabilities are, as opposed to what transpires in reality. It must also be recognized that the investigator visiting these clinics represented a source of prestige. As a clinical psychologist, I was an "expert" on American mental health. American standards of treatment are aspired to by many of those interviewed.

Several considerations mitigate the impact of this tendency to give socially desirable responses. First, staff with diverse points of view were sought out to secure as many "biased" perspectives of agency functioning as possible. A more realistic picture emerged when these viewpoints were blended together. Second, the questionnaires were complex. They asked for specific examples of a certain practice and its availability and desirability. When inconsistencies in these three levels of appraisal were apparent, they are pointed out in the text. Third, with regard to resource deficits, most respondents were quite open in revealing that many of the thirty-one items were indeed serious problems in their clinics. Interviewees responded differentially to these thirty-one problems. Some were deemed quite serious; others were not considered important deficits. This demonstrated an intention to fill out the questionnaire objectively.

Moreover, with each interview I worked hard to establish rapport and trust. Anonymity was promised to help create an atmosphere of open and honest exchange. I sought to demonstrate an awareness of—and a genuine concern for—the problems of the care providers. They seemed to respond, with few exceptions, with sincere answers. In fact, many interviewees were quite frank about the limitations they saw in their systems, especially those trained overseas. They seemed to welcome the opportunity to talk with a researcher interested in their opinions.

The case studies describe the *structure* and *organization* of psychiatric services. These data represent the *potential* resources for providing psychological care, not the actual quality of care provided. Thus, the information errs consistently on the side of optimism. It is a conservative or stringent test of the research hypothesis that Western standards of psychiatry are not feasible in these developing nations. In other words, if the systems fall short of the established criteria of "modern" psychiatry—

even when given the benefit of the doubt based on available structure (i.e., number of hospitals, specialty units, manpower resources, etc.)—it strengthens the conclusion that the Western model is inappropriate.

Finally, there may be questions about sampling bias with regard to those interviewed. Indeed, there was an unmistakable tendency toward interviewing psychiatrists and those who spoke English. In fact, 42 percent of the total Southeast Asian sample had received advanced professional education abroad. These were a select group with regard to training experience, international perspective, and motivation to talk with a visiting psychologist. On the other hand, their opinions had considerable value. They appeared quite interested in discussing this topic and well-suited to critically evaluate the status of their facilities. Furthermore, these experienced professionals were able to quickly grasp the nature of the survey and formulate their perspective without difficulty. In essence, these persons are the transmitters of modern psychiatry in their home cultures. Their professional goals reflected that aim. Their experiences and dilemmas in the enterprise are the heart of the case studies.

chapter 3

The Mental Health System of Taiwan

Against the backdrop of Taiwan's dynamic development since World War II, an equally impressive national mental health program has emerged. This program owes its origins to Professor Tsung-yi Lin, a planner and administrator of remarkable foresight, who has become an internationally distinguished leader of psychiatry through influential roles in the World Health Organization and the World Federation for Mental Health.

Lin returned from medical training in Japan immediately after the war to inherit a psychiatric system devoid of personnel and consisting of no more than a few buildings housing unattended psychotics. All Japanese psychiatrists employed by the former colonial administration were repatriated. The government was preoccupied with reorganizing the nation's political, economic, and educational spheres. Fellow health professionals were burdened by the immediate tasks of combating acute infectious diseases and restoring public health services to the prewar level (Tseng 1978). Traditional indifference, ignorance, and prejudice about formal psychological care remained strong among both professionals and lay people.

In Lin's favor, though, was the rare opportunity to begin carte blanche. He could create his own vision of a rational mental health program unconstrained by the precedents of traditional custodial treatment that were the legacy in many former colonial Southeast Asian settings. A pioneer in social psychiatry, Lin conceived the mental health program as a three-stage plan developing over twenty-five years (Lin 1961). The first stage called for psychiatry's integration into medicine as a respectable discipline within a medical school curriculum. Secondly, mental health content should be integrated into general public health practice. Lastly, principles of mental health should be instilled into the nation's educational scheme.

From its early onset, Lin sought to mold a program oriented toward the community. Its services were to be dispensed through the public health system of general hospitals, health stations, and even schools. He emphasized day care, home care, and rehabilitation programs backed up with inpatient facilities. Concurrently, he focused on getting mental health education into the general medical curriculum for physicians and nurses and on teaching to general practitioners as opposed to creating a few specialists. Lin's conception was to initiate a psychiatric system strongly formulated along noncustodial lines. Ideally it would be accessible to the public, diffused through existing health networks, and responsive to Chinese health care attitudes and local problems.

Initial Foundations

The first task in generating Taiwan's mental health program was to develop a Department of Psychiatry and Neurology within the National Taiwan University Medical School Hospital (NTUH). The neurological component was essential to undermine opposition from the other medical branches and gain respectability. A psychiatric center was established at NTUH and became the birthplace of modern psychiatry for the nation: the source of innovation in services, therapeutics, research, and teaching.

The early duties of Lin and his core staff were threefold. First, a curriculum was set for educating psychiatric nurses and undergraduate medical students. After a modest beginning, two American consultants helped to launch the teaching component by making it a mandatory clerkship and having half of the students intern in psychiatry during their final year. The second function was to open an outpatient and small inpatient service to the public. According to Tseng (1978), people requesting care quickly flooded the center. Lastly, a survey was undertaken between 1946 and 1948 to ascertain the magnitude of psychological disorder in the community.

The prevalence study had enormous implications for planners. It suggested that 10.8 individuals out of every 1,000 required some psychiatric attention and that 95 percent had no contact with modern treatment whatsoever. Lin used these data both to contradict the notion that Chinese culture moderates psychopathology and to argue for the relevancy and continued expansion of his program. This was a rare example of an epidemiological survey and study of existing community resources becoming the basis for determining an educational and community mental health program (Lin 1961). This research theme continued with epidemiological studies of aboriginal mountain tribes, high blood pressure, and a fifteen-year follow-up of the original groups. Investigations were also done of child development and the effects of family attendance on the psychiatric ward.

Bilateral and international input into the mental health program was also crucial to its development. A fully operational and modern Department of Psychiatry presumably required upgrading the educational experiences of Lin and his colleagues. It was deemed essential for teaching staff to secure advanced training abroad in different specialties then return to build a postgraduate program. Aid came in the form of WHO fellowships and assistance from the American Bureau of Medical Aid to China.

Seeking what he considered the best overseas training possible, Lin initiated ties with Harvard University and went there in 1950 to study neurology. Upon his return, other faculty were encouraged to develop their specialized interests within clinical psychiatry. Lin was enthusiastic about the conceptual orientation of the Boston group, which at that time included Harry Stack Sullivan, Gerald Caplan, and Erich Lindemann. Hsien Rin was sent to Harvard in 1955 and was soon followed by Chenchin Hsu and Chu-chang Chen, who studied child psychiatry and group psychotherapy respectively. More than a dozen trainees in psychology, psychiatry, social work, and nursing followed these initial sojourners over the next fifteen years. They studied in London, Boston, and elsewhere in the United States. Most were funded through WHO, but the United States Agency for International Development (AID) and the East-West Center were also sponsors. Returning staff became graduate instructors and were called upon to direct new service projects within their specialties.

International assistance played other roles, too. Consultants to the medical school lent their weight towards integrating psychiatry more firmly into the general curriculum. In 1955, Dr. Charles Gundry carried out a WHO survey for Taiwan. He recommended that the child psychiatry division be enlarged to function as a demonstration center for child guidance: to serve as a teaching, training, and research center in child psychiatry (Hsu 1972). As a consequence, the Taipei Children's Mental Health Center (TCMHC), affiliated with the Department of Psychiatry and Neurology, was opened in 1956. Shortly thereafter, Hsu spent two years training at the Judge Baker Guidance Center and Harvard University Children's Medical Center. Funds to build TCMHC and a new 400-bed mental hospital in Kaohsiung and to train its personnel were provided by the United States International Cooperation Administration Mission to China (ICA).

Expansion of Services

Taiwan's Provincial Health Department (PHD) drafted a Ten-Year Health Plan in 1964. In that report, Dr. Lin summarized the mental health program's previous eighteen years, projected its goals for the next ten years, and described some difficulties. Mental health services and activities had expanded on several planes. Graduate education was organized in 1956 based on the themes of local training to meet the sociocultural needs of Chinese patients, theoretical eclecticism, and multidisciplinary teams for service delivery (Lin 1961). In 1954, the Child Mental Health Division began looking for ways to work with teachers in an early identification and primary prevention capacity. A mobile clinic begun in 1959 stimulated teacher interest in acquiring mental health concepts to deal with problem children. This interest grew into a series of seminars. One year later, a special demonstration program, the East Gate Project, was set up with two objectives. The first was to teach basic knowledge and skills in mental health to all teachers of the school; the second was to train leaders to establish counselors' offices (Hsu and Lin 1969).

The pilot project brought governmental attention to the need to fund counselor training and work with children with learning disabilities. By 1964, twenty-six schools were affiliated with TCMHC and were receiving consultation in handling problem children.

On the research plane, the preliminary epidemiological survey (which had sampled 20,000 subjects in three communities) was replicated. New findings showed a significant increase in all categories of disorder except schizophrenia. These were partially attributed to life stress associated with the massive arrival of immigrants from the mainland that had taken place since the first survey in 1946.

In 1964, Lin's perspective of the future called for a complete integration and expansion of mental health services into the public health program, benefiting the entire population served by the provincial and local health systems. This required intensifying University Hospital's use as a national training center for psychiatrists, psychologists, social workers, and nurses. It was hoped that teams of trained workers could be placed at key points in the existing public health system. Provincial general hospitals would add psychiatric units as personnel became available. These would function as centers for domiciliary, preventive, and clinical activities. Mobile mental health clinics would meanwhile serve the public through visits to general hospitals and health centers until specialized units could be added. Organizationally, the local health stations and public health centers would coordinate their services with the newly created acute care units in the general hospitals. Mental hospitals at Kaohsiung and Chikou would serve as regional centers to provide long-term treatment. Rehabilitation for chronic cases would be carried out at the 600-bed sanitorium to be built at Yuli. A second children's mental health center was planned for completion in 1972 in Kaohsiung. Like the TCMHC, it would focus on the prevention of disorder through programs in the schools and public health centers.

Problems salient to Lin in 1964 were personnel and funding shortages and TCMHC's temporary status, which made it difficult to carry out teaching and research duties there. More serious was the absence of a medical officer in the Provincial Health Department to direct implementation of this plan. This shortcoming, which remains today, underscores the limited political weight Lin was able to amass for advancing the interests of national mental health programing. In his report, Lin urged the PHD to assume responsibility for planning and carrying out the program, training the various workers, and supervising direct services. He stated, by way of justification, that, "since mental health is a public health problem, PHD should be able to secure the funds required" (Lin 1964a: 177).

Public and Private Health Systems as the Context for Mental Health Services

None of the three levels of health administration for the country—National Health Administration, Taiwan Provincial Health Department (including county and city services), and Taipei City Health Department—contains an administrative bureau, division, or committee responsible for mental health programs. Responding to Lin's plea, the Department of Health did establish in 1968 a Committee for Mental Health at the provincial level. Its aim was to undertake planning commensurate with the Ten-Year Mental Health Project. The committee, composed of Provincial Health Department administrators, consultants from NTUH, and superintendents of the public mental hospitals, met occasionally until August 1972 and was mainly involved in training mental health personnel. In 1972, however, it was disbanded and its functions theoretically integrated into the operations of a related PHD department (National Health Administration 1976).

The low priority assigned psychiatric care is further reflected in the fact that it was the eleventh and last priority item considered in the Ten-Year Health Plan. In the budget, it was the sixth priority among the programs listed (Lin 1964a). Its total ten-year cost was estimated at $5,762,736. This figure can be compared with the highest budget item, medical care, predicted at $27,091,131.

The place of psychiatric care can be better appreciated by knowing the overall public health system in which it functions. All health bodies are under the executive branch (yuan) of the national government (fig. 3.1). The National Health Administration (NHA) has a functional, although not directly administrative, relationship to both the Taipei City and Provincial Health Departments (THD, PHD). All three departments have separate budgets, although they share some sources of funding. It is

Figure 3.1
Administration of Taiwan's Health Organization
June 1977

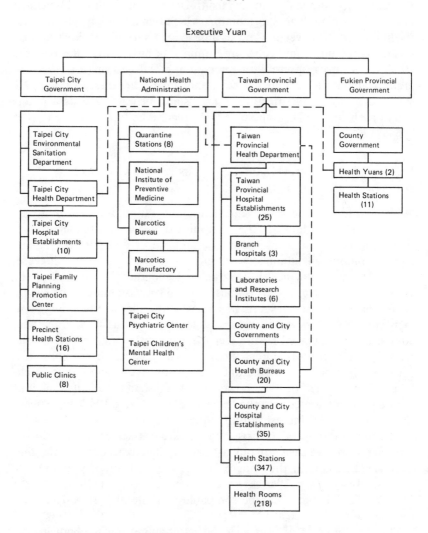

Key: ———— Administrative responsibility
     – – – Functional relationships

Source: *Health Statistics: General Health Statistics, Republic of China, 1976.* Taipei: National Health Administration, 1977.

worth noting that at the national level, health has a lower administrative position and lower priority than, for example, education, which operates at the ministerial level.

The delivery system includes twenty county and city health bureaus, 347 local health stations with 216 branch village health rooms, 423 mobile health units, twenty-six provincial hospitals, eighteen county and city hospitals, and various disease hospitals and control stations (fig. 3.2). The provincial bed capacity is 9,052; 3,700 (41 percent) are situated in Taipei. Within this network, there are three mental hospitals located at Yuli, Taipei, and Kaohsiung. Bed capacity for these three facilities is 2,600, or 29 percent of the total available for general health.

Administratively, Taipei city is divided into sixteen districts and serviced by a health station for each area. Four general hospitals and four other specialty facilities serve the metropolitan area under city jurisdiction. Taipei sponsors one mental hospital, the 150-bed Taipei City Psychiatric Center (TCPC), plus the TCMHC, which offers outpatient and day-care services.

Additionally, the military operates eleven veteran's hospitals in affiliation with the Veteran's General Hospital, a modern and prestigious 1,500-bed compound in Taipei. Among the veteran's hospitals and the army general hospitals, it is estimated that there are some 3,800 psychiatric-designate beds (NHA 1976). Several of these facilities, notably at Puli and Peitou, are used primarily as long-term care centers for chronic patients.

This public health program is by no means the complete health picture in Taiwan. The majority of people use private practitioners. There are approximately 8,563 hospitals/clinics in the private sector with more than 18,600 beds. More than 2,000 private beds are in Taipei alone. In terms of psychiatry, sixty private mental hospitals and clinics exist with an accumulated 1,750-bed capacity. Private care takes two forms (Kleinman 1980). The Taipei City Health Department grants a token subsidy ($1 per patient per day) to a number of small institutions providing care for impoverished public patients. With such minimal resource allocation, conditions in these settings are bleak. They function more like prisons or warehouses than hospitals, since patients abandoned by their families often are incarcerated for life with minimal treatment (Kleinman 1980: 201). In stark contrast, elite-class patients can attend special clinics and hospitals, charging fees comparable to those in the American system. Here patients receive contemporary Western therapeutics from Taiwan's most prominent psychiatrists.

Health planners are very much concerned about the typical maldistribution of services. Tsuei (1978) points to Taipei as the vortex of both general and specialty health services for the country—at the expense of rural

Figure 3.2
Organization of Taiwan Provincial Health Department
June 1977

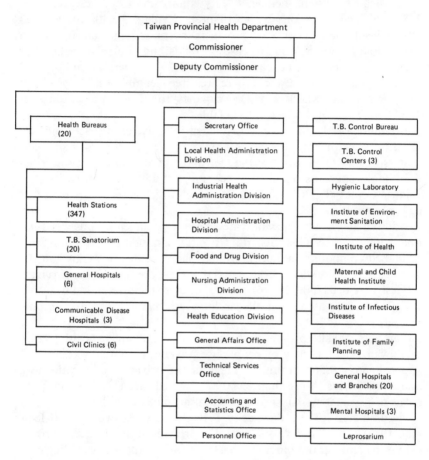

Source: *Health Statistics: General Health Statistics, Republic of China, 1976.* Taipei: National Health Administration, 1977.

areas. Not only are ten city and five large private hospitals concentrated there, but all three government medical schools (each affiliated with a large teaching hospital) are located in Taipei. Of the 32,452 medical beds in the country, 7,172 (22 percent) are found in this one metropolitan area holding 12 percent of the populace. In other terms, Taipei has 34.7 beds per 10,000 people. The rest of the nation has only 17.7. Moreover, Taipei has over twice as many physicians per 10,000 population as the rest of the country: 13.9 versus 6.0 per 10,000. Interestingly, 80 percent of the population employ nongovernmental physicians to treat their ailments.

In addition to the three provincial mental institutions and one city hospital with a total of 2,750 public beds, the three major teaching hospitals in Taipei have approximately 100 beds altogether. Therefore, 3,000 beds are associated with active therapeutic intervention, while 5,000 beds in veteran's hospitals and other private hospitals receive "chronic" cases. Translated into global population terms, there are 5,533 persons for each therapeutic bed and for all classes of psychiatric care, one bed per 2,075.

About 100 trained psychiatrists practice within these settings. This contrasts with the almost 10,000 licensed general practitioners. Taiwan has only two Ph.D.-level clinical psychologists. These figures strongly underscore psychiatry's tenuous position even within the government's medical service framework.

Budgetary Allocations

Another indicator of mental health priority is its monetary allocation within national and public health budgets. In 1975, the national, provincial, and Taipei City budgets for public health amounted to .08 percent, 4.03 percent, and 6.03 percent of their respective total budgetary allocations (NHA 1976). The following year, a total of $58 million (including foreign aid contributions) was expended on health among all levels of government. The Taiwan provincial government—with $38 million to spend—has almost 60 percent of the total health budget. This compares with an overall national budget of $4.5 billion, including more than $1 billion spent for defense alone. Therefore, about 1.29 percent of the national expenditure went to health concerns (Europa 1977).

Lin first calculated the Mental Health Program's budget in the 1964 Ten-Year Health Plan. He saw an initial capital outlay of $350,000 for constructing a custodial care hospital at Yuli, setting up fifteen-bed acute care wards in provincial hospitals each year, and opening a new children's clinic in Kaohsiung in 1972. By FY 1975, the complete operating budgets for the mental health program were projected at $810,000.

However, actual expenditures in 1976 far exceeded these earlier estimates (see Health Statistics, NHA 1977). The Provincial Taipei Mental Hospital alone required $3,626,000. Yuli and Kaohsiung Hospitals spent

$913,132 and $725,649 respectively. TCPC, whose opening caused a cutback in expansion of TCMHC, expended $365,187 during the same period. These four facilities account for a surprisingly significant 9.71 percent of the overall health allocation.

These figures reflect both the extraordinary burden of long-term custodial care and the expense of operating teaching facilities—major functions of Kaohsiung Hospital and TCPC. Not included are NTUH, Tainan's Department of Psychiatry, and the community mental health centers at Taipei, Kaohsiung, and Taichung.

OTHER FACTORS INFLUENCING THE DELIVERY OF SERVICES

Additional factors at the national level also influence the nature and quality of mental health services. These involve availability of insurance, training opportunities, "brain drain" problems, and the perceived need for psychological resources identified through epidemiological surveys.

Insurance

Insurance or third-party payment governs the behavior of both health care providers and those seeking help. Insurance providers have the power to decide who the clients are plus which types of personnel receive payment for their services. A national health insurance for multiple categories of citizens is not available in Taiwan. People are generally responsible for their own medical needs except for "indigents," who receive government-subsidized treatment (NHA 1976). The other exceptions to this generalization are government employees and certain laborers. These individuals, amounting to about 10 percent of the population, receive free medical attention as beneficiaries of two insurance plans. The remaining 90 percent (excluding military personnel) must personally pay to visit a physician, including a psychiatrist.

Although the TCPC does have a new program to accept a few low-income patients, the specialized services of psychiatric hospitalization and consultation are restricted to the slim percentage of Westernized upper-middle and upper classes who can afford them. Within this system, economics dictates treatment policy. Those with limited finances can only afford brief, drug-oriented interventions with minimal hospitalization. Wealthier, educated families conform well with the Western-trained psychiatrists' orientation and are willing to financially support the psychocentric and biomedical therapeutics offered them.

Training Opportunities

Until the early 1970s, NTUH was the only training ground for Taiwan's mental health manpower. Its core staff was responsible for determining the country's course of action in this area: it researched program needs, conceived service delivery components, and educated a multidisciplinary group to operate the clinics.

The orientation transmitted by Taiwan's first psychiatrists to their students originated from contact with the social and community psychiatry formulations of Harry Stack Sullivan and Gerald Caplan. The educational relationship with American psychiatry, a source of advanced training, consultation, and funding, gave psychiatry at the National Taiwan University a "contemporary" character from the beginning. It was contemporary, that is, as defined by the American preoccupation with psychoanalytic theory and sociocultural aspects of psychiatry. This contrasts with the Kraepelinean or "descriptive" approach adhered to by the European-influenced psychiatric educators throughout Asia.

NTUH continues to dominate psychiatric education in Taiwan although its early driving force, Tsung-yi Lin, departed for the director's position of the WHO Mental Health Division in the mid-1960s. Now, however, psychiatric residency is available at the psychiatric unit of the Tri-Service Hospital (serving the army, navy, and air force); TCPC, directed by a NTUH professor, Eng-kung Yeh; Veteran's General Hospital; and at the provincial mental hospital in Kaohsiung.

Even with these new training centers opening up, academic psychiatry remains tightly constricted. Critical problems arise because there are few positions and little institutional pressure to create new ones. Lin had sought to circumvent this problem through creation of psychiatric units in government hospitals, but the idea never materialized.

The key question is where to place professionals when existing university departments are restricted in size and number by limited resources. The growth in the number of individuals receiving credentials, some of them trained in prestigious schools overseas, creates the demand for assignment to responsible positions commensurate with educational status. Such opportunities simply do not exist for more recent graduates. Adequately funded positions in private hospitals and rewarding governmental assignments are also scarce because of psychiatry's relatively low priority. Under these conditions, it is more advantageous for qualified personnel to leave the country. In fact, many have left over the last ten years.

Brain Drain

A number of factors have combined to make "brain drain," the loss of well-educated mental health workers, a severe problem for Taiwan.[1] The lack of jobs within prestigious institutions like NTUH is a major one. Another factor is that almost a score of the brightest students were sent abroad. Many earned degrees qualifying them to work in their host country. Returning to Taiwan, they were sometimes placed in the awkward position of working under former teachers who were educationally less "sophisticated" than themselves. Yet, because of the age-related seniority system, the older staff were able to maintain their more powerful positions. Consequently, some returnees were frustrated in efforts to try out newly learned skills or teach their specialties.

On a different plane, Tsung-yi Lin's departure left a leadership vacuum difficult to overcome. He was a powerful, authoritative figure. Nationally and internationally recognized, Lin was capable of gaining support for the discipline's expansion within Taiwan. A successor had not been cultivated prior to Lin's departure. In the transition, the program's momentum and attractiveness to new students began fading. Factionalism emerged over the question of whether psychiatry and neurology should be split into separate departments. In this atmosphere, the opportunities overseas became more attractive. Especially vulnerable were those who felt their advancement chances limited and saw more possibilities for professional and personal freedom abroad.

A final influential factor is the political uncertainty of Taiwan in the face of withdrawal of political recognition by the world community. Taiwan's fading political position has pushed its professionals outside the circuit of communication and knowledge exchange fostered by international agencies. This lack of stimulation and support from abroad cannot help but reduce the development and innovation of its programs.

Epidemiological Surveys

The last factor shaping the character and quality of Taiwanese psychiatry is the intensive survey documentation of psychological problems and research pinpointing the social stresses presumed to be their determinants. Taiwan, perhaps more than any other country in Asia, has made direct use of epidemiological findings to promote and plan its mental health program. This is attributable to the fact that Tsung-yi Lin, Hsien Rin, and Jung-ming Chu, principal investigators in the three major epidemiological investigations, were also the key figures in conceiving and implementing the country's system of mental health care (Lin 1953; Lin et al. 1969; Rin, Chu, and Lin 1966).

In appraising the psychiatric needs of Taiwan, these researchers gave full attention to the linkage between the sociocultural variables and patterns of disorder. The identification of high-risk groups led them to examine closely the effects of migration stress, sex and sibling rank, rural versus urban residence, and the consequences of giving up traditional value orientations under pressure of modernization (e.g., Chance, Rin, and Chu 1966; Chu 1972; Ko 1975; Lin et al. 1969; Rin 1969; Rin et al. 1966; Rin, Schooler, and Caudill 1973).

Several findings highlight the impact of culture on rates of disorder. For example, Rin (1969) found that the highest proportion of psychophysiological reactions were among youngest-born females, while the eldest sons were overrepresented among psychotic inpatients. Extreme family role differentiation by age and sex were used to explain these phenomena. The youngest girls are the object of intrafamilial tension and aggression. They are sometimes put up for adoption in times of economic hardship. Predictably, female suicide attempts account for 77 percent of the total cases at Taipei's suicide treatment center (MacKay Counseling Center 1976). Older brothers, on the other hand, enjoy the most privileged offspring position. Encouraged to be dependent, they are pampered, overindulged, and unprepared for later high-pressure situations. School competition is the first major stressful experience for males; entrance into a good university insures subsequent attractiveness to employers.

NTUH epidemiological studies also showed that groups undergoing rapid social change did have elevated rates of psychoneurosis, although no positive correlation emerged between change and psychosis (Rin, Schooler, and Caudill 1973). Comparing those individuals who fled to Taiwan during the mass migration of 1949 with native Taiwanese Chinese, the former group showed more susceptibility to neurosis. The Taiwanese had a greater proportion of mental retardation. For the migrants, being a female and dramatically losing one's socioeconomic status were strong predictors of neurotic symptoms. Also at risk were men who abandoned their traditional value system for identification with modern modes of thinking without sufficient knowledge of modern social life or intercultural contact. Men with modern values plus higher intercultural contact and men who clung to a traditional value core although interacting with modern society fared much better.

Apparently, the strict security control and prevailing tensions associated with the omnipresent "threat" from the mainland foster a social norm of defensive and distrustful behavior (Yeh 1972). Psychological security is found only within family and primary kinship groups. Insecurity is felt with most "outsiders." "One must be cautious about his own behavior and be vigilant against others to keep from being cheated" is a typical attitude. Yeh sees this as generating a "paranoid society." It is particularly evident in the delusional—yet somehow real—themes of students in therapy.

Taken together, these studies served both to advance the disciplines of transcultural and social psychiatry and to form the basis for requesting new treatment programs for high-risk groups. In recent years, programs for counseling college students, adolescents, and suicidal individuals have joined the already operating adult and child treatment centers in

Taipei (Tseng 1978). The provincial government has also begun three community mental health centers. The first one started in 1974 at Hsin-chuang, Taipei County. Taipei City has initiated a mental health project to deliver services through the city's health stations. It is under the supervision of staff from five psychiatry departments. From the perspective of rational planning, the direct link between research and services found in Taiwan is both exemplary and rare.

PSYCHIATRIC RESOURCES AVAILABLE: SELECTED EXAMPLES

This section presents an analysis of the services undertaken at selected sites using the framework depicted in table 2.1. The variables in this scheme describe the components of a modern mental health delivery system as planned in the United States or recommended by WHO experts. They provide a framework for portraying therapeutic resources in all three countries investigated in this survey.

Table 3.1 summarizes major residential treatment centers, including private as well as city- and province-funded facilities. Those identified as teaching facilities provide training for psychiatric manpower. Table 3.2 lists important outpatient and counseling centers, including those where staff were interviewed for this survey. This list is not exhaustive, but it accounts for the well-established and publicly visible counseling services on the island.

Intensive interviewing was done at TCPC, NTUH, Northern Area Community Mental Health Center (NACMCH), Tri-Service Department of Psychiatry (TSP), and Jen-Chi Charity Mental Hospital. Visits were also made to the Taipei City Community Mental Health Project, Professor Chang Counseling Center, Hua-Ming Counseling Center, and Mac-Kay Hospital's Life-Line Suicide Counseling Center. This case study is based on data from questionnaires and other information gathered in these visits, as well as on recorded conversations with eight physicians, four psychologists, three counselors, three social workers, and two psychiatric nurses from ten diverse agencies (table 3.3).

FRAMEWORK FOR MENTAL HEALTH RESOURCE STATUS
Comprehensive Services

The first attribute of a mental health system is comprehensiveness, i.e., the availability of diverse services, specialty units, and treatment modalities covering the entire spectrum of client population needs. Community mental health programs in the United States are required by the 1975 Public Law 94–63 and National Institute for Mental Health policy to

TABLE 3.1 Major Residential Facilities in Taiwan

	Size (beds)
Government	
Provincial Taipei Mental Hospital	900
Provincial Yuli Mental Hospital	1,400
Provincial Kaohsiung Mental Hospital (teaching)	200
Tainan General Hospital Department of Psychiatry	100
Veteran's and Army General Hospitals with Psychiatric Units (throughout Taiwan)	3,800
*Taipei City Psychiatric Center (teaching)	150
*National Taiwan University Hospital (Taipei, teaching)	40
*Tri-Service Hospital Department of Psychiatry (Taipei, teaching)	25
Veteran's General Hospital (Taipei, teaching)	20
Private	
MacKay Hospital Department of Psychiatry (Taipei)	50
*Jen-Chi Charity Hospital (Taipei)	182
Yu-Shan Hospital	50
Jen-Ai Charity Hospital (Taipei)	230
Chu-Huei Charity Hospital	200
Other private hospitals	1,038
Total	8,385

*Interview sites

TABLE 3.2 Major Outpatient and Counseling Centers in Taiwan

Government
  *Taipei Children's Mental Health Center
  *National Taiwan University Hospital Children's Day Care Center (Taipei)
  Veteran's General Hospital Adolescent Mental Health Project (Taipei)
  *National Taiwan University Hospital Psychiatric Day Care Program
  *Northern Area Community Mental Health Center (Taipei)
  Kaohsiung Community Mental Health Center
  Taichung Community Mental Health Center
  *Taipei City Community Mental Health Project (via 16 district health stations)

Private
  *Professor Chang Adolescent Counseling Center (Taipei)
  *Suicide Life-Line; MacKay Hospital Counseling Center (Taipei)
  *Hua-Ming Counseling Center for Family and Youth (Taipei)

*Interview sites

TABLE 3.3 Personnel Administered Questionnaires 1, 2, and 3 (Taiwan)

	Number of staff completing			
	Questionnaire			Open-ended
Facility and staff	1	2	3	interviews
Taipei City Psychiatric Center (TCPC)				
Psychiatrist	1	2	2	1
Nursing director		1	1	
Social worker		1		
National Taiwan University Hospital (NTUH)				
Psychiatrist	1	1	3	2
Social work (director)		1	3	1
Psychologist			2	1
Occupational therapist			2	
Psychiatric nurse			2	
Taipei Children's Mental Health Center (TCMHC)				
Psychiatrist	1			1
NTUH Children's Day Care Center				
Psychologist (director)				1
Tri-Service Hospital (TSP)				
Psychiatrist	1	2		
Jen-Chi Charity Hospital				
Psychiatrist (chief)	1	1		
Psychiatric nurse		1		
Northern Area Community Mental Health Center (NACMHC)				
Psychologist (chief)	1	1	2	
Professor Chang Adolescent Counseling Center				
Psychologist			1	2
Life-Line				
Social worker				1
Hua-Ming Counseling Center				
Counselor				2
Veteran's General Adolescent Mental Health Project				
Physician				1
Total	6	11	18	13

provide twelve essential services and support functions. These define the concept of "comprehensive" for federally funded facilities. Table 3.4 lists these criteria plus additional supporting functions related to agencies: research, evaluation, planning, and teaching.

Specific treatment modalities that may be drawn upon for case management are listed in table 3.5. These two lists are complementary: the first reflects the breadth of client populations served, and the second shows the depth of therapies available to them.

Are the mental health centers in Taipei offering comprehensive psychiatric care? The answer appears to be a qualified yes. The full range of care is available, but only if the various programs are taken together as a composite system. The question of integration and referral among these centers is complex. It is reviewed later under the rubric "Interinstitutional Continuity of Care." For discussion purposes, the patterning of services can be analyzed as though there were some degree of integration and wholeness to the system.

The prestigious NTUH complex and the more recently developed TCPC are by far the most comprehensive care providers in Taiwan. These two key teaching hospitals are identical in what they do and do not offer. All inpatient facilities visited had outpatient departments, neurological assessment, and—except for Jen-Chi—carried out consultation and education functions. TSP was the only site without a day-care program. NTUH's day-care center is the most developed. It was initiated in 1952 by the present chairman of the Psychiatry Department, Chu-chang Chen (1971).

Neurological and diagnostic assessment are well established at the teaching centers. The Department of Psychiatry and Neurology at NTUH devotes half of its beds to neurological cases, continuing the historical association of these two disciplines. Training, education/consultation, and research are active components of the hospital departments. NTUH coordinated the mental health personnel development project planned by the Committee for Mental Health in the early 1960s. Staff were also assigned to educate elementary school teachers in early identification and management of behaviorally dysfunctional and mentally retarded pupils. Recently, public health nurses and social workers received specialized instruction for manning Taipei's sixteen health stations. Research has ranged from the seminal investigations of psychopathology in selected towns to more recent studies of cortical lesions and malformations, drug trials, suicide, effects of acupuncture on neurotic disorders, and assessment of developmental disabilities in children.[2] Consultation is an important link between the psychiatric departments and a number of counseling centers and education agencies in Taipei. The community mental health centers are mandated to conduct education

TABLE 3.4 Availability of Comprehensive Services in Taiwan

Service function	NTUH Complex	TCPC	TSP	Veteran's General	Jen-Chi	NACMHC	Three counseling centers
Inpatient	+	+	+	+	+	−	−
Outpatient	+	+	+	+	+	+	+
Emergency	+	+	+	+	−	−	+
Partial hospitalization	+	+	−	−	+	−	−
Transitional living	planned	planned	−	−	−	−	−
Follow-up	+	+	−	−	−	+	+
Children's service	+	+	−	+	−	−	−
Geriatric care	−	planned	−	−	+	−	−
Drug abuse	−	−	−	−	+	−	−
Diagnostic	+	+	+	+	+	+	−
Neurological	+	+	+	+	+	−	−
Suicide prevention	−	−	−	−	+	+	+
Educational	+	+	+	−	−	+	+
Mental health research	+	+	+	−	−	−	−
Program evaluation	−	−	−	−	−	−	−
Teaching/training	+	+	+	+	−	−	inservice only

+ indicates available
− indicates unavailable

TABLE 3.5 Treatment Modalities Available in Taiwan

Modality	NTUH Complex	TCPC	TSP	Jen-Chi	NACMHC	Three counseling centers
Electroconvulsive therapy	++	+	+	+	–	–
Physiotherapy	+++	–	–	–	–	–
Drug	+++	+++	+++	+++	++	–
Psychotherapy	++	+	++	++	+++	++
Behavior modification	++	+++	+++	–	+	+
Group therapy	+++	+++	+++	++	+	++
Family therapy	++	–	–	++	++	++
Occupational therapy	+++	+++	+++	+++	–	–
Work therapy	+++	–	–	+++	–	–
Other	ex-patient club, play therapy	milieu therapy	recreation	dancing needlework cooking	home visits	crisis intervention

+++ often
++ sometimes
+ seldom
– never

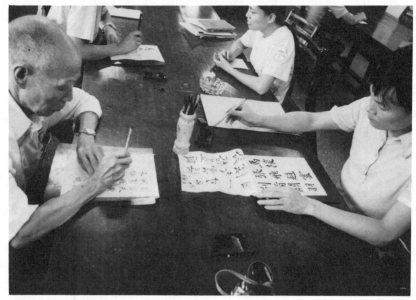

A recreational therapist, *left,* demonstrates traditional calligraphy at National Taiwan University Hospital's day-care program for chronic cases.

seminars within community organizations and at public meetings in their areas.

Evidence of strength in clinical tasks was found in the areas of occupational therapy (OT), group work, and chemotherapy. Chemotherapy is by far the most widely employed intervention modality and is usually expected by patients. Besides drug treatment, ward activities appeared well structured. The patients are kept busy with such OT tasks as folk dancing, singing, arts and crafts, calligraphy, recreational sports, and making small objects for sale. NTUH has some patients in clerical tasks or gardening assignments around the hospital prior to discharge, enabling them to gain prevocational work competency. Belonging to a group is an important and reinforcing facet of Chinese socialization, so this format has been seized upon for therapeutic talk sessions by ward psychiatrists. C. C. Chen and Agnes Wu at NTUH facilitate an ongoing encounter group whose members include day-care patients and former inpatients.

Limitations among these agencies are also apparent. There were no geriatric, transitional living, or substance abuse units. Jen-Chi Hospital did, however, house many older patients and some drug dependents. The City of Taipei manages an Anti-Narcotics Institute, but no information was found on its operations. Informants did not view narcotics addiction as a significant problem: it is discouraged by a mandatory death sentence for those found selling heroin.

Psychological assessment other than elementary differential diagnosis is conspicuously absent since very few psychologists work within the medical teaching centers. Applied behavioral analysis is done only within the Children's Day Care Center (NTUH). Neuropsychological test batteries for assessing cortical dysfunction have yet to be developed. The three community mental health centers do give their outpatients psychological tests. Therefore, some use is made of personality, intelligence, and aptitude scales, and especially Ko's Mental Health Questionnaire (T. H. Ko's modification of the Minnesota Multiphasic Personality Inventory).

Follow-up services are restricted to those who make return visits to hospital outpatient clinics. Manpower numbers prevent home visits or active efforts to initiate contact with discharged patients. One suicide prevention program in Taipei operates out of MacKay Memorial Hospital and has telephone, walk-in, and emergency counseling functions. This center appears to have a well-trained and enthusiastic staff. It is linked to other city facilities through a referral network and has close contact with the other hot-line group, at Professor Chang Counseling Center. Lastly, program evaluation has not gained the attention of Taiwanese professionals. Nor is therapy outcome research regularly undertaken in these settings (e.g., Ko 1974).

Chemotherapy, previously mentioned as a clinical strength, can also be viewed as a limitation of the system. Drug assignment dominates to the point of excluding alternative forms of therapy. Except for the private counseling and community mental health centers, the traditional medical approach is stressed. It emphasizes physical interventions—drugs, shock, and hospitalization.

The contravening option, considering client psychosocial conditions and using a social-influence or educative model, is to some extent offered by the counseling centers. This difference can be attributed to the types of patients seen since these centers work with less-impaired individuals. Behavior therapy, as practiced by British and North American professionals, is represented only by Yang's work at the Children's Day Care Program at NTUH and a simple token economy system on one ward at TCPC. Although families frequently participate in case management and are encouraged to maintain close contact with doctor and patient during hospitalization, nothing akin to the Family Therapy Movement exists in Taiwan. On the other hand, several faculty at NTUH are interested in this approach and it may become popular in the future (C. C. Chen et al. 1975).

Preventive Orientations

The second mental health resource variable concerns the presence of prevention programs. Intimately tied to the community mental health ideology, prevention programs aim to eliminate conditions adverse to "normal" psychological development and secure coping resources for individuals at "risk" of disorder. Theoretically, this occurs when practitioners leave their offices and employ their skills in changing stressful elements affecting oppressed minority groups and institutional life. Prevention usually takes the form of consultation, education, and experimentation in settings like schools, social welfare agencies, prisons, primary medical care clinics, parenting groups, and so forth. Action at this level presumably mitigates the pressure for direct services as the rate of new cases declines. Yet, it requires additional personnel to cover both clinical and educational functions.

Preventive services expected at accredited mental health programs cover four areas (Errion and Moen 1976). *Public Information* dissemination requires the use of news media and public forums to motivate people to take responsibility for their own health and the health of others. *Public Education* is more specific; it is aimed toward risk groups, such as expectant mothers, instructing them in how to avoid psychological problems. Organizations and agencies dealing with large populations are offered *Public Consultation* services. Lastly, *Ecological Changes* are those activities focusing on people's interaction with their environment. The level and magnitude is significantly enlarged to include action at the social, economic, and political systems level. Action here would include efforts to assist groups to achieve political power, the development of neighborhood and community organizations, or work on poverty relief projects to stem the dehumanizing effects of economic uncertainties.

Prevention services undertaken among the sites visited are displayed in table 3.6. It is difficult to use this schema accurately because it requires much finer discrimination among types of prevention work than those made by professionals in Taiwan. In fact, although some projects may be conceptualized as preventive, they may not actually be labeled as such and are included here only by investigator inference.

Inferences are unnecessary, however, regarding the work of the community mental health center and the three counseling clinics. Their expressed objectives are public information, education, and consultation. The NACMHC is most strongly associated with these service areas. It has a public education specialist (a B.A. psychologist) who plans lectures on such topics as family and interpersonal conflict, problems of adolescents and of child rearing, and development of self-concept. In one month

TABLE 3.6 Availability of Prevention Programs in Taiwan

Prevention type	NTUH complex	TCPC	TSP	Jen-Chi	NACMHC	Three counseling centers
Public information	+	+	−	−	+++	+++
Public education	++	++	−	−	++	+++
Public consultation	+++	+++	+	−	+++	+
Ecological change	+	+	−	+	+	−

+++ often
++ sometimes
+ seldom
− never

alone (June 1977), there were seven community lectures with 600 people in attendance. In 1976, 128 families composing an entire village were individually contacted for mental health discussions. Offers for intensive help and education were not well accepted, so staff decided that approaching the community through such structures as the schools was more fruitful.

Targets of consultation by NACMHC include factories, neighborhood groups, public health nurses, and school teachers. Parent education contacts form a major service area. An annual publication by the center is sent to the Department of Public Health for teacher education. Additional educational materials are planned for distribution among the public. Most clients are attracted through newspaper advertising and community lectures.

Professor Chang and the Suicide Life-Line are also active in educating the public about their services. Each targets its own high-risk population, either adolescents with problems or those contemplating suicide. These centers are less involved in educational work with other agencies or community groups.

NTUH and TCPC have strongly emphasized consultation with organizations in contact with potential cases. NTUH began more than twenty years ago to send its mobile clinic out for guidance sessions with public health nurses. It was soon broadened to include school teachers through the East Gate Project. Now, other educational programs, the police department, and the pediatrics section of NTUH are involved. NTUH has roots in nearly all social welfare/counseling centers in Taipei. Its staff either developed or now offers regular consultation to NACMHC, Life-Line, Professor Chang, and the Adolescent Mental Health Unit at Veteran's General Hospital, and others. TCPC, under Professor Yeh's guidance, has helped train 200 public health nurses and social workers as mental health specialists. These workers now occupy the Taipei district health stations and operate a small community mental health clinic within one of them. Specialists are trained to direct attention toward schools in particular. They also assist social welfare workers and private general practitioners. This program has continued the community extension service that was previously carried out by TCMHC.

Jen-Chi and TSP concentrate completely on direct services, although TSP does send personnel to the surgical departments of its hospital for selected cases.

Ecological change as a service area is weakly developed. The only signs of institutional change as a function of intervention were efforts to make teachers more sensitive to the psychological needs of children and access given poor families to the resources of Jen-Chi and TCPC. Projects for social action and economic or political change among risk populations are not considered within the purview of mental health care.

Continuity of Care within the Facility: Manpower

This resource variable focuses on manpower strength and the capacity for multiprofessional "team" contact with clients. The full team approach to staffing—including psychiatrist, psychiatric nurse, psychologist, social worker, and occupational or rehabilitation counselor—provides a continuity of care within the agency. A multidisciplinary team is better suited for meeting the diverse and changing needs of a patient. Continuity is evidenced in the smooth intrateam referral process and a well-coordinated plan of treatment for each individual. A simple measure of manpower contact availability is the ratio of therapeutic personnel to inpatients and outpatients.

All categories of staff are well represented at TCPC and NTUH, but present to a lesser extent in the other settings (table 3.7). Psychiatrists are numerically the strongest of the treatment staff. After a large drop in numbers, social workers and occupational therapists appear to be second. Psychologists are least employed. Nurses are found in varying ratios to patients, from 1:2 to 1:6 in residential facilities.

The concept of multidisciplinary team involvement is most developed within the NTUH complex and TCPC. Both have emphasized training

TABLE 3.7 Multidisciplinary Teams and Manpower Availability in Taiwan: Staff Numbers and Staff-to-Patient Ratios

Profession	NTUH psychiatry	NTUH child day care	TCMHC	TCPC	TSP	Jen-Chi	NACMHC	Total
Psychiatrist (including residents)	15	1	2	15	5	4	.5	42.5
Psychologist	1.5	1	1	3	1	0	2	9.5
Nurse	15	1	1	50	9	22	1	99
Social worker	3	0	1	5	1	1	1	12
Occupational therapist	3	1	0	10	0	4	0	18
Beds	26			250	25	180		
Daily outpatients	60	26	10	50	20	20	±7	
Total new outpatients per year	3,434		673	581			±250	
Total outpatients per year	17,394			8,063			1,393	
Inpatients per therapeutic staff	1.8			7.5	2.85	20		
Outpatients per therapeutic staff	4	8.7	5	3.3	4	5	1.75	

nonmedical professional staff for support roles. However, these ancillary personnel remain secondary to the psychiatrist. Intake interviews, treatment plan formulation, and most major decisions are left to the physician. He brings ancillary personnel into a case as he sees fit. Typically, a psychologist is called in if a question of testing arises. The patient's family is occasionally referred to the social worker. Occupational therapy staff become involved before discharge or run day-care and rehabilitation activities under supervision.

The few highly trained social workers and psychologists are given teaching roles within the hospitals. Outside the medical structure, they become extremely active in counselor training, group psychotherapy, designing new services, and consultation to a wide range of social service agencies. TSP and Jen-Chi rely far less on multidisciplinary staff, although the former does provide a practicum for psychology students. Jen-Chi has an active occupational rehabilitation program with four OT staff, but is without the services of a psychologist and has no capacity for follow-up care.

The manpower potential is reflected in the figures at the bottom of table 3.7. Staff/patient ratios index the system's capacity for giving patients access to care providers. NTUH and TSP, with their small inpatient wards, obviously maintain the highest potential for staff availability. Jen-Chi has the lowest ratio of inpatients per therapeutic staff with 20 to 1. The other set of ratios examines the number of daily outpatients in relation to manpower (primarily psychiatrists). These numbers all seem satisfactory. Even NTUH with its enormous yearly attendance, 17,395, still has ample staff to see outpatients. NTUH averages one psychiatrist per four clients per day.

However, these figures are extremely conservative. On any given morning, one therapist may see between ten and thirty patients since outpatient duty is taken on rotation by just a few physicians. The majority of senior personnel are in resident supervision, outside consultation, research, administrative tasks, and pursuits other than outpatient care— a task assigned resident psychiatrists.

Continuity of Care: Interinstitutional

A second continuity of care resource variable involves the coordinated linking of services among different agencies. Continuity of care is achieved when a common relationship is maintained with an individual throughout an uninterrupted sequence of services (Errion and Moen 1976). The referral process within a facility, among different care providers, or between agencies should always aim for a standard of continuity. Strong linkage among institutions establishes a well-integrated refer-

Figure 3.3
Taipei City Referral Pathways

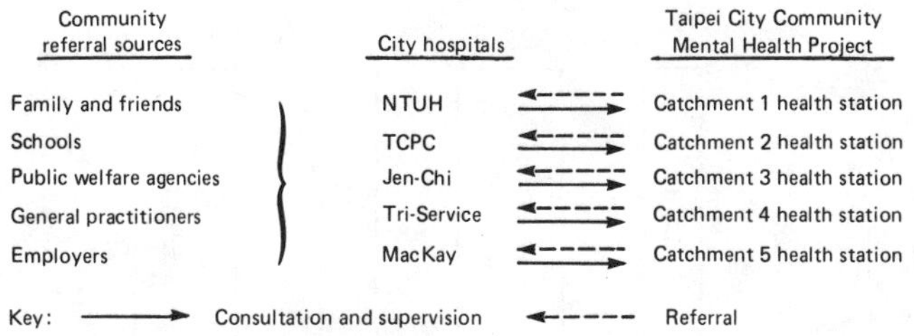

Community referral sources	City hospitals		Taipei City Community Mental Health Project
Family and friends	NTUH	◄----→	Catchment 1 health station
Schools	TCPC	◄----→	Catchment 2 health station
Public welfare agencies	Jen-Chi	◄----→	Catchment 3 health station
General practitioners	Tri-Service	◄----→	Catchment 4 health station
Employers	MacKay	◄----→	Catchment 5 health station

Key: ———→ Consultation and supervision ◄----- Referral

ral network when all necessary elements are merged into a unified service system.

A survey of sites showed that family and friends were by far the most frequent community referral source, followed by schools, the public welfare agencies, general practitioners, and employers. Police and priests were listed as "seldom" or "never." Referrals from the folk system were also extremely rare.

These community sources feed into the five major city hospitals (fig. 3.3). These hospitals, in turn, supervise clinical services within their five respective catchment areas of the newly founded Taipei City Community Mental Health Project (TCCMHP). The duties are performed by psychiatrically trained social workers and public health nurses within the sixteen health stations. The health stations not only receive consultation from their supervising hospitals, but have a working channel of communication for referring cases. Professor E. K. Yeh at TCPC has spearheaded the effort to unify the five hospitals as a formal supervisory unit for the TCCMHP.

NTUH occupies a central position based on its historical role in the evolution of Taiwan's programs (fig. 3.4). NTUH personnel maintain active consultation responsibilities at the four counseling centers listed, several of which they helped to create. The NACMHC was founded by two NTUH psychologists, Y. H. Ko and S. K. Yang, among others. It refers clients for additional treatment to either TCPC or NTUH and has a part-time psychiatrist consultant from Veteran's General Hospital. NTUH, with its small inpatient ward, must rely on other residential institutions for long-term patients and those who are uncontrollable. Yu-Shan, a small private mental hospital, occasionally houses obstreperous patients under the care of NTUH doctors. Jen-Chi and TCPC are sometimes given long-term referrals.

The provincial mental hospitals and army general hospitals are the last

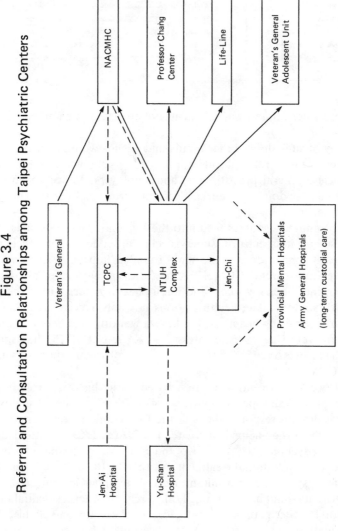

Figure 3.4
Referral and Consultation Relationships among Taipei Psychiatric Centers

NACMHC

Professor Chang
Center

Life-Line

Veteran's General
Adolescent Unit

Veteran's General

TCPC

NTUH
Complex

Jen-Chi

Provincial Mental Hospitals

Army General Hospitals

(long-term custodial care)

Jen-Ai
Hospital

Yu-Shan
Hospital

Key: — ─ ─► Referral of patients
————► Consultation

stop for chronic, unresponsive patients coming out of Taipei clinics. TCPC has a substantial number of yearly admissions referred from another private hospital, Jen-Ai. It receives fewer referrals from NTUH but maintains an extremely close working relationship with that department since E. K. Yeh retains a professorship there. Also, several NTUH residents are assigned to TCPC. Its child program is being assisted by Professor Hsu from the TCMHC.

The relationship patterns and channels of communication that have evolved historically determine to a large degree the referral pathways just cited. These channels are conduits for institutions to assist one another in expanding and strengthening their respective programs and passing along those clients whose needs are more effectively met elsewhere. Personnel from the major city hospitals have come together since 1975 to work as a supervisory unit ensuring a viable mental health program through the health stations. This feat is based on personal relationships and a prevailing spirit of cooperation and identity. The hospitals involved range from a private charity institution to facilities under the administration of the national and city governments and the armed forces.

It is difficult to judge whether an individual client is able to traverse the various components of Taipei's mental health system in a smooth and well-connected fashion at all times. But given the relatively large number of links among these diverse institutions and their professionals, it seems credible to suggest that an individual with financial resources has a good chance of moving through the system with an uninterrupted sequence of appropriate services.

Continuity with Community Care-giving

Continuity with community care-giving refers to the relationship between the service agency and those individuals who assume primary responsibility for the patient in her home or work environment. Typically, these individuals are family members, friends, employers, or community agents such as school teachers, police, village officials, and religious leaders. Their involvement with the service system may be prior to, during, or after the patient's direct contact with agency personnel. This variable seeks to determine the ways in which the agency uses community persons during intervention and their degree of involvement. The assumption is that greater involvement of significant others and community agents permits a smoother transition for the patient back into her social environment after discharge. By extending its treatment effects into the community through the assistance of significant others, the agency promotes continuity of care.

Six alternatives for providing continuity of care into the community were found in Taiwan (table 3.8). The first of these is the active follow-up of discharged patients. Follow-up takes two forms: either the client maintains contact with the agency as a regular outpatient or a public health nurse/social worker makes home visits. NACMHC was the only agency where home visitation was a major treatment policy. NTUH complex and TCPC sometimes followed-up their former inpatients but only through outpatient clinics. Jen-Chi lacked personnel for an active follow-up program. As a military hospital, TSP found it impractical to maintain contact with patients since they were either sent back to their bases or discharged from the service and returned home. Follow-up programs were especially difficult for those clinics with clients coming from distant parts of the island. These individuals were usually discharged into the care of doctors in their home towns.

A second means of promoting continuity of care into the community is

TABLE 3.8 Six Alternatives for Providing Continuity with Community Care-giving in Taiwan

Alternatives	NTUH Complex	TCPC	TSP	Jen-Chi	NACMHC
Active patient follow-up especially by social worker	++	++	−	−	+++
Educate or utilize family members as part of treatment plan	++	++	+	+	++
Relative stays in hospital with patient	+	+	+	+	N/A
Treatment within home or village setting	+	+	−	−	+++
Community agents assist in treatment (teacher, employer, village leader, M.D., police, etc.)	++	+	+	−	++
Participation in community activities during hospitalization encouraged	++	++	+	++	N/A

+++ always
++ sometimes
+ seldom
− never

to invite relatives to participate in the treatment process. This is accomplished by educating relatives in how to help deliver care. Sometimes family members assist by living in the hospital. All four residential facilities made some provisions for family members to stay with the patient. They requested this if the patient was critically ill, suicidal, senile, or uncontrollable. NACMHC was particularly interested in carrying out family educational activities and focused on parent training for child-rearing problems. The child division of NTUH is also interested in parent involvement. Child therapists there model techniques of behavior modification for home use by the parents. Sixty percent of the parents meeting with therapists are mothers while 20 percent are fathers.

Social workers at TCPC work with the family to find mutual treatment goals. Often this comes only after the family's confidence has been won by the physician. At Jen-Chi, a psychiatric explanation of the patient's condition is sometimes conveyed to family members, although their active involvement in case management is rare. This is also the situation at TSP where "education" is done through informal interviews and discussions. Even though family participation at TSP is problematical because patients come from outlying areas, visitation is strongly encouraged.

Treatment within the home or village setting after discharge or in lieu of hospitalization is quite rare except at NACMHC, which provides active outreach into homes, schools, and neighborhoods. In general, manpower is too precious for home treatment, and it is out of the question for areas outside of Taipei. The newly established TCCMHP is bringing services a little closer to the neighborhood level. NTUH's long-standing school consultation is aimed towards the same goal, but on a limited scale.

Staff at the two teaching hospitals and NACMHC report using community agents to assist in treatment. Those who do cooperate with the agencies are public health nurses and social workers at the district health stations, teachers, and occasionally the general practitioners who initially referred the patient. Employers, village leaders, and the police are seldom called upon to work with the agency.

Lastly, continuity of care in this domain is thought to be promoted by encouraging inpatients to participate in ongoing community activities, celebrations, or trial home visits. Except for TSP, staff do report occasional encouragement to keep patient attention on events outside the hospital. At TCPC, home visits are used as reinforcers in a kind of token economy system. Outings are made once per week at Jen-Chi to various points of interest in Taipei, such as fairs or temples. TSP has an option of giving recovering patients a weekend pass.

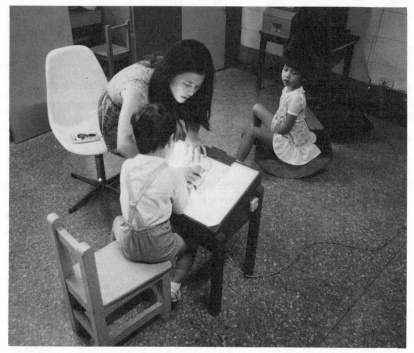

Child behavior modification program at National Taiwan University hospital.

Accessibility of Facilities

Accessibility is measured by the ease with which an individual in need may successfully use psychiatric services. This is accounted for by a number of factors. The most important one is simply the existence of facilities handling particular problems. Hospital accessibility, for example, is quite good within Taipei and Kaohsiung, even for specialty care, but practically nonexistent throughout the rest of the island. Except for government employees and certain laborers, though, insurance reimbursement is unavailable for those requesting psychiatric consultation. Indigent cases without family support are likely to be abandoned in warehouselike institutions. Accessibility is being strengthened in Taipei with the training and supervision of district health station workers by TCPC and the other supervisory hospitals. Similarly, the numerous private counseling centers, phone-in services, and community mental health centers strive toward ease of access for clients. However, once again, these programs are restricted to a few urban enclaves.

Staff perceptions of their agencies' accessibility can also be cited.

TCPC patients are seen to have difficulty getting to the facility primarily because it is on the outskirts of Taipei and the road leading to the hospital is under construction. The outpatient clinic is located more conveniently at a general hospital near the center of town. There was only a short wait to get into the hospital at the time of the survey. The government recently initiated a program to provide funds for the treatment of a few indigent people.

Staff interviewed at NTUH saw the long waiting list for hospitalization and the cost to the client's family as a "moderately serious problem."[3] NTUH is conveniently situated in the heart of Taipei. Therefore, location accessibility is good except for those who travel from outlying counties. Jen-Chi also has an excellent location. As a charity hospital, it does serve poor clients, but there is a moderate problem with a waiting list. Access to the NACMHC is seen by staff to be quite good on all dimensions except cost—viewed as a "moderately serious problem." TSP staff do not view accessibility as a major concern either: the military personnel are simply assigned there for treatment.

Two principal accessibility issues face Taiwan. First is the fact that the average citizen must pay for mental health care out of his own income. Secondly, there are only a few highly desirable and respected inpatient facilities. These institutions (NTUH, TCPC, Veteran's General, and a few others) each contain very limited bed space. All are located in Taipei. Outpatient and counseling services for certain problems are becoming generally more available and are well attended. However, they operate on limited funding, with limited manpower, and they serve only a few urban areas. It is obvious that most Taiwanese who need therapeutic assistance receive such help from alternative sources.

Staff Evaluation of Resource Strength

The final resource variable attends to staff perceptions of resource strength. Staff were asked to make judgments about the seriousness of twenty-one potential resource problems. These global evaluations may be used to confirm or qualify previous statements about Taiwan's mental health resources based on other data.

Table 3.9 presents responses from ten professionals confirming earlier statements about resource deficits in the system. First, the overall sense of low national priority and lack of budgetary support for present and future programs are found in items 1, 2, and 3. In terms of manpower, there is clear agreement that trained administrators and follow-up personnel are lacking. There is slightly less agreement that serious problems arise from lack of diagnostic and treatment staff. TSP and Jen-Chi are the only institutions indicating no problems in this area. The lack of inte-

TABLE 3.9 Staff Perceptions of Resource Deficits in Taiwan (*N*=10)

Potential problem	Problem seriousness			
	Very serious	Moderately serious	Slightly serious	Not a problem
1. Lack of help from government		30%	50%	20%
2. Not enough money for present treatment program		60%	30%	10%
3. Not enough money to develop future treatment programs		40%	20%	40%
4. Not enough trained administrators	30%	50%		20%
5. Not enough diagnostic staff	10%	30%	20%	40%
6. Not enough treatment staff	20%	30%	10%	40%
7. Not enough follow-up staff	50%	40%	10%	
8. Lack of relationship with other institutions	30%	20%	10%	40%
9. Other professionals don't support the program	20%	30%	20%	30%
10. Long waiting list		50%		50%
11. Not enough rooms to separate different kinds of patients		40%	20%	40%
12. Lack of building space	20%	10%	20%	50%
13. Too many patients	40%	20%		40%
14. Lack of money for equipment and research	20%	30%	30%	20%
15. Library is not good enough	20%	20%	30%	30%
16. Little information about new treatments and new research findings	10%	10%	50%	20%
17. Lack of epidemiological data regarding mental problems	10%	40%	50%	
18. Staff relations are not good			30%	70%
19. Not enough treatment supplies		20%	40%	40%
20. Lack of transportation services	10%	40%		50%
21. Low success rate of treatment	10%	20%	60%	10%

gration with other institutions and poor support from other professions are less uniformly problematic. Yet, at least 50 percent of those interviewed saw them as very or moderately serious.

Another dimension involves crowdedness and space restrictions. Staff at TSP, NACMHC, and TCPC tend not to view these as problems. The other institutions report waiting lists, patient load, lack of building space, and not enough rooms to separate different types of patients as "very serious" or "moderately serious" concerns. Research resources is a fourth dimension showing clear deficits. There is a consensus that research equipment, library materials, research findings about new treatments, and epidemiological data of community disorders are unavailable. Problems of this sort may be a consequence of personnel and funding shortages. Moreover, direct services take precedence over research, and Taiwan is cut off from the information flow of new therapies evolving in other countries.

The four remaining items deserve comment. Few workers admitted any difficulty with staff relations. Interestingly, two of the three respondents who did indicate it as a "slight problem" were chief administrators. An absence of treatment supplies was not viewed as too serious, except by a NACMHC psychologist and by a head nurse at a teaching hospital. Personnel carrying out nonmedical activities feel an absence of supplies that they deem important.

Except for Jen-Chi and TSP respondents, the lack of transportation services was viewed as a "serious" issue. Transportation availability relates to agency accessibility. Having buses or cars available permits staff to make home visits and agency consultations and assists patients in getting to the clinic. Lastly, 90 percent of the subjects indicated their frustration with the system by reporting that low success rate of treatment was to some extent a problem. This finding may be the most important indicator of staff attitude toward the resource deficits found in their work settings. Presumably, with an adequate structure for intervention, this opinion would be less uniform.

COMMUNITY INTEGRATION AND ACCEPTANCE OF THE MENTAL HEALTH SYSTEM

Another key characteristic of a mental health system is its acceptance as an integrated part of the recipient community. Measurement of acceptance is ideally carried out through community survey techniques. Attitudes toward the agency, consumer satisfaction, and knowledge and use of agencies are general indices of community acceptance. Unfortunately, this avenue of data collection was unavailable to me during the brief site visits. Community acceptability was therefore measured through the opinions of staff members: perceptions of how acceptable their programs are in terms of community involvement in treatment and agency review.

One means of integrating a service into the community is to involve relatives and friends in the intervention process. The clinics could structure their programs so that family or community people play active roles in goal setting, treatment selection, service delivery, and rehabilitation. Several instances shown in table 3.8 reflect community participation in service delivery and rehabilitation. This occurred most often with child cases: parents and teachers were taught improved ways of handling behavior problems. On some occasions, family members "live in" with hospitalized relatives, assisting in daily care. Assessment of client problems through family interviews is common; intervention plans using family therapy is rare. At NTUH, the family is requested to assist in getting employment for day-care clients as the goal of rehabilitation. NACMHC is most active with indirect methods: parents, community agents, and others are used as sources of social influence for the client.

Selection of therapy and goals of treatment are additional ways in which relatives and others could participate in therapy. Staff were asked to indicate which persons helped in treatment and goal selection. Not surprisingly, the power to make these decisions rests almost completely with the physician. Other professional staff add their opinions upon physician request. At TCPC, staff report that oftentimes they do try to involve family in the treatment selection process; this never occurs at Jen-Chi. NTUH and NACMHC report some involvement of family, friends, and teachers. Folk healers, policemen, clergy, and priests were rarely mentioned as invited participants. It appears that intervention is viewed primarily as the physician's domain. Community members close to the patient are useful in some phases of assessment and their cooperation is seen as important for success, but there are few formal ways in which they are brought into the decision-making and service-delivery process.

Besides giving case management input, community decision making could also entail participation in planning program policies and goals. Community integration is thought to be enhanced by formal avenues of agency accountability to the opinions of social leaders. This may take the form of having interested community leaders consult with administrators about their perceptions of local needs or establishment of a formal community advisory board to shape the direction of agency development.

There was no evidence of formal or informal input from nongovernmental sources into the operations of public mental health facilities.

Agency development and direction appears to be in the hands of the chief administrators who work arduously to maintain funding options for their current operations and future plans. Private counseling services, like Life-Line, are more responsive to community-expressed needs. Their governing bodies are a mixture of laymen and medical personnel.

Another way of looking at an agency's integration with its social context is to survey staff perceptions of whether or not their clinic is viewed as a treatment place of choice by potential clients. Community acceptability is a critical issue recognized by all staff interviewed (table 3.10). There is strong agreement that mental health services are outside of general community awareness and that agency functions are a mystery. This lack of knowledge is coupled with a strongly held opinion that psychiatric clinics are stigmatized and used only as a last resort. Moreover, once the patient is brought in for help, there is a sense that patients and their families have little faith in treatment efficacy. Only the Jen-Chi group maintain that this community attitude is not a problem. However, responses to item 4 uniformly assert that hospitalization and psychiatric treatment results in patient stigmatization. Ninety percent of all respon-

TABLE 3.10 Staff Perceptions of Agency Acceptability in Taiwan (*N*=10)

	Seriousness of problem			
Questionnaire item	Very serious	Moderately serious	Slightly serious	Not a problem
1. Community people don't know about or understand the treatment program.	30%	60%	10%	
2. Community people have a bad opinion of the treatment program and use it only as a last chance.	50%		30%	20%
3. Patients and their families don't believe the treatment will help.		20%	60%	20%
4. Patients returning home have problems because people know they were in a mental hospital.	50%	30%	20%	
5. People with traditional beliefs about mental problems won't use the treatment program.	30%	60%	10%	
6. People go to "folk doctors" instead of using the treatment program.	20%	70%	10%	

dents saw this as a "very serious" or "moderately serious" problem. This consensus is one of the strongest for any question in the survey.

Items 5 and 6 reveal why staff feel that their programs are not accepted: individuals maintaining traditional beliefs about mental problems eschew modern clinics and prefer folk doctors. It may be that folk healing, available in the neighborhoods or local temples, does not carry the stigma of being a "psychiatric treatment for the insane." Perhaps folk medicine is more closely interwoven with the individual's life style—more clearly understood and less threatening. Regardless of the rationale, however, 90 percent of the staff deem these two problems as "extremely serious": (1) tradition-minded patients turn to folk services for assistance and (2) families avoid any sort of contact with the mental health system until their member becomes violent or unmanageable.

CULTURAL CONTINUITY AND ACCOMMODATION OF MENTAL HEALTH SERVICES

The third key characteristic defining the status of a mental health system is culture accommodation. Unique cultural patterns demand the "indigenization" of psychiatric services for members of that culture. Accommodating elements of the service delivery system to the recipient community builds culture continuity of care and ensures greater therapy acceptance. In Taiwan, culture accommodation appears to proceed along five dimensions.

Recognizing the Supremacy of the Chinese Family

Taiwanese psychiatrists recognize the preeminent position of the Chinese family group in the lives of its members. Operating as a "health management" team, the family assumes responsibility for choosing and implementing the treatment modality most suited to the ill member's condition (Lin and Lin 1981). Only after intrafamilial resources prove inefficacious will outsiders be consulted. Even then, decisions about whom to consult and when to comply or change practitioners remain within family purview (Kleinman 1980).

For most families, it is a radical departure from familiar sources of healing to bring their sick member to a Western-style psychiatrist. This exposes them to the possibility of intense shame that would envelop the family should the person be diagnosed as mentally ill. Popular moral and religious beliefs ascribe "madness" to incorrect life within the family and misdeeds by one's ancestors, respectively. The mental illness label exposes family shame to outsiders, stigmatizing the kin group even more than the person labeled disturbed. It is within this context of fearfulness and anticipated disgrace that the kinfolk deliver unto the psychiatrist their ailing relative. Moreover, the disquieting possibility emerges that a family will reject and abandon some uncontrollable and "chronic" cases to institutional confinement (Lin and Lin 1981).

In recognizing the family's central role and the pressures operating on it, the agency workers devise a strategy to ensure its cooperation. It is well understood that without the family's cooperation and commitment to the therapy plan, professional efforts would remain ineffective. TCPC psychiatrists work to gain rapport and trust by first relieving the unspoken fears that treatment involves a shameful public record, punishment, and shock. The physician takes an authoritative yet understanding position. He or she explains the nature of therapy and promises not to divulge family secrets.

The resistance to intrusion by outsiders, such as the therapist, into the "sacred bastion" of the clan is sometimes overcome by first gaining family confidence through a demonstrable improvement in the patient and then inviting the relatives in for a conference. At TCMHC behavior modification and medication are quickly applied for immediate results. The parents' confidence is secured before attempting to move into family-assisted models of intervention which are known to be unpalatable since they imply a psychosocial etiology to the child's problem.

Other settings, biased by the biomedical ethos of Western training, attempt to take full responsibility for patient development. TSP staff, for example, indicated that relatives may ultimately interfere with therapeutic instructions. Psychiatrists reported that some Chinese mothers are especially overprotective of their servicemen sons. They bring them charms to wear and give advice contrary to the doctor's orders. On these occasions, relatives are asked to stop their visits unless willing to cooperate. By denying the traditional matrix of family obligation, such institutional practices increase the risk of severing the only set of enduring supportive ties available to Taiwanese for resolving health maladies. If the family abandons its health care responsibilities, the ultimate recourse is the predatory system of ill-run "warehouse" institutions or vagrancy.

Accommodation Response to Popular Indigenous Conceptions of Disorder

The family "health management team" handles illness and its consequences according to an interwoven network of popular beliefs and values. Illness discourse characteristically contains several parallel sets of interpretations—both secular and sacred—to explain a particular illness episode. For example, Kleinman (1980:199) observed that etiology is often discussed according to the balance of polar opposites in the body— hot/cold, yin/yang, or whether disorder causality lies "within the body" or "outside the body." The family knows that the Chinese herb doctor or

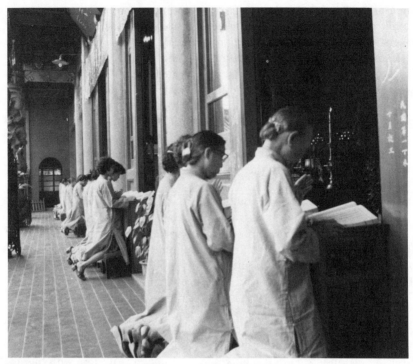

Temple counselors in Taipei offer prayers before turning to the long lines of peti-
tioners seeking advice on matters of health, fortune, and personal relationships.

Western-style physician offers technological interventions appropriate to
"within the body" disorders. Practitioners of sacred healing are required
to handle the supernatural forces implicated in "outside the body" sickness. Although the mental health professionals interviewed recognized
the importance of dealing sensitively with relatives and patients who
maintain these attributions, few professionals have researched the nature
of these conceptions as a prerequisite for training and practice.

On the other hand, physicians at NTUH do feel that it is important for
professionals to be aware of the circuitous route traversed by some
patients before reaching the clinic. The psychiatrists know that they may
just be one in a series of "healers" seen by the family. Families will often
take their ill member to a series of providers—fortune tellers, temple
priests, pharmacists, as well as Chinese-style and Western-style doctors—
to insure a cure (Kleinman 1980:188–189). One NTUH professional suggested that to establish rapport in such cases, it helps to assure the family
that they have a right to do what they feel is best. They are sometimes
given permission to take the patient to folk healers if they so choose.

When patients are brought to modern clinics, conceptions of disorder that they express to the Western-style practitioner are often biogenic in line with their expectations of the staff's biomedical orientation. The relatives report that there is something wrong with the patient's brain, or he has "weak nerves." An enuretic child is thought to have weak kidneys or bladder; "elevated liver fire" evokes tension and agitation. Tseng's (1975) research showed that 70 percent of NTUH's outpatient population complained chiefly of somatic symptoms. Physical distress, naturally, is the socially recognized and accepted signal for psychological dysfunction because it precludes implicating and disgracing the familial/ancestral nexus in the problem's etiology (Lin and Lin 1981). Hence, "emotional problems" are deemed irrelevant and exceedingly difficult for Chinese to discuss openly (Tseng 1975).

Following from these organ-centered notions of disorder is the expectation of a quick, physical cure. Western drugs are seen to work quickly, or not at all (Kleinman 1980). The family will frequently list the problems as they define them, then turn the patient over to the doctors expecting a 100 percent cure that will enable the person to return to work and social obligations. Neurologists are chosen over psychiatrists. Demands are made that EEG readings or a brain scan be performed to find the locus of damage.

Faced with these conceptions of psychopathology, the most common strategy is a resigned acceptance of the fact that families mix therapeutic resources. Under these conditions, it appears wise not to take a negative view of folk practices or confront patients who hold religious or biogenic explanations of their problems (Tseng 1975, 1976). Psychiatrists at NTUH and TCPC agreed that to directly deny the veracity of patient beliefs was counterproductive. The attitude was either to ignore such ideas or to gently educate patients about the differences between modern and folk medicine and get them to consider psychological roots of behavior.

If the medical regimen was "interfered with" by folk practices, or they appeared to be "harming" the patient and draining her finances, then staff felt compelled to encourage the patient to stop visiting native healers. The more seasoned professionals recognized that, at minimum, knowledge of folk conceptions and cultural expressions of disorder such as culture-bound syndromes is useful in working effectively with traditional clients (Chang, Rin, and Chen 1975).

Providing Expected Therapeutics

Similarly, culture accommodation involves staff efforts to provide treatment modalities expected by recipients. Since many complaints are couched in a somatic idiom, physical/somatic interventions are the client's treatment choice when consulting the scientific doctor. Since problems are seldom expressed publicly using psychosocial attributions, patients do not see talk as a form of therapy. If patients receive talk therapy only, then they are reluctant to pay and have little confidence in its success. This reinforces psychiatrists' use of drugs or vitamins and placebos—even when they would prefer not to—to make the patients feel satisfied.

Recently, traditional Chinese medicine and pharmacopoeia have been given governmental attention through the support of the China Medical College in Taipei. As part of this renewed interest in Chinese medicine, researchers have begun to look at the effects of acupuncture on hospitalized psychiatric populations. At TSP, patients with clinical depression were administered acupuncture treatment. There is no information on the efficacy of this approach nor on whether or not patients view it as a desirable therapy.

Except for experimentation with acupuncture, there are no examples of psychiatric institutions offering any components of the popular folk healing sector within which the majority of lower- and middle-class Taiwanese find solutions to their health complaints. The potency of various indigenous healing modalities could well be lost if folk practitioners were invited to operate within a biomedical setting without their customary control of the treatment context. Therefore, it would be a disservice to folk medicine and the clients it serves to advocate any form of accommodation that entails co-opting indigenous healers or integrating them into formal psychiatric care.

On the other hand, mental health professionals cannot ignore: (a) the enormous manpower contained within the popular health sector and its accessibility to the populace;[4] (b) the breadth of therapeutics this sector delivers and its intimate matching of cure with problem conceptualization; and (c) the consistent evidence of treatment efficacy at least equal to Western-style intervention and patient satisfaction levels that are frequently more favorable for folk practitioners (Kleinman 1980:290–292). At minimum, staff should acquire a comprehensive understanding of the indigenous care system, learn to value it as an allied resource, and cultivate contacts with respected practitioners who would be willing to take referrals. Unfortunately, accommodation along these lines falls well beyond the clinical reality envisaged by adherents to medical standards taught from Western textbooks.

Accommodation through Staff Qualities and Mannerisms

Certain staff attributes and personal manners were reported as important for gaining patient and family cooperation. For example, a consideration for hiring personnel at the NACMHC was fluency in Fukienese, the dialect of native Taiwanese. Linguistic matching was also considered important at NTUH Child Division, where the two psychiatrists were competent in three major Chinese dialects plus Japanese.

The therapist's manner is considered critical for evoking confidence and reducing client resistance. First, the family's authority in managing the illness needs recognition. Time should be spent allaying their concerns regarding the disorder's social consequences. With this, the family receives its due respect and etiquette remains intact—a condition all too rare in disease-oriented scientific medicine. Therapists are expected also to be figures of authority, actively dispensing fatherly approval and disapproval (Hsu 1976). They must be direct in their explanation of the problem, offering specific formulae for curing. Assurance and hope are especially looked for from doctors to relieve the suffering, along with a proclamation that treatment will completely cure. Scientific or technical explanations and honest doubts about efficacy disappoint the patients and their relatives. Unfortunately, staff report that their enormous caseloads preclude adherence to these known principles of proper patient-therapist transaction. Yet, as Kleinman (1980) observed, physicians continue treating patients as if they had little time for discussion even when their waiting rooms are empty.

Furthermore, the Western psychotherapeutic goal of encouraging open and direct expression of feelings and desires is inappropriate in the Chinese context (Tseng 1975). Chinese are not taught to openly express their personal feelings in public, particularly negative emotions like hostility or anger—or sexual desires (Tseng 1975). Tseng (1975) advises that the first goal is to make the client feel comfortable in relating to the therapist; then gradually begin an inquiry about his life, environment, and history.

Another cultural attribute in the accommodating therapist's repertoire is sensitivity to nonverbal communication. In American and European cultures where psychotherapy developed, verbalizations are deemed the most mature and successful avenue of human communication. People are socialized to express themselves somewhat freely since childhood. This contrasts with Chinese norms, in which nonverbal, subtle, and reserved self-expression are considered virtuous (Hsu 1972). The therapist's techniques and approach to clients must be suitably modified to account for these preferences. Along similar lines, use of local or slang terms indicating "madness" is strictly taboo; it is considered insulting by patient and family.

Accommodation in Ward Activities

The final important way in which inpatient treatment adjusts to Chinese culture is to allow relatives to reside on the hospital ward near their ailing family member. Tseng and Hsu (1969) reported that up to one-fourth of the inpatients at NTUH were attended by relatives, either full- or part-time. This practice sometimes results in a very close working relationship between staff and family. At most of these hospitals, elderly, ill, or unmanageable patients will have an amah (female attendant) stay with them twenty-four hours per day.

Another approach to accommodation is to make ward activities similar to important social functions outside the hospital. TCPC initiated a self-governing system where patients establish the rules of the ward and assign jobs to each resident. Since economic productivity is a critical social role, TCPC has a contract with a private company to make plastic toys. This gives patients the opportunity to earn money through occupational rehabilitation. NTUH's day-care program focuses on developing similar skills. It offers prevocational guidance. Patients are assigned hospital jobs such as typist, clerk, gardener, or plasterer and earn a small income. Day-care staff encourage families to find suitable jobs for patients ready for release. Of the first twenty-two patients released from the program, 50 percent were able to find some sort of job through family assistance (Chen 1971). Occupational therapy at NTUH also includes familiar Chinese pastimes such as calligraphy, tea making, and landscape painting.

STAFF PERCEPTIONS OF CULTURE ACCOMMODATION

Staff members see it as fairly common to give inpatients the opportunity to make choices and to participate in outside community activities (table 3.11). They also feel that the inpatient setting is structured to include elements of community life and that family often help on the ward. These attitudes add weight to the previous descriptions of ward events.

However, staff report an even stronger effort to adjust their personal manner to fit client expectations and to accept the beliefs of tradition-minded patients (table 3.12). All those questioned endorsed the statement that "staff should adjust their personal manner to fit the expectations of patients from different social backgrounds."

In contrast, accommodation practices such as hiring staff with certain social backgrounds and involving native healers rarely occur. Interestingly, 50 percent of the respondents reported problems arising because patients and staff differ in their ethnic backgrounds. NACMHC is unique in that staff are hired on the basis of their linguistic ability to relate easily with their clients through the Taiwanese dialect.

The data in table 3.12 are from twenty professionals representing all disciplines at the different clinics. It is remarkable that even with such

TABLE 3.11 Perceptions of Institutional Accommodation
Practices in Taiwan (*N*=8)

Accommodation practice	Percentage of staff endorsing accommodation item	
	Always/ sometimes	Seldom/ never
1. Native healer involvement in patient care		100
2. Staff accept beliefs of traditional patients	57	43
3. Staff adjust their personal manner to fit patient expectations	71	29
4. A policy exists to find staff whose backgrounds are similar to those of the patients	33	66
5. Inpatient activities are similar to their activities outside the hospital	66	33
6. Patients make choices about their daily activities	66	33
7. Patients are encouraged to participate in community activities outside the hospital— work and recreation	83	17
8. Patient's family helps with hospital care	20	80
9. Problems occur because patients and staff have different social backgrounds	50	50

diversity, 85 percent or more of the respondents endorsed three-fourths of the accommodation statements.

Many of the items given uniform endorsement are consistent with previous descriptions of clinic accommodation. However, some interesting discrepancies emerge. Although 95 percent agreed that community leaders should help in planning and directing facility activities, this policy did not exist anywhere. Staff also disagreed that it is useless to consult with native healers. However, folk healer involvement was a practice alien to modern medical settings. Moreover, with respect to therapeutic modalities, the ultimate decision making rested with the physician. This contrasts with the expressed sentiments that the patient and his family should help choose the treatment type (item 6) and strong disagreement with the item stating that the doctor alone should decide treatment outcome (item 10).

Four culture-accommodation dimensions were not endorsed. The issue of hiring staff whose social backgrounds are similar to patients did not

TABLE 3.12 Staff Endorsement of Culture Accommodation Dimensions in Taiwan (*N*=20)

Accommodation statement	Percentage of staff endorsing statement
1. Staff should know the traditional names for mental disorder.	100
2. Staff should adjust their personal manner to fit the expectations of patients from different social backgrounds.	100
3. While in the hospital, patients should remain isolated from activities in the community.	100% disagree
4. Staff should know the traditional healing practices for mental disorder.	95
5. Community leaders should help in planning and directing facility activities.	95
6. The patient and his family should help choose the type of treatment given.	95
7. Patient activities in hospital should be similar to their activities in community.	90
8. Patients should go to larger central hospitals for their treatment.	90% disagree
9. What is considered the appropriate outcome of treatment should be different for different cultures.	85
10. The doctor alone should decide treatment outcome goals.	85% disagree
11. What is considered "normality" is the same for all cultures.	85% disagree
12. It is useless to consult with native healers since most cannot help people with mental disorders.	80% disagree
13. It is best to hire staff whose social backgrounds are similar to those of patients.	65
14. Only those trained in scientific treatment techniques are qualified to help people with mental problems.	35% disagree
15. Staff should try to correct or reeducate patients who maintain traditional beliefs and customs about mental disorder.	25% disagree
16. It is useless for staff to know the traditional beliefs about causes of mental disorder.	5% disagree

seem that important except at NACMHC. Only 35 percent disagreed that scientifically trained workers were the most suitable practitioners. Those expressing the strongest disapproval of this conclusion were nurses, occupational therapists, and social workers. Furthermore, only this same small group failed to support the notion that patients maintaining traditional beliefs should be reeducated. Finally, all except one psychologist agreed that there is no value in knowing the traditional beliefs about the causes of disorder. This seems incongruent with other responses showing full agreement that staff should know traditional names of disorder and folk practices. Yet, knowing conceptions of causality may genuinely be seen as less useful than knowing folk names for psychopathology and folk interventions.

Accommodation in Taiwanese psychiatric institutions is both circumscribed and superficial. No serious interest is shown in researching Chinese cultural idioms pertaining to psychopathology or in translating such insights into training young professionals. Certainly no effort has been made to forge a referral link between Western-style services and the more-accessible system of folk practitioners. When authorities fail to value this sector's wealth of resources, the cost of this denial falls most heavily upon the person in distress and upon the family struggling to fulfill its health management responsibility.

NOTES

1. Although 1,508 physicians have immigrated in the last twenty years (Kleinman 1980: 293), no published statistics document the number of mental health professionals departing. Nevertheless, Professor Hsien Rin of NTUH considers manpower loss to be a problem of enormous magnitude.

2. See *Bulletin of Chinese Society of Neurology and Psychiatry,* 1, no. 1 (1975) for a full listing of research.

3. "NTUH sets different hospital charges based on class of room occupied (first, second, third, etc.). The basic charge [prior to 1978] on the psychiatric ward is $1.25 per day for food, $2 per day for room, and everything else, including medication, is extra" (Kleinman 1980:13–14).

4. Manpower in the popular health sector offering various forms of psychological help far outweighs available Western-style personnel. Taiwan in 1974 had 1,592 licensed Chinese-style doctors; an estimated 800 temple-based shamans *(tâng-ki)* in Taipei alone saw between five and fifty clients per day (Kleinman 1980; Kleinman and Sung 1976). A partial list of other folk specialists includes Chinese-style (herbal) pharmacists, streetside fortune tellers, physiognomists, Taoist priests, and temple-based interpreters of *chou-ch'ien* (bamboo fortune sticks). Most indigenous healers are unlicensed and illegal. For more complete explanations of their practices, see Ahern 1978; Kleinman 1980; Kleinman and Lin 1981; Tseng 1976, 1978; Wu 1982; Li 1976; and Hsu 1976.

chapter 4

The Mental Health System
of the Philippines

The mental health system of the Philippines has evolved in the context of a socioeconomic structure in which the public sector has been kept purposely small and in which efficient, long-range planning for national development has been crippled. Politicians tend to focus on highly visible "pork barrel" projects that elevate their personal status with the voters and maintain the status quo (Woolley et al. 1972). Without revenues and capital formation in the public sector, infrastructure components such as roads, airports, railroads, and public services have suffered, although the government has now begun to redress this historical imbalance through international financial assistance and increased budgetary allocations.[1]

In this atmosphere, the position of social welfare, health, and mental health matters is tenuous at best. Public revenues for this domain are minimal, and nongovernmental agencies are left to provide whatever services they can. Such official attention as is given to mental health appears to be little more than a conscious effort to create an image of good will and religiously inspired concern for individual well-being, motivated as much by political reasons as by genuine desire to solve social ills. During the rule of Ferdinand Marcos as president, this governing style evolved into an artform. First Lady Imelda Marcos, in particular, adopted a highly public posture of support for various health and social welfare projects.

Unlike Taiwan, there is no central figure in the evolution of Philippine psychiatry. The earliest major institutional development was the creation of the Insular Psychopathic Hospital, opened in Mandaluyang near Manila in December 1928, thirty years after the beginning of American colonization. Later renamed the National Mental Hospital (NMH), this facility was built to house the "insane" from throughout the Philippines (J. Castaneda 1974), replacing the "Insane Department" of San Lazaro

Hospital. In 1935, it became the only government treatment facility when the Manila Sanitorium closed. The initial capacity of 400 beds was quickly filled, an event that was often repeated, requiring the construction of more and more wards.

By the time World War II came, there were 3,000 inpatients. Starvation and mistreatment under Japanese rule led to hundreds of patient deaths and their removal by families. By the end of the war, only 445 remained. Eric Berne (1950) visited this hospital two years after the war and found the population up to 1,813 patients cared for by ten physicians and twenty nurses. He reported electroconvulsive shock as the principal therapeutic modality, applied via an outmoded Japanese apparatus. At that time, there were no psychiatrists outside of government employment.

By the mid-1950s, it became apparent that the patient population could not be handled in one institution. The solution to ease overcrowding was to build branches and extension clinics in other parts of the archipelago. This approach continues today, although it has never achieved its mission because of lack of support and resources (J. Castaneda 1974).

A reorganization in the Department of Health (DOH) during 1958 led to the creation of the Mental Hygiene Division (MHD) within the Bureau of Disease Control. The intended purpose was to formulate policies, develop plans and programs, and carry out research germane to mental hygiene. Then, in 1962, bolstered by the presence of MHD, a national mental health program pushed in earnest for the decentralization of the National Mental Hospital at Mandaluyang. The principal objective of this plan was regionalization of services, placing the burden of distribution on the eight Regional Health Offices. This move was in line with a general DOH effort to integrate public health services with hospital-based care, so it was natural to include mental health in the overall integration scheme (Aragon 1977).

Decentralization, aimed at realigning the inefficient centralized administration of psychiatric treatment, resulted in NMH losing its executive control over mental hygiene units. These became the responsibility of the eight regional health directors. A five-year program was initiated following a set of recommendations to: (1) limit the number of inpatients to a maximum of 2,000; (2) transfer selected patients to general hospitals near home; and (3) establish a series of regional mental hospitals, psychiatric units in general hospitals, halfway houses, and mental hygiene clinics. The MHD was to provide technical support by training physicians and nurses to work in these new services and facilitate decentralization through coordinating contact between NMH and the DOH Bureau of Medical Services.

The plan to phase out NHM congestion through the integration of mental health care with the public health system has been slow in its implementation and is far from successful. In 1977, NMH, with an official capacity of 3,500 beds, housed some 8,000 inpatients.

The tenuous nature of this plan is revealed by several facts: (1) there are very few specially trained workers: (2) their role at the local level is nebulous; (3) they are often health officers who return to old jobs without concentrating on psychiatric problems; and (4) success hinges on regional directors, who may have little knowledge of, and give little attention to, mental health concerns.

While the public sector was beginning to experience the massive overburdening of its lone residential facility, a private agency was formed—the Philippine Mental Health Association (PMHA). PMHA's goals are to promote mental health activities, educate the public on the issue, and provide a wide range of clinical services. In 1951, it pioneered a nationwide educational movement through promotion of the first annual National Mental Health Week. This became an official yearly event in 1957 through presidential decree. It also initiated the first community mental health clinic in the Philippines in 1951, later adding both rural and urban-based rehabilitation services.

PMHA provides the main stimulus for mental health research through the publication of two periodicals and since 1965 has awarded about twenty research grants. Several grants have gone to the MHD to assist epidemiological surveys. The first MHD epidemiological field investigation was followed up six years later through a PMHA grant to examine the status of eighty-six identified cases. These two field surveys, pointing toward an incidence rate of 36 per 1,000 (including mild dysfunctions), are heavily relied upon by government planners in discussions of psychological impairment and service needs for the country. In addition to research support, PMHA has sought to coordinate its educational and clinical activities with the MHD, thereby promoting decentralization, and to aid that government unit with training professionals for public health psychiatric projects.

PUBLIC AND PRIVATE HEALTH SYSTEMS AS THE CONTEXT
FOR MENTAL HEALTH SERVICES

The DOH envisions its national mental health program as part and parcel of the public health system. In order to appreciate what this entails, it is necessary to sketch an overview of the public health program and its position within the government.

Medical care in the Philippines is provided by the DOH, the Philippine Medical Care Commission, and chartered municipal and private agencies. The DOH, located in Manila, has responsibility for all public health services and additionally supervises and consults with private care-givers throughout the country. Since the majority of Filipinos cannot afford private care, concentrated exclusively in urban centers, the burden of health delivery falls upon the DOH. At the time of this 1977 survey, the DOH was operating under a 1973 organizational scheme consisting of sixteen divisions under the secretary of health and his under secretary. One division, the Bureau of Health and Medical Services, contained the Disease Control Unit under which the Mental Hygiene program operates. Curative and preventive services are administered through eleven regional offices. Each regional health director supervises provincial health officers under whom are a number of municipal health officers and rural health workers. The rural health units and municipal clinics form the base of the health delivery system.

The 1975–1978 Health Plan lists as its priorities an increase in life expectancy, reduction in population growth and infant mortality, upgrading nutrition, expansion of the national insurance program, and a focus on health disabilities associated with growing urbanization (DOH 1975). These goals are to be met through a concentrated effort to expand and upgrade the rural health infrastructure (National Economic and Development Authority (NEDA) 1977). This means building scores of new rural health units and creating neighborhood *barangay* health stations on a massive scale with community, emergency, and regional hospitals. Integrated into these units from the *barangay* to the central level are the three principal programs of health, nutrition, and family planning. Presumably, a mental health program is included, yet it is not mentioned in the national development documents (e.g., NEDA 1977), nor did psychiatric specialists serve on the national health planning committees.

Manpower targets to operate the rural health system in the immediate future call for 2,300 physicians, 2,300 nurses, 9,300 midwives, and the training of 3,102 family planning outreach workers. Eventually, 54,365 *barangay* workers are also to be added (NEDA 1977). One measure to fill the manpower gap is the Rural Health Practice Program instituted in January 1974 (Pilar, Boncaras, and Santos 1976). It requires medical and nursing graduates to serve in rural areas for six months; it is expected that some of them will choose a career in rural health care. In essence, the current theme is greater health coverage to low-income rural, depressed, and slum regions with an expressed interest in community participation and reliance on local resources. Additionally, the government policies call for a strong involvement of the private sector in the same processes (Pilar, Boncaras, and Santos 1976).

Funding. National health development has never been a priority consideration in the Philippines, as is reflected in financial allocations. From 1970 to 1976, the DOH's share of the national budget decreased from 4.5 percent to 3.05 percent. Public spending on health as a proportion of the

GNP has also declined from 0.40 percent in 1974 (Europa 1977). Although the expenditure has gone up numerically ($96.5 million in 1976), this is offset by population growth, inflation, and the devaluation of national currency, which has resulted in scarcity of medical supplies and equipment (DOH 1975). Health ranks fifth behind other government functions such as defense, education, agriculture, and infrastructure expansion. According to the latest five-year development plan (FY 1978–1982), 21 percent of the national budget in 1978 went to social service considerations: education and manpower; health, nutrition, and family planning; housing; social welfare; and community development (NEDA 1977). Approximately 15 percent of this allocation ($200 million) was earmarked for health, nutrition, and family planning; half went toward curative and preventive services. In the context of these expenditures, it is interesting to note that funding for the National Mental Hospital was $4.93 million in 1977—about 5 percent of the total health budget.

In short, all social service programs in the Philippines compete for a relatively small ($870 million) national budget. The share given DOH, $200 million for 1978, must go toward infrastructure development, manpower training, salaries for new positions; and special projects for nutrition and family planning. Mental health considerations fall secondary to these priorities, with very little trickling down except for maintenance of existing facilities, employee salaries, and some retraining of public health workers in mental case management. Under these conditions, the burden falls upon the private sector for active promotion and expansion of treatment centers.

Service delivery components and network. Characteristic of developing nations, ratios of physicians and hospital beds to population in the Philippines are one-third and one-fifth, respectively, of those typically found in developed countries. Specifically, there are approximately 13,480 physicians, or one per 3,150 population in 1975 (WHO 1977c), and 68,000 beds, or one per 662 population in 1977 (DOH 1977). Statistics for 1977 showed a total of 1,027 hospitals, 356 public and 671 private, which evenly divided between them the 68,000 beds (DOH 1977).

Total health manpower—including physicians, nurses, dentists, midwives, traditional birth attendants, and so forth—consists of some 42,523 workers (WHO 1977c). Professional training takes place in the country's nine medical schools: five in Manila and four in Cebu City. Approximately twenty-four schools offer a B.A. in nursing, while forty-four hospital programs exist for nursing degrees (Diesfeld and Kroger 1974). Dispersion of these professionals and treatment centers is a critical problem. Almost 22 percent of all hospital facilities, including the largest ones, are centered in Manila. An estimated 37 percent of all physicians and 46 percent of all nurses are located in this same area (Vreeland et al.

1976). Based on this estimated maldistribution of personnel, Manila would have one M.D. per 600 citizens, while rural areas maintain a ratio of 1:9,000 (Vreeland et al. 1976).

In some rural districts, however, 1974 manpower ratios held one M.D. per 30,264 and one nurse per 32,529 (Pilar, Boncaras, and Santos 1976). Rural health unit personnel in 1977 were estimated at 2,152 physicians and 2,810 nurses; 17,898 nursing and medical students were assigned to the Rural Health Program (Pilar, Boncaras, and Santos 1976). Psychiatric specialists number approximately 180. Most of them practice in the Metro-Manila district. The NMH is the country's single largest employer of psychiatrists.

Originally, the DOH conceptualized health delivery in terms of preventive services, to be undertaken by the rural health units, and curative medicine handled through hospitals of varying size and specialization. In practice, the rural health units and the nearly 2,000 city health department clinics offer both preventive—community disease control, environmental sanitation, maternal and child health, health education, etc.— and general clinical care as recommended by WHO guidelines.

The health teams that operate within these local units generally comprise four types of workers—midwife, sanitary inspector, rural health physician, and public health nurse (Woolley et al. 1972). The recent trend is to add family planning, nutrition, and (possibly) mental health workers to the roster. Rural health units (primary level) are intended to be the initial entry point in the public health system, screening and referring to city or provincial hospitals (secondary level) those patients needing hospitalization. More specialized care is available upon referral from these facilities to regional hospitals (tertiary level) in the eleven health regions. At the apex of the referral system are specialized treatment units in Manila associated with university medical schools (World Bank 1976). Once inpatient care is terminated, the patient is supposed to be referred back to the rural health unit for follow-up care.

A number of problems beset this public health structure. First, administrative communication is quite difficult. It originates at the central level in Manila and travels down through the eleven Regional Health Offices to the sixty-five Provincial Health Offices before reaching the rural health units and *barangay* health stations (Pilar, Boncaras, and Santos 1976). Secondly, the referral process doesn't work smoothly since patients would rather return to the hospitals that treated them for outpatient care than to the local rural health unit. Moreover, patients and their families complain of shortages of personnel, beds, and medication, asserting that clinic hours are arranged for staff convenience and are irregularly met. Private clinics are preferred but unaffordable (Vreeland et al. 1976).

A 1973 survey found severe deficiencies in the infrastructure and resources available to the rural health units (World Bank 1976). Vacancies were noted in 23 percent of the M.D. and 46 percent of the nursing positions. Lack of interest in rural care was blamed on unsatisfactory working conditions: lack of supplies, physicians having to carry out nonprofessional functions, low salaries (earnings one-half of what was possible in private practice), and the lack of cultural amenities in rural zones.

Other problems plague the Philippine health situation. The medical training available in Manila is inappropriate for patterns of rural disease. There, workers confront pervasive communicable illnesses (gastroenteritis, tuberculosis, etc.), malnutrition, poor environmental sanitation, malaria, schistosomiasis, and so forth. The teaching orientation of the North American-educated faculty, however, emphasizes high technology and hospital-based, uneconomical curative medicine. The majority of graduates go abroad for specialized training, viewing as uninteresting the simple tasks required of a rural physician. Perhaps fewer than 50 percent of the trainees return as the country can only support a limited number of specialists (World Bank 1976).

A statement by Woolley et al. (1972) expresses a gloomy summary of the health picture:

> It appears that the Philippines is losing ground in meeting the health needs of a rapidly growing population. The situation presented by rising costs and the need for continuing expansion of facilities would be difficult under the best conditions. These problems are greatly aggravated, however, by misallocations of resources, lack of logistical support, ill-defined programs, overlapping and ill-defined responsibilities of health workers, lack of usable data with which to establish priorities, and particularly the lack of an overall policy in the health sector (Woolley et al. 1972: 57).

Mental health provisions within the Department of Health. In 1974, DOH sponsored the First National Workshop in Community Mental Health Nursing with WHO assistance. The director of NMH reviewed its existing treatment measures and called for a new direction that would not limit care to institutions alone, but include contact with patient communities and family support environments (J. Castaneda 1974). F. C. Castaneda, chief nurse at NMH, urged serious consideration of the model under which she had recently trained in the United States—the comprehensive community mental health center approach. Noting the absence of a comprehensive program, Castaneda strongly encouraged consideration of the American model as a tool to redevelop services in the Philippines. A preventive orientation would help reduce the caseload at NMH. Under new coordinated direction, all existing service units in the Philippines would be linked and mandated to deliver care at the neighborhood level. Further recommendations called for (a) integration of psychiatric services into basic health care given by the rural health units and provincial general hospitals and (b) community mental health training for physicians in the rural and provincial health system.

MHD's official orientation to service delivery is contained within its publication, *Manual of Operations on the Control of Mental Disease* (Aragon 1977). It suggests case management strategies adopted from the National Workshop on Community Mental Health that entail linking outpatient departments with life in the community to provide continuous care. Hospitalization will be short-term and only as a last resort. To maintain the patient in the community and prevent relapses, conjoint involvement of the family, rural health unit, and Department of Social Services and Development is stressed. Ideally, the patient would be followed up with a coordinated program of drug therapy and vocational, social, and educational rehabilitation (Aragon 1977: 9). The economic advantage of patient containment within community environments is stressed. A significant point is the proposed assignment of a mental health consultant to the regional offices to be responsible for coordinating these activities.

Services directed by the Department of Health. Psychiatric treatment under the DOH is delivered either through the NMH and its extension facilities or by psychiatric units under the administration of provincial and city health offices ultimately responsible to the Regional Health Offices (fig. 4.1). These two systems receive separate funding. In 1977 they were each allocated 35 million pesos for operating expenses (E. Aragon, personal communication).

Although a national program presumably began in 1958 with the order to decentralize NMH, almost twenty years passed before the DOH officially spelled out through a departmental circular (Department Circular no. 35, January 20, 1977) what the agencies' functions were in the "Control of Mental Disorders Program" (Aragon 1977: Annex II). That circular specified that the NMH shall "provide services for the prevention, treatment, and rehabilitation of the mentally ill; conduct case studies on the nature and treatment of mental disorders and shall serve as a center for manpower training of mental health workers in the government service" (Aragon 1977: Annex II, 3). At present, NMH has branch hospitals and clinics in eleven locations throughout the Philippines with bed space for approximately 2,500 patients (see table 4.1). NMH in Mandaluyang has an official bed allocation of 3,500 (actual occupancy 8,000), bringing the total number of public psychiatric beds to roughly 6,000 with well over 100 percent overcrowding.

These numbers suggest public psychiatric bed availability of one per

Figure 4.1
Organization of the Bureau of Health and Medical Services

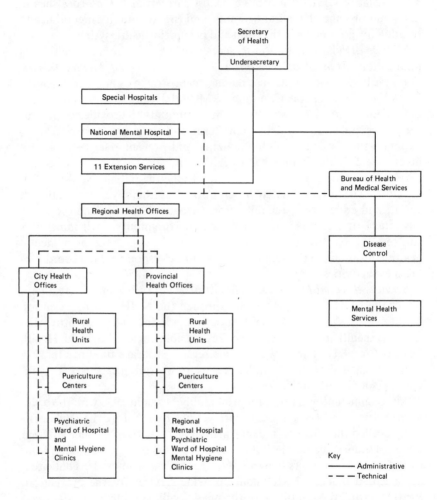

After E. Aragon, *Manual of Operations on the Control of Mental Disorders.* Manila: Department of Health, Republic of the Philippines, 1977.

TABLE 4.1 Major Residential Facilities in the Philippines

	Number of beds
Publicly funded	
*National Mental Hospital, Mandaluyang, Rizal (teaching)	3,500 (officially)
NMH extension services	
Mariveles, Bataan	850
Davao Regional Mental Hospital	600
Camarin Branch, Caloocan City	300
Tuguegarao Hospital, Cagayan	200
D.S. Rodriguez Hospital, Caddan, Pili, Camarines Sur	200
Batangas City	200
Andres Bonificio Hospital, Cavite	150
Southern Islands Hospital, Cebu City	60
Zamboanga City	20
Tagbilaran, Bohol	5
Davao Medical Training Center, Nervous Disease Pavilion	?
Baguio City Psychiatric Unit	?
*Victoria Luna Medical Center, Quezon City	81
*University of the Philippines, Philippines General Hospital Manila	15
Laguna Provincial Hospital, Sta. Cruz, Laguna	?
Rizal Provincial Hospital Mental Hygiene Unit	?
Total	±6,300
Privately funded or non-Department of Health facilities	
St. Lukes Hospital, Quezon City (teaching)	50
*University of the East, Ramon Magsaysay Memorial Medical Center, Quezon City (teaching)	15
*Veteran's Memorial Hospital, Quezon City (teaching)	90
*Medical City, Rizal	44
*University of Santo Tomas Hospital, Manila (teaching)	36
*Philippine Mental Health Association, Half-Way House, Pinagpala, Dasmarianas, Cavite	20
Cebu Community Hospital, Neuropsychiatric Unit	?
Total	±336

*Interview sites

8,800 population. The number of psychiatrists working in these settings is uncertain, although figures for NMH alone show sixty physicians and thirty-five psychiatric residents. Neki's survey (1973a) found a ratio of five psychiatrists per one million population, placing the total specialist population at 200. A large portion of these are engaged in private practice and university teaching.

The second DOH system of psychiatric services is administered through the public health organization. According to DOH Circular no. 35, the regional health officers are "to administer, direct, coordinate, and implement the policies and plans of the Mental Health Program through the field health agencies." The administrative officers under the directors, the provincial city health officers, "shall be responsible for the administrative direction, supervision, coordination, and control of the plans and policies of the Mental Health Program within his province or city as the case may be" (Aragon 1977: Annex II, 3).

Presumably, assigned to each regional officer is a mental health consultant. His position is to assist the officer in implementing the "disease control program"; "supervise the psychiatric units, hospitals, and outpatient clinics; participate in training new workers; conduct pertinent research; and, in general, coordinate all mental health activities within the region" (Aragon 1977: 4). An important function of the officer is to make arrangements to provide technical training of public health workers in the discipline of psychiatric treatment. The training officers of the Regional Health Office Training Centers are pressed into service for this function.

A number of mental hygiene clinics, psychiatric outpatient clinics, and day-care units are under the jurisdiction of the Provincial Health Offices. Manila has one mental hygiene clinic; Quezon and Pasay City, also within the Metro-Manila region, have four such centers. All three of these districts use NMH for inpatient requirements. Scattered throughout the rural areas are seven mental health clinics and psychiatric outreach programs attached to general hospitals (see table 4.2). The regional mental hospitals and psychiatric wards that serve as extension services for NMH also receive administrative direction from the regional health officers. These mental health units and wards are instructed to take only psychiatric emergencies and those needing short-term hospitalization.

Mental hospitals are to provide transitional services for long-term patients—halfway homes or sheltered workshops. Under this scheme, the rural health units are expected to cooperate and coordinate their activities with the mental health program. Rural health unit duties include receiving discharged patients from NMH or regional hospitals and providing follow-up and crisis intervention aid. Other functions include

TABLE 4.2 Major Outpatient Facilities in the Philippines

Publicly funded
1. Jose R. Reyes Memorial Hospital, Manila
2. Manila Health Department, Mental Hygiene Clinic
3. Pasay City Health Department, Mental Hygiene Clinic
4. Quezon City Health Department, 14 district mental hygiene clinics
5. Palomar Health Center, Department of Health, Manila
6. Rizal Provincial Hospital, Pasig
7. Calcoon City Health Center
8. Tacloban City Outpatient Clinic
9. Bohol Outpatient Clinic
10. Cagayan de Oro Outpatient Clinic
11. Legaspi Extension Services, Albay Provincial Hospital
12. Camarine de Sur Provincial Hospital Outpatient Clinic
13. Iloilo City Mental Health Unit, Pototan
14. Batangas Outpatient Clinic
15. Cabanatuan Outpatient Clinic

Privately funded
*1. Philippine Mental Health Association, Clinical, Diagnostic and Research Center, Quezon City
   PMHA chapters with clinical services: Baguio, Cebu City, Butuan, Davao, Dagupan, Zamboanga, Cabanatuan
2. Drug Abuse Research Foundation, Quezon City
*3. Institute of Maternal and Child Health, Manila
4. U.S. Veteran's Administration Outpatient Clinic, Ermita, Manila
5. Various university student counseling centers

*Interview sites

keeping an updated registry of all cases in the district, engaging in case-finding via school examinations or clinic consultation, health education campaigning, and assisting in the transportation of patients needing short-term hospitalization to the nearest psychiatric ward.

While this integrated system of referral, treatment, and follow-up is outlined on paper, its implementation is still sparse and incomplete. One instance where it was begun on an experimental basis in 1968 is Davao City. The regional mental hospital there has been able to link itself with various rural health units to coordinate patient release and supervise follow-up intervention.

The MHD was given the task of overviewing the nation's mental health program and rendering technical assistance to the aforementioned dual systems of treatment delivery through program development, research, and training. Curiously enough, however, once given this mandate by the DOH, the MHD was never given the funding, logistical support, or administrative power to carry out its role. Research surveys undertaken by the Division have relied upon PMHA for their funding. In 1971, this state of affairs prompted one official to remark in the DOH Annual Report:

> Since there is no money to set up field mental hygiene services, the activities of the Division staff had been concentrated on continuous planning, clinical consultation in conjunction with research activities, evaluation and improvement of the very limited existing resources and facilities, limited training activities, advisory and consultative services, and active coordination with various agencies (DOH 1971).

The influence of MHD for the development of a governmental therapeutic program is questionable. It took DOH twenty years from the inception of MHD to come out with a manual of operations stating specifically what its duties are and the responsibilities of the other public health officials are to the MHD program. Regional officers are expected to carry through the policies and plans promulgated by the MHD. Gaining the full cooperation of the regional officers and officials at the provincial, city, and *barangay* level is another matter altogether. MHD has no direct authority over these individuals.

The regional mental health consultants are the instruments of program implementation, yet their numbers are few and, as yet, they have very sparse manpower and resources to work with. Moreover, it may be that health officials in general are not only apathetic to the program but actively reject it. This is based on the negative connotations of the subject and their fear of dealing with the "mentally ill." Supporting this, one study of general health workers who had been given special training in psychological treatment showed that most did not employ this knowledge once they returned to their jobs (Manapsal 1974).

On the other hand, certain MHD accomplishments can be noted. The MHD manual of mental disease control includes several officially drafted policy statements regarding decentralization, "disease control," and guidelines for handling psychiatric emergencies in general practice. Secondly, the MHD has worked hard in developing training seminar curricula for educating general health personnel in psychiatry. Lastly, the Division has detailed avenues through which personnel should work to identify potential cases. Among them are school children screenings, visits to guidance clinics in puericulture centers, and referrals from *barangay* officials.

Private Sector

Private psychological services, concentrated in Metro-Manila, are available to the 20 percent of Philippine society who have the economic resources to use them. Economic parameters are important determinants of the system of private psychiatric care, since professionals practice their specializations only where the local economy has the strength to support them. Mental health care within the private sector is characterized by the clustering of small psychiatric inpatient units in university and general hospitals in Metro-Manila and the expanding system of outpatient clinics offered by Philippine Mental Health Association chapters. The PMHA is an example of a nongovernmental institution offering social services on a national scale. There are fourteen PMHA chapters, nine of which render some degree of psychological counseling, testing, and intervention (see table 4.2). The association operates on a budget of one million pesos (FY 1976). Funds are secured through the charity sweepstakes, national membership dues, client fees, and sales from its rehabilitation centers.

The national headquarters in Quezon City offers the fullest range of clinical services, including an industrial therapy program drawing day-care patients from NMH. In the early 1960s, a rural-oriented rehabilitation center was built in nearby Cavite; it offered released NMH patients both halfway house accommodations and training in agricultural skills. An early evaluation study of the Cavite program by Reyes (1970) showed that almost 25 percent of the residents left "completely recovered," while another 50 percent showed definite improvement on behavior rating scales.

A focal point of PMHA chapters is education. An estimated 290,000 people were reached in 1976 through 280 programs, press releases, radio, workshops for youth and professionals, film showings, lectures, and a national conference on urbanization and mental health (PMHA 1976). Aggregate statistics for 1976, combining chapters, showed 4,192 psycho-diagnostic tests, 2,293 psychiatric consultations, and 1,587 clients given social work assistance. The two rehabilitation centers each had about thirty monthly trainees, altogether serving 146 clients.

PMHA operations in the same year included consultations to government and private groups to assist program planning; development and support of twelve student mental health clubs in Metro-Manila; creation of an outreach program for high school dropouts; and funding of four research projects on such topics as aggression and the effects of television viewing on children.

Although PMHA appears to be the most dynamic agency in mental health promotion in the Philippines, it has not endeavored to provide

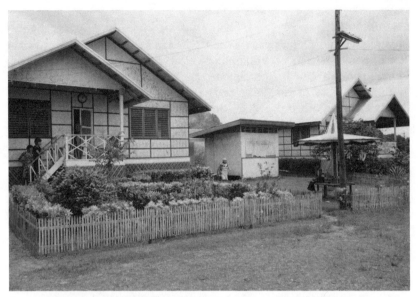

The Philippine Mental Health Association rural rehabilitation center in Cavite, Luzon, involves patients in farming occupations.

hospital-based treatment. Patients requiring hospitalization must turn to a number of small inpatient units situated in private general hospitals and university medical centers. If eligible, they may use non-DOH governmental facilities like V. Luna Medical Center, operated by the armed forces, and the American-funded Veteran's Memorial Hospital (see table 4.2). Altogether, there are six such facilities in Metro-Manila with a total of about 350 beds. There is, moreover, a special "pay ward" at NMH housing up to 200 more patients. While few in number, these units represent the "best" psychiatric care available in the Philippines, extending to acute cases a reasonably up-to-date regimen of medical intervention and rehabilitation.

OTHER FACTORS INFLUENCING THE DELIVERY OF PSYCHIATRY IN THE PHILIPPINES

Medicare Insurance

A key influence on the provision of psychological services is the Philippine National Health Insurance scheme. In 1969, the first phase of the Medicare System came into existence through passage of the Philippine Medical Care Act. It covered all employees under the Social Security System and Government Services Insurance System. In 1974, Medicare was extended to employee dependents, taking in almost 50 percent of the population. This coverage included periods of medical confinement and surgical expenses, but completely excluded psychiatric care. Such exclusion underscores and reinforces the alienation of psychiatry both within the medical context and within the society as a whole.

Insurance coverage of psychological care would boost the interest of care providers in the discipline while permitting greater access to existing private clinics by middle-class families who cannot now afford them. (The poor would still remain unserved.) As it is, the intensive treatment opportunities provided by a handful of private practitioners and private residential settings in Metro-Manila will remain the exclusive domain of the well-to-do Filipino.

Influence of Overseas Training

International contact also has played a part in deciding the nature of Philippine psychiatry. The Americanization of professional training is perhaps the most obvious example. Most of NMH's first psychiatrists and the founders of psychiatric instruction at the University of the Philippines Medical School—Horacio Estrada, Baltazar-Reyes, Lourdes Lapuz—received their specialist training in the United States. Maguigad (1964), in his summary of Philippine psychiatry in the mid-1960s, noted that 35 of the 167 psychiatrists were certified or eligible for certification by the American Boards Examination. Moreover, the predominant theme running throughout the National Workshop on Community Mental Health Nursing in 1974 and articulated most forcefully by F. C. Castaneda (trained in psychiatric nursing at the University of Maryland) was how best to adopt the principles of community mental health evolving in the United States.

Participation by the WHO Mental Health Division in the Philippines has been somewhat limited in comparison with nearby countries. This is surprising since the headquarters for the Western Pacific Region are located in Manila. Manuel Escudero, one of the first regional advisors, sought to introduce changes into the pattern of administration, diagnosis, and recruitment of personnel at NMH, but met with little success. An attribute of NMH that made it less amenable to change was the practice of appointing its chief administrator on the basis of political merit rather than knowledge of the field.

WHO has, however, provided fellowships for specialist training abroad and has gotten involved in several research projects. The most recent one, entitled "Collaborative Study on Strategies for Extending Mental Health Care," is headed by the chairman of psychiatry at the University of the Philippines (PGH), Lourdes Ladrido-Ignacio (See Climent et al. 1980).

Brain Drain

UNESCO estimates that 40 percent of the physicians registered during the past ten years have departed the country (UNESCO 1975). Mejia, Pizurki, and Royston (1979) describe the Philippines as a major "donor" country which has "suffered heavy net losses of physicians (outflow minus inflow). The percentage ratio of losses in relation to the 'stock' or total number of physicians remaining, was 67 percent."

Several conditions are responsible for this: (1) the Philippines has a higher M.D. and nurse "stock" than is the average for its level of GDP per capita and is producing more than the economy can absorb; (2) the focus of the medical system is on the private sector—government services are an insignificant employer of physicians; (3) health education is in English with employment opportunities available in English-speaking nations; (4) training is geared to disease patterns found in affluent societies, quite dissimilar to local conditions, thus credentials are more useful for work abroad; (5) given the country's low economic capacity, it is unlikely that many more people could afford to use the services of these health workers had they remained at home; and (6) the government has shown little interest in stemming the flow of these professionals to distant shores.

Epidemiological studies

Psychiatric services have not been planned with reference to empirical findings. To date, the MHD has undertaken only one epidemiological survey in a Central Luzon barrio (Manapsal 1969). Six years later, a team of MHD investigators returned to follow up the progress of the eighty-six cases identified earlier from the sample of 2,360 residents (Manapsal et al. 1974). This single survey has become the basis by which planners have set the prevalence rate for disorder at thirty-six cases per 1,000 population, or conservatively, 1.4 million affected persons nationwide.[2]

Identified cases primarily express their problems through somatic complaints; 44 percent had gone to general practitioners, 5 percent to native healers, 15 percent saw both types, and only 10 percent had sought assistance from a psychiatric specialist. This last figure is not surprising as it required a journey to Manila to attend the nearest mental hygiene clinic. The only other relevant information comes from a handful of studies describing the presenting problems of two mental hygiene clinics (Aragon 1977: Annex VII), monthly admissions to NMH (Sena 1974), and the progress made by residents at PMHA's halfway community in Cavite (Reyes 1970).[3]

An issue requiring empirical documentation concerns negative public attitudes toward psychological disorder, a problem identified by Manapsal (1974). Her initial impression is that families' feelings of shame toward disordered relatives and their belief that the illness is incurable results in abandonment of members in mental hospitals even when the person could be handled as an outpatient. This certainly bears research attention. Moreover, the finding that 50 percent of NMH's 400 monthly admissions are previous patients deserves explanation (de Guzman 1974). These figures could reflect family reluctance to commit themselves to home care or be an indictment of follow-up services. There may be a breakdown in the referral system whereby the rural health units are failing to pick up discharged patients.

PSYCHIATRIC RESOURCES AVAILABLE: SELECTED EXAMPLES

The public and private residential treatment centers in the Philippines and the major outpatient clinics—including both the mental hygiene clinics administered by the Department of Health and the clinical services of PMHA chapters—are summarized in tables 4.1 and 4.2. These lists are not exhaustive, but they do show the major treatment centers. Information is least available for private clinics and wards outside the Metro-Manila district.

Intensive interviews were conducted at seven residential facilities and one nonresidential clinic in Metro-Manila (table 4.3). Unstructured interviews and program descriptions were gathered at six additional agencies in the region. In all, this case study is based on conversations with approximately fifty mental health professionals from psychiatry, psychology, social work, and nursing working almost exclusively in the major psychiatric centers in Metro-Manila.

FRAMEWORK FOR MENTAL HEALTH RESOURCE STATUS

Comprehensive Services

Again applying the seven-variable framework for describing resource status, the first element examined is comprehensiveness, i.e., the degree to which the Philippine system provides a full spectrum of clinical programs.

Given the assumption that there is fluid referral among the programs, an average adult psychiatric case who can afford private care has access to almost the entire spectrum of services expected from a "modern" comprehensive system. Readily available among the eight settings are inpatient, outpatient, emergency, diagnostic, neurological, and to a lesser extent, partial hospitalization and follow-up care (table 4.4). Entering one of the centers, a patient can expect to be given chemotherapy, occu-

TABLE 4.3 Personnel Administered Questionnaires 1, 2, and 3 (Philippines)

Facility and staff	Number of staff completing Questionnaire			Open-ended interviews
	1	2	3	
National Mental Hospital (NMH)				
Psychiatrist (director)	1	1	1	1
Consultant psychiatrists		2	3	2
Psychologist		1 (chief)	4	
Social worker		1 (chief)	3	
Nurse		1		
University of the Philippines, General Hospital (PGH)				
Psychiatrist	1	2	7	1 (director)
Nurse (chief)			1	
Victoria Luna Medical Center (VL)				
Psychiatrist	1 (chief)	1 (chief)	2	
Psychologist		1 (chief)	2	
Nurse			2	
Veteran's Memorial Hospital (VMH)				
Psychiatrist	1 (chief)	2	4	
Psychologist		1 (chief)	2	1
Social worker		1	2	
Nurse			2	
University of the East, Ramon Magsaysay Hospital (UERM)				
Psychiatrist (chief)	1	1		
Psychologist		2		
University of Santo Tomas Hospital (UST)				
Psychiatrist	1	1	2	
Chief nurse		1	1	
Medical City (MC)				
Psychiatrist	1	1	1	
Chief nurse		1	1	
Philippines Mental Health Association (PMHA)				
Director/social worker/ psychiatrist	1			
Psychiatrist		1		1
Psychologist			2	
Social worker/OT			5	

TABLE 4.3 *(continued)*

| | Number of staff completing | | | |
| | Questionnaire | | | Open-ended |
Facility and staff	1	2	3	interviews
Department of Mental Hygiene				
Director			1	1
Region III Provincial Health Center				
Regional director				1
WHO Regional Headquarters				
Regional adviser for mental health				1
Bay Laguna Comprehensive Health Center				
Physician				1
PMHA Half-Way House, Cavite				
Social workers				3
Totals	8	22	48	14

pational therapy, and individual, group, and family therapy on an "often" or "sometimes" basis (table 4.5).

General ward milieu and various work assignments around the hospital are the other therapeutic components frequently cited. Psychotherapy is either supportive or follows a psychoanalytic orientation, given the American ego-psychology training of the professors of psychiatry in the university departments. The Ramon Magsaysay Hospital of the University of the East (UERM), however, practices Integrated Medical Psychology, a school of thought founded by the former director, Professor Zaguirre.

Family and group work is surprisingly popular. Its form ranges from ward community and patient government sessions at NMH and the University of Santo Tomas Hospital (UST) to drug dependency groups and youth-parent relationship training at PMHA. Routine screening at PGH enables social workers to assign appropriate families to therapeutic sessions given by experienced resident psychiatrists. UST staff take advantage of family members staying with their relatives (so-called watchers) to conduct family discussion and education groups.

Interestingly, psychodiagnostics (termed neuropsychological testing—N.P.) has grown extremely popular since the early 1970s. Government

TABLE 4.4 Availability of Comprehensive Services in the Philippines

Service function	NMH	PGH	VL	VMH	UERM	UST	MC	PMHA
Inpatient	+	+	+	+	+	+	+	−
Outpatient	+	+	+	+	+	+	OT only	+
Emergency	+	+	+	+	+	+	+	−
Partial hospitalization	−	+	−	+	(referral)	−	+	+
Transitional living	(referral)	−	−	−	(referral)	−	(referral)	+
Follow-up	+	+	−	+	+	−	−	+
Children's services	+	+	−	−	planned	−	−	+
Geriatric care	−	−	−	−	−	−	−	−
Drug abuse	−	−	planned	+	−	(referral)	−	+
Diagnostic	+	+	+	+	+	+	+	+
Neurological	+	+	+	−	+	+	+	formerly
Suicide prevention	−	−	−	+	formerly	−	+	−
Educational	−	−	−	+	−	−	−	+
Mental health research	−	+	+	−	−	+	−	+
Program evaluation	−	−	−	−	−	−	−	sometimes
Teaching/training	+	+	−	+	+	+	−	+

+ indicates available
− indicates unavailable

TABLE 4.5 Treatment Modalities Available in the Philippines

Modality	NMH	PGH	VL	VMH	UERM	UST	MC	PMHA
Electroconvulsive therapy	+	++	+++	+	+	++	++	−
Physiotherapy	++	−	++	++	−	+++	+	−
Drug	+++	+++	+++	+++	+++	+++	+++	+++
Psychotherapy	+++	+++	+	+++	+++	+++	++	+++
Behavior modification	+	−	−	+	formerly	planned	−	−
Group therapy	+++	++	++	+++	+++	++	++	+++
Family therapy	++	++	+	+++	+++	++	+	+++
Occupational therapy	+++	+++	−	+++	+++	+	+++	+++
Work therapy	++	−	+++	+	−	−	+	+++
Other	milieu	milieu	work on ward	assertion training	hypno-therapy	−	milieu attitude	home visit

+++ often
++ sometimes
+ seldom
− never

agencies (e.g., the police) and private companies routinely request psychological testing for personnel hiring, placement, and promotion. UERM and PMHA psychologists are frequently called upon to administer these tests. Partial hospitalization usually takes the form of a day-care program where outpatients return to participate in sheltered workshop and occupational therapy projects. Follow-up services are generally extended via regular outpatient contact. NMH has activated a mobile unit to extend domiciliary care in the Manila area. On a limited basis, home visitation is also a part of the social workers' schedule at the Veterans Memorial Hospital (VMH) and PHMA.

Finally, characteristics of institutional care can be compared. It should be noted that although the small private teaching units like UST and UERM do offer reasonably intensive therapeutic contact, they are not necessarily comprehensive. VMH, on the other hand, has the greatest capability in terms of function and treatment types. This might be explained by the fact that it was set up as an American Veterans Administration hospital in 1955 and receives its budget from the U.S. government. Except for the absence of acute inpatient care, PMHA has more depth than other facilities sampled. It alone has developed an extensive halfway house rehabilitation program and child and youth development services and has undertaken program evaluation. In contrast, Victoria Luna (VL) and Medical City (MC) hospitals are the least comprehensive of the centers visited. VL is the only psychiatric facility for active military personnel. It caters only to the restricted needs of soldier-patients. MC is ostensibly a ward for private practitioners to hospitalize their patients. It does have an active day-care/occupational therapy program, but, unlike PMHA's clinic, is not set up to provide comprehensive services for the general public.

Limitations in efforts to provide comprehensive services are also discernible. First, there is no program for the elderly, nor for autistic or mentally retarded children. NMH's three wards for adolescents and PMHA's recently initiated Children and Youth Development Center are the only intervention services addressed to childhood populations. Private programs for the mentally retarded are, however, found elsewhere.[4] Suicide prevention or telephone hot line services were not a part of institutional operations, nor could any be located in the descriptions of the other programs available in the country (Amor 1975). Only two sites were involved in drug abuse treatment: PMHA had a counseling group and VMH offered detoxification services. Interestingly, when MC's psychiatric unit first opened, its population was 90 percent drug-abuse patients from upper-class families. VMH was planning to begin a drug rehabilitation program once its staff received training from Clark Air Force Base personnel, who now operate this type of service. The other

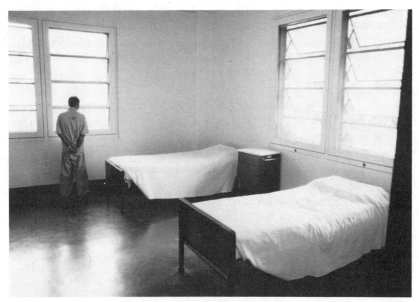

A Philippine veteran observes the world beyond his hospital bedroom.

facilities sometimes receive consultation from and refer drug cases to the Drug Research Foundation of Quezon City.

Transitional living units are another scarce resource. PMHA's halfway house in Cavite, Pinagpala, draws referrals from the other institutions, especially NMH. It has a capacity for about fifty men and twenty women. A handful of private transitional living units, plus the Department of Social Welfare's Halfway Home for Released Prisoners and Recovered Mental Patients, are scattered around the Metro-Manila area. These, however, are simply boarding homes without active rehabilitation objectives.

Other deficits are apparent in the areas of mental health education, consultation to other social service agencies, research, and program evaluation. Consultation and education action is restricted to VMH and PMHA. The former gives consultation to the VA clinic and homes for disabled children and the elderly; its clinical psychologist supervises psychologists at PMHA. The latter allocates the largest portion of its budget (25 percent) to education and information programs. PMHA has also developed extensive consultation relationships with social service groups.[5] The other sites are called upon to give outside educational lectures or consultations, but do so only upon special request.

Research inquiry is peripheral to the function of these programs and evidence of formal ongoing program evaluation was absent. Research undertaken is usually drug trials or "end-of-the-year" studies turned in by psychiatric residents. Exceptions to this were investigations at PGH concerned with the adaptation of hemodialysis patients, malnutrition in child development, and the WHO collaborative study on strategies for extending mental health care. PMHA has sponsored nineteen research projects. Ones not previously mentioned are on such topics as parents' attitudes toward their children's disabilities; evaluation of popular American personality tests; and Marsella's studies of dwelling density and sociocultural stressors on psychopathology.

All of the major treatment modalities are well represented among the sites visited, with the exception of behavior modification. As in Taiwan, chemotherapy is the foremost treatment of choice, used "often" in all settings. Moreover, there is some reluctance to use electroconvulsive therapy (ECT). Nevertheless, it remains a relied-upon option in all facilities except PMHA. It is curious that behavior modification has not become an established treatment regimen. The long-term chairman of the Psychology Department at the University of the Philippines was one of B. F. Skinner's early students at Harvard and participated in the original experiments laying down the principles of operant conditioning. However, Professor Alfredo Lagmay focused his curriculum on experimental psychology. Eschewing applied clinical training, he focused instead on training academicians.

VMH recently began looking into the use of token economy on one of their wards. While visiting VMH, in fact, I was invited to give an in-service training consultation on this topic. The chief psychologist at Jose Reyes Memorial Hospital has been spearheading the movement to introduce token economy at UST, VMH, and other residential treatment centers. Finally, it is apparent that work therapy is not offered within the three university teaching units—PGH, UERM, and UST.

Preventive Orientation

The presence of preventive mental health programs is the second resource variable in the framework. Table 4.6 lists the four key prevention components and indexes their presence within the institutions.

Half the institutions make some formal effort to disseminate public information. They use the media and various gatherings to motivate people to become concerned about mental health issues that may affect them. When such action occurs at NMH, PGH, and VMH, which is seldom, it typically involves staff personnel being invited to community seminars as resource persons, or staff may become involved in workshops designed for workers from other social agencies. PMHA expends 25 percent of its budget on public information and education, the most highly developed and longest-standing components of its program. In

TABLE 4.6 Availability of Prevention Programs in the Philippines

Prevention type	NMH	PGH	VL	VMH	UERM	UST	MC	PMHA
Public information	+	+	–	+	–	–	–	+++
Public education	–	–	–	–	–	–	–	++
Public consultation	+	+	–	+	–	–	–	+++
Ecological change	–	–	–	–	–	–	–	+

+++ often
++ sometimes
+ seldom
– never

1976, for example, PMHA information and education activities reached an estimated 290,000 people.

National Mental Health Week, a highlight of the year for PMHA, directs national attention to this area through seminars, workshops, and press releases. The theme of the 1976 Mental Health Week was "Mental Health and Economic Growth."[6] At other times during the year, PMHA organized orientation lectures, forums on approaches to psychiatric treatment, and film presentations, and presented its annual conference.

Public education, the second type of prevention activity, aims instructional experiences at identified high-risk groups. Except for PMHA, none of the sampled sites had ongoing public education programs. This condition is also reflected in table 4.4: suicide prevention services are unavailable from these agencies.

Through the Pangkalahatun Center in Quezon City, a series of "Life Enrichment Seminars" is held by PMHA for out-of-school-youth. The problem of an excessive number of high school dropouts was recently given a high priority by Philippine political leaders, including the mayor of Metro-Manila, Imelda Marcos. The PMHA seminars, accredited by the Department of Education and Culture as nonformal education curricula, are aimed at assisting those in this "risk" group to recognize and develop their individual potential. Through group dynamics training, social values are transmitted to the youth, encouraging social responsibility and service. The overall goal is to get them employed or back into school. Along similar lines, at least twelve high school mental health clubs have been established in Manila. These use peer counseling and leadership training activities.

Those institutions offering public information also offer public consultation, rendering technical assistance to other social agencies dealing with large populations. NMH offers to nonhealth workers—schools, police, local governments—one-month seminars on mental health. It also supported the National Workshop on Community Mental Health Nursing and follow-up sessions called Echo Seminars. The psychiatry professors at PGH are well known throughout the Philippines and are called upon for consultation on their own. In 1977, however, four psychiatric residents went to a regional hospital in Tacloban, Leyte, as consultants to educate other residents. VMH provides regular visitations to at least three agencies: the outpatient clinic of the Veterans Administration, Golden Acres home for the elderly, and a residential facility for developmentally disabled children.

The extent of PMHA public consultation goes beyond that of these other institutions. Besides its assistance to government groups, schools, and private organizations, trainers from the Education and Training Committee organized quarterly training sessions for the different PMHA chapters as well as other community mental health workers in the provinces. The trainers are also called upon to give in-service training to guidance counselors and school physicians at city schools.

Ecological change consists of diverse efforts at the social, economic, and political systems level to introduce changes that enhance psychological competency. As a rule, the institutions visited did not envisage their role as change agent for sociopolitical institutions. Nor were they concerned with enhancing the status of poverty-stricken peoples or assisting in the building of neighborhood and community groups that could mobilize their members' resources.

In certain respects, however, PMHA is concerned to a limited degree with ecological change. In 1976, through public forums and publications, PMHA sought to bring into public consciousness the relationship between national economic growth and psychological well-being, and the implications of increasing urbanization (e.g., Faraon 1976; Ignacio 1976). Oftentimes, though, messages regarding optimum mental health conditions communicated by PMHA extol values and ideals reflecting the vision held by present political leaders, i.e., Marcos' "New Society." The national development value of considering psychological conditions was spelled out by one speaker at the National Mental Health Week seminar series:

> If the New Society is to succeed, economic planners and policymakers must be reoriented in their thinking so that they can see the importance of providing for the development of good mental health hand in hand with their plans for the development and growth of the economy because mental health is the most effective answer to the dangers posed by the revolution of rising expectations in the overall development effort (Sanvictores 1976:21).

Furthermore, PMHA may be viewed as contributing to ecological change, albeit on a limited scale, to the extent that it seeks to develop high school clubs, recruits Manila dropouts, and works through the *barangay* organization (the neighborhood political unit seen as the foundation of the New Society) as its primary community contact.

Continuity of Care within the Facility: Manpower

The presence of various categories of professionals and the ratios of these to patient populations are rough indices of intrainstitutional continuity of care. They denote the agency's potential for smooth patient referral among professionals at different stages of contact.

Among sampled sites, the different categories of professionals are unevenly distributed (table 4.7). Numerically, psychiatric nurses far outnumber other staff types. They are especially noticeable in high concen-

TABLE 4.7 Multidisciplinary Teams and Manpower Availability in the Philippines: Staff Numbers and Staff-to-Patient Ratios

Profession	NMH	PGH	VL	VMH	UERM	UST	MC	PMHA	Total
Psychiatrist (including residents)	95	12 (10 PT*)	3 (3 PT)	7	3 (5 PT)	11	5	1 (1 PT)	137
Psychologist	20	(2 PT)	7	3	2	0	0	2	36
Nurse	500	12	4	11	6	16	13	0	562
Social worker	26	2	0	2	2	0	0	5	37
Occupational therapist	100	2	0	1	1	0	2	3	109
Beds	3,500 (8,227 patients)	15	81	90 (45 patients)	15	36	44 (31 patients)	None	
Monthly outpatient contacts	60/day	65	32	93	180	80	None	450	
Total outpatients	3,500							1,055	
Inpatients per therapeutic staff	11.11	.47	5.06	3.60	.88	1.33	2.20	41 (out-patients)	

*Part-time staff

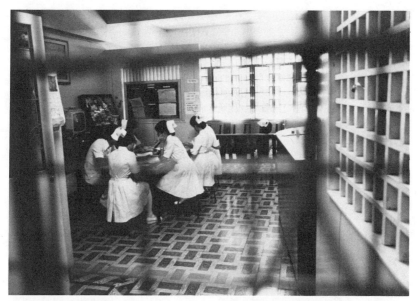

Patients' view of a nursing station at a university hospital in Manila.

trations at NMH. Nurses were more numerous than other professionals in the majority of inpatient facilities. Their ratio to beds ranged from 1:20 and 1:16 at VL and NMH respectively to 1:1.2 at PGH. Psychiatrists were the second largest group, appearing in adequate numbers across most facilities, except perhaps at PMHA and NMH. The ratio of inpatients to psychiatrists at NMH was 1 per 86. Occupational therapists are the third largest group. This finding is misleading, though, since more than 90 percent of these workers are employed at NMH, two sites have none, and the rest have only one or two at best. Social workers and psychologists are numerically the smallest categories of staff. VL, UST, and MC are without the services of social workers. The latter two private institutions also do not have staff psychologists.

However, it should be recognized that the number of occupational therapists at NMH who actually have specialized training in that discipline are far fewer than the 100 listed. Given this consideration, it becomes clear that each facility employs psychologists, social workers, and occupational therapists—if they have them at all—in approximately equal numbers.

The concept of multidisciplinary contact with inpatients is well established at NMH, PGH, VMH, UERM, and PMHA. Hence, the likelihood of continuity of care within these settings is good. Division of labor and assignment of responsibility follows conventional hospital setting lines for the multidisciplinary team members. The exception is PMHA, where nonmedical professionals have full authority over their respective projects.

Typically, psychiatrists (usually residents) screen for organic conditions, prescribe medication, diagnose, carry out individual and group psychotherapy, and are sometimes involved in family education sessions. Psychologists are primarily involved in psychological testing (I.Q., projective, personality, aptitude) to support physician diagnoses. This activity has dramatically increased the caseload recently as companies and government bodies have begun to rely upon psychological screening for hiring and promotions. However, in some places, like NMH, UERM, and PMHA, psychologists are running individual, group, and ward community psychotherapy sessions by themselves and as co-therapists with residents. At PGH and UERM, psychologists are given teaching roles. They explain the use of tests to residents, consult on group psychotherapy, and supervise psychology interns.

Social workers enact a broad variety of roles across agencies. Some coordinate discharge and follow-up patients through home visits, make referrals to the Provincial Health Offices, or help patients find jobs. Others are active on the wards, doing intake interviews, case histories, screening for family therapy, guidance counseling, and offering education services for families with inpatients. At PGH, social work consultants supervise residents in family therapy. PMHA social workers run the outreach center, design and run the educational seminars for mental health workers, handle the youth programs, and engage in individual, group, and family counseling at the rehabilitation centers.

Occupational therapists are active on the four rehabilitation wards at NMH, run the outpatient program at MC, and, of course, are responsible for the two well-used rehabilitation centers administered by PMHA. The residential treatment centers that operate on a multidisciplinary team basis—NMH, PGH, VMH, and UERM—also call upon team members to assist in discharge decision making. This is in contrast with MC, where the admitting psychiatrist alone decides whether his patient has improved enough for discharge.

The conservative estimate of manpower potential as reflected in the contact possibilities between staff and patients is shown at the bottom of table 4.7. Unfortunately, data are available only for inpatients. In most instances, these ratios are extremely small, suggesting a good chance for contact and continuity of care among team members. They range from 1:0.47 at PGH to 1:11 at NMH, with 1:3.5 as the average. The size of these ratios is attributable to the numbers of available psychiatric nurses and adequate supplies of full- and part-time psychiatrists working in small university teaching units.

In contrast, NMH is grossly understaffed when nurses are subtracted from the totals. With only one psychologist per 400 patients, one psychiatrist per eighty, and social workers in a ratio of 1:310, it is assumed that active team care is restricted to a small percentage. Indeed, the hospital is organized into sections that include the acute and first admissions (treatable) and the continued treatment or chronic, long-staying patients (untreatable). The latter constitute the overwhelming majority of residents.

Under these conditions, it is difficult to imagine individual psychotherapy undertaken with any but a handful of highly selected (and paying) inpatients. Social work efforts to provide follow-up care, do home visitation, and check the progress of trial home stays are perhaps merely token gestures in light of the total needs. It is this set of circumstances that has brought forth the twenty-year plea for decentralization of this facility, the largest mental hospital in Asia.

Continuity of Care: Interinstitutional

Well-established referral pathways among psychiatric agencies allow them to function as a unified service system and afford the individual an opportunity to maximize her contact with diverse services. A mapping of the referral process and the linkage patterns among selected sites in Metro-Manila are presented in figure 4.2.

Community sources referring patients initially into the network were pinpointed in the administrator interviews. Ten referral agents and their importance for each facility are listed and rank-ordered at the top of figure 4.2. Family, friends, and employers are the most active of community referring agents. Traditional healers, priests, and police are least frequent. It is important to note that physicians and other psychiatric personnel and agencies are also important sources. This suggests viable ties both to allied medical workers and among fellow mental health professionals. Clearly certain sites like NMH and PMHA have strong ties with the police and school systems while others do not. None of the agencies reported receiving direct referrals from traditional healers like herbalists and shamans.

The two foci of this referral network are NMH and PMHA, although for somewhat different reasons. Considering NMH first, the reason for its overcrowding is strikingly apparent. It is the recipient of referrals from a host of sources: numerous Department of Health clinics, rural as well as urban, the courts, private hospitals, and the military hospital. In essence, NMH is a dumping ground for long-term, chronic patients who cannot be handled successfully among the acute, intensive, and short-term units.

Conversely, according to decentralization, NMH is supposed to be discharging patients back into facilities being developed in their home prov-

Figure 4.2
Referral and Consultation Relationships
among Metro-Manila Psychiatric Centers

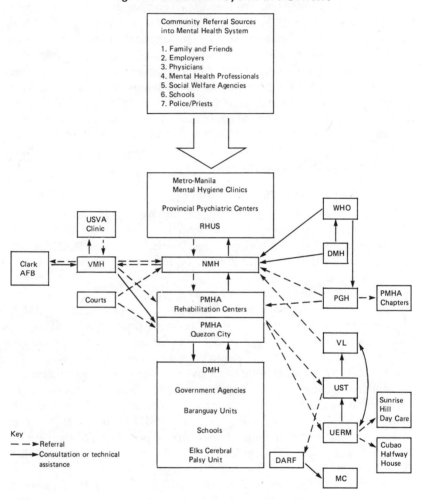

Community Referral Sources
into Mental Health System

1. Family and Friends
2. Employers
3. Physicians
4. Mental Health Professionals
5. Social Welfare Agencies
6. Schools
7. Police/Priests

Metro-Manila
Mental Hygiene Clinics

Provincial Psychiatric Centers

RHUS

USVA Clinic

WHO

DMH

Clark AFB

VMH

NMH

PGH

PMHA Chapters

Courts

PMHA
Rehabilitation Centers

PMHA
Quezon City

VL

UST

DMH

Government Agencies

Baranguay Units

Schools

Elks Cerebral
Palsy Unit

UERM

Sunrise
Hill
Day Care

Cubao
Halfway
House

DARF

MC

Key
- - - ► Referral
———► Consultation or technical
assistance

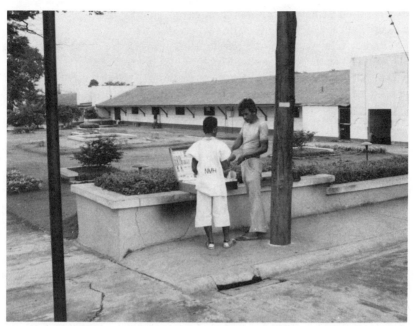

A patient buys cigarettes from a vendor at the National Mental Hospital in Mandaluyang, the Philippines' largest mental hospital.

inces. Moreover, it uses the PMHA Cavite facility for patients suitable for rural, live-in rehabilitation. Others are sent to the day-care industrial rehabilitation program at Quezon City. The technical capabilities of VMH are utilized for EEG and EKG assessment of certain NMH patients. Consultation ties exist between NMH and PMHA, the MHD, and the WHO Regional Office for the Western Pacific. These latter two organized with NMH the 1974 workshop on community mental health nursing and subsequent follow-up sessions.

PMHA, the second focus of the system, has an elaborate set of linkages not only with other psychiatric clinics but with government agencies, schools, courts, and community groups. Their rehabilitation programs are the targets of referrals from VMH, NMH, and PGH. In provincial areas, PMHA chapters are the only sources of clinical intervention and are relied upon by local physicians. PGH makes referrals to such chapters when they discharge inpatients living in these areas. From time to time, PMHA uses the small, private units at UST and UERM to hospitalize referred patients. Furthermore, its key function of consultation and technical assistance can also be noted in channels of communication between it and the host of other groups, including MHD and

NMH. Interestingly, VMH psychologists supervise the psychologists on the staff at the Quezon City national headquarters.

Other active centers in the relationship network are apparent. Besides its contacts with NMH and PMHA, VMH gives drug referrals to the Clark Air Force Base drug treatment program. VMH receives technical assistance from Clark on this topic and takes referrals from the U.S. Veterans Administration clinic in Ermita, Manila. The two university units, UERM and UST, have a consultation relationship with one another; both assist VL, the army psychiatric program. UERM makes use of its psychiatric director's day-care facility, Sunrise Hill, and also the Department of Social Welfare's Halfway Home in Cubao, Quezon City. UST refers drug cases to the Drug Abuse Research Foundation (DAR), which has one residential and several day-care programs. DAR is working closely with MC to prepare its staff for treatment of substance-abuse clients.

The World Health Organization over the years has tried to advise NMH administrators—beginning with Manuel Escudero's efforts—as well as work through MHD. At present, WHO contact has been mostly centered on PGH and the collaborative research being done through University of Philippines psychiatrists.

These lines of communication and referral are the only evidence available for assessing interinstitutional continuity of care. Do agencies effectively pass along clients whose particular needs are more appropriately met or followed up by allied institutions? In terms of NMH and its interchange with the general health system administered by municipal health offices, this continuity is what is expected, but it may be lacking in most instances except in Davao. Getting into NMH appears to be a lot easier than getting out; the sources for inward referral are more numerous than those receiving patients being referred out. Like the wards of NMH, the rehabilitation opportunities of PMHA seem quite visible among different sectors of the network, private and public, and are well used, although not to their maximum.

U.S. military-connected Filipinos have access to perhaps the most comprehensive care available via VMH, the U.S. Veterans Administration clinic, and their relationship with Clark Air Force Base and PMHA. Those who can afford the private university units or are able to be seen at PGH can take advantage of these adequately developed programs. Those with good incomes are apt to receive proper referrals, either to drug abuse, day-care, or halfway care programs. Those without adequate incomes have the handful of mental hygiene clinics, but referral options are restricted to NMH or one of its extension facilities. On the issue of consultation, there is a small core of recognized, long-standing experts who move fluidly among several institutions. They assist in the development of specialized care and strengthen the staff capacity of these sites.

Moreover, PMHA and groups like the Philippine Psychiatric Association and the Division of Mental Hygiene have sought to bring the professional community together through annual conferences, workshops, seminars, joint research projects, and special celebrations.

However, a formal organizational connection among the institutions—as found among Taipei's five major psychiatric hospitals—and their attempt to create a communitywide treatment project has not coalesced in Metro-Manila. MHD, the most plausible proponent of such an organization, is without the power base to suggest it. PMHA, which has the viability to suggest more formal ties among the service providers, has no administrative access to the public health system. Public health would naturally need to be included to make such an organizational setup of value to the general public.

Continuity with Community Care-giving

Continuity of movement from the institutional setting back into community environments is heightened when the service agency encourages or relies upon the participation of various community agents (family members, teachers, employers, religious leaders) in the treatment and discharge process. It also arises to the extent that agency personnel carry out their therapeutic functions in those settings where the patient lives and works.

In some instances, continuity is maintained by giving the family the responsibility for bringing the patient back for periodic consultations at the outpatient clinic. This is the case for NMH, PGH, and UERM (table 4.8). When this is not possible, NMH has a mobile unit for Metro-Manila offering domiciliary service. This service, like the one at VMH, is manned primarily by social workers. However, for both institutions, the professional time permitted for doing this is restricted. The scarcity of manpower versus need makes the task seem almost futile. VL, UST, and MC don't offer this alternative. VL either sends the patients back to their military units, discharges them from the service, or places them for long-term care at NMH. UST simply refers their discharge cases back to the admitting physicians.

A characteristic of these programs was their formal and informal strategies for getting the family involved in patient care. Another was their working against what was perceived as a natural tendency for the families to turn over complete responsibility for patient improvement to the medical personnel. PGH and VMH were perhaps the best organized: In the former, all families are screened for suitability of family therapy and often permitted input into treatment decisions. VMH has routine weekly family education sessions as well as social worker-led groups for parents, spouses, and full family participation to discuss patient behavior and

TABLE 4.8 Six Alternatives for Providing Continuity with Community Care-giving in the Philippines

Alternatives	NMH	PGH	VL	VMH	UERM	UST	MC	PMHA
Active patient follow-up especially by social worker	+	+	−	++	+	−	−	
Educate or utilize family members as part of treatment plan	+	+++	−	++	++	+	+	++
Relative stays in hospital with patient	−	+++	−	−	++	−	+	
Treatment within home or village setting	++	−	−	+	−	−	−	++
Community agents assist in treatment (teacher, employer, village leader, M.D., police, etc.)	+	+	−	+	+	+	−	++
Participation in community activities during hospitalization encouraged	+	+	+	+	++	++	+	

+++ always
++ sometimes
+ seldom
− never

assist in problem solving in home situations. Family "watchers" who stay twenty-four hours with most cases at PGH—and selected ones at UERM—are keys to relative-assisted treatment. Watchers are educated by psychiatric residents and nurses through group meetings in how to assist in the intervention process while on the ward and in how to handle the patient upon return home.

Other less-formal involvement of families was also noted. At NMH, they were sometimes given specific information regarding home care as part of the discharge plan. Staff encourage family visitation only after the hostility toward the admitted member dies down. Visitation is also encouraged at VMH, where picnics with relatives on hospital grounds are frequent. MC sets aside one hour per day for visitation. PMHA attaches significance to family education and therapy with its clinic clients and employs this approach as an integral part of its two rehabilitation programs. Only VL, which by necessity must start treatment of military patients in the absence of contact with family, is unable to draw upon familial assistance in the treatment regimen.

Intervention involving professional services carried into the home or village settings was rare. Only two residential programs gave examples of such action, which was infrequently carried out. NMH, through its mobile clinic, sends social workers into the homes of patients in nearby neighborhoods who are unable to come to the outpatient department at the hospital. Social workers at VMH are allotted four hours per week to use hospital transportation to do home visitation and keep watch on trial home stays of recently discharged cases. At PMHA, home visits for the full range of clinical care offered by social workers are a routine service.

In short, the extension of treatment into the living places of people in need is generally unavailable. Since it is a function apparently assigned exclusively to social workers, its absence may be tied to the scarcity of these professionals. On a more global plane, the addition of NMH extension services and the expressed desire to include mental health components in rural health units and provincial hospitals is a step toward placing such services closer to the home environments.

Getting community agents like teachers, employers, and general practitioners is another alternative that is available but used only on a "seldom" basis. If any community agent is used, it is likely to be a public health nurse or school teacher who was involved in the referral of the patient to the institution. PMHA, more than any other site, draws upon such individuals in treatment planning. In addition to teachers and public health nurses, PMHA has sought to work closely with school counselors and clergy when making referrals. Moreover, it has begun to set up peer counseling programs for high school youth.

At all sites visited, the residential programs encourage their patients to participate in various community activities, whether work or recreation, but this is not done with any regularity. Perhaps the most common outing would be to attend a dance or fiesta. Staff at VL did report that some of their patients participated in a kind of Olympic sports meet for disabled and handicapped persons. While many staff reported that "sometimes" patients did go out and participate in community events, the existence of a program for regular off-grounds excursions for recreation, religious worship, or work was not mentioned.

Accessibility of Facilities

Availability and ease of access to existing mental health resources are the two components of the "accessibility" variable. As earlier noted, psychiatric services exist in the public sector via the National Mental Hospital, its eleven extensions, the municipal mental hygiene clinics, and whatever care is able to follow from specialized training filtering down to the public health worker. The private sector has its own system comprising self-employed practitioners, small units in general and university hospitals, assorted specialty clinics, and the fourteen chapters of the PMHA scattered about the islands. A PMHA directory of Philippine agencies engaged in the promotion and development of mental health lists 117 programs touching on various aspects of therapeutic assistance (Amor 1975).

However, the use of these sites by those in need is governed by such factors as the agencies' proximity to their users, cost, hours of operation, whether there is bed space available, and policies regulating admissions.

Staff generally considered location as a "slight problem," except in reference to those patients who must travel from outlying areas to seek assistance. Excluding those at VL and VMH, who are drawn from throughout the Philippines, the majority of inpatients live in or near Metro-Manila. NMH does have a sizable minority, however, who are referred from the provinces. This problem has prompted DOH intentions to establish one mental hospital in each region and a small (ten to fifteen beds) inpatient unit in each provincial general hospital. Because of the lack of such facilities at present, NMH staff label location as a moderately serious problem.

National health insurance, Medicare, does not extend to psychiatric treatment. Thus, private treatment is restricted to those who can afford it. Private hospitals are required to allow 10 percent bed occupancy for charity cases. The extent to which this is adhered to is not known. UERM was the only private facility visited that reported service delivery to low-income patients. The expense of private care varies among settings, with the most expensive found at MC. Daily costs there ranged between $14 and $17, depending on dormitory versus semiprivate room status. While

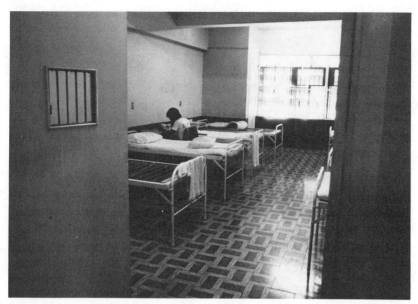

Eight patients share this typical room at a Manila University psychiatric unit.

PMHA charges a nominal fee for clinical care, NMH is required to accept all those needing institutionalization. Families sometimes contribute for medicines not supplied by the hospital. PGH, VL, and VMH are also without fee requirements. Because of the possibility of receiving some charity cases, most staff felt that it was "often" or "always" possible for people with little money to use the treatment program.

The consensus among staff sampled was that long waiting periods were either not a problem or only an occasional "slight" problem. Even PGH with its fifteen-bed capacity for the entire University of the Philippines did not complain of pressure for bed space. In fact, the impression was given that the services were underused. VMH was only half full at the time visited; neither was MC at capacity. PMHA's halfway house was operating well below its capacity and awaiting more referrals. In contrast, NMH, functioning at 200 percent overcrowding, is required by policy to take in those needing hospitalization immediately without waiting for vacancies. NMH is uniquely open to overcrowding.

Other institutions have screening criteria or conditions that limit the flow of users. VL and VMH take only military personnel. The former receives men who are routed there from unit commanders, while the latter only takes in those enlisted in the American army prior to Philippine independence. Both sites are only interested in short-term, acute cases. PGH admissions come only from other sections of that hospital, especially the emergency room. UST and MC cases only have access to the ward through private physicians who have a relationship with those units.

These findings suggest differential ease of access based on facility characteristics and the client's status and residence. Well-to-do Filipinos can visit the PMHA clinic in Quezon City or a score of private psychiatrists in Metro-Manila. These practitioners usually have some tie with one of the private general hospitals and can easily hospitalize more severe cases on a psychiatric ward without the worry of a waiting list. Low-income individuals in need can choose from five municipal mental hygiene clinics in Metro-Manila or a dozen NMH extension services in the outlying health regions. Although some charity beds are available in several of the small private units, most who require hospitalization end up in the grossly overcrowded and undermanned NMH system. Only Filipino men who served in the United States armed forces are eligible for the most comprehensive psychiatric program available, operated and funded by the Veterans Administration.

Specialized psychiatric resources are overwhelmingly concentrated in Metro-Manila. Rural people unable to journey to Manila or to find psychiatric intervention through their Regional Health Offices have no access whatsoever to professional therapeutics. Rural health units are criticized for not actually reaching rural populations; most are situated in large towns or cities. Formal care for psychological distress is even more remote for provincial citizens since it is seldom, if ever, even a part of rural health unit operations.

Staff Evaluation of Resource Strength

There is a moderate amount of diversity in staff opinion regarding resource strengths, not only across the sites visited but among workers within the same settings (table 4.9). It seems clear that there are worries for future funding, although worries for present monetary insufficiencies appear slightly less intense. Governmental uninvolvement is given as a problem by just half of the respondents; most of those who view it as unimportant are employed by private clinics like UERM and UST.

Concerning manpower, no clear pattern unfolds: responses are almost evenly divided problematic/nonproblematic for each relevant item. A careful examination of individual institutions, however, tells a different story. NMH and VL, both government facilities, consistently report manpower shortages, especially among administrators, treatment, and follow-up staff. These perceptions are congruent with the actual manpower numbers reported (see table 4.7). PGH, VMH, UERM, and UST, on the other hand, consistently report minimal or no problem in these same areas. These perceptions are congruent with their therapeutic staff

TABLE 4.9 Staff Perceptions of Resource Deficits in the Philippines (N=22)

Potential problem	Problem seriousness			
	Very serious	Moderately serious	Slightly serious	Not a problem
1. Lack of help from government	19%	33%	14%	33%
2. Not enough money for present treatment program	23%	32%	32%	13%
3. Not enough money to develop future treatment programs	32%	36%	27%	4.5%
4. Not enough trained administrators	40%	10%	15%	35%
5. Not enough diagnostic staff	24%	19%	14%	43%
6. Not enough treatment staff	27%	27%	14%	32%
7. Not enough follow-up staff	27%	23%	18%	32%
8. Lack of relationship with other institutions	14%	18%	23%	45%
9. Other professionals don't support the program	27%	9%	23%	41%
10. Long waiting list	45%	4.5%	36%	54%
11. Not enough rooms to separate different kinds of patients	41%	18%	18%	23%
12. Lack of building space	32%	9%	23%	36%
13. Too many patients	41%	14%	23%	23%
14. Lack of money for equipment and research	54.5%	14%	23%	9%
15. Library is not good enough	36%	14%	4.5%	45.5%
16. Little information about new treatments and new research findings	9%	13%	14%	64%
17. Lack of epidemiological data regarding mental problems	27%	32%	18%	23%
18. Staff relations are not good	9%	4.5%	27%	26%
19. Not enough treatment supplies	27%	32%	32%	9%
20. Lack of transportation services	27%	14%	18%	41%
21. Low success rate of treatment	4.5%	14%	54.5%	27%

per inpatient ratios (table 4.7). But, they are still out of line with reality in the area of follow-up care, in which each is extremely understaffed. Interestingly, PMHA and MC follow NMH and VL in complaining of severe understaffing.

Linkages among institutions and acceptance of mental health programs by other personnel are not viewed as difficulties by a substantial majority of respondents. Apparently the multiple ties shown in figure 4.2 are satisfactory to most workers with the possible exception of those at NMH and PGH and the one physician interviewed at PMHA. Moreover, VL staff felt particularly alienated from their fellow professionals. This may reflect how their unit is viewed within the context of the army hospital.

A feeling of space availability carries over consistently for VMH, UERM, UST, and MC. Complaints of overcrowded buildings, lack of special quarters, and generally too many patients are voiced by the three governmental sites—NMH, VL, and PGH. NMH staff are particularly homogeneous in their perceptions of overcrowdedness.

The existence of only a few cursory epidemiological studies of psychiatric disorder is viewed as problematic. About 70 percent are concerned also with the absence of money to carry on research. Poor library facilities are not bothersome except at NMH and VL. All respondents, with five exceptions (two of them at VL), do not see being out of touch with new therapeutic innovations or research data as troublesome at their clinic.

Staff relations are seen as good—or mostly all right—across the eight locations. Supplies sufficient to carry out treatment intervention (medication, occupational therapy equipment, psychological tests) are somewhat unavailable. Transportation service provided by the facility is not an issue except, once again, for the government-sponsored programs. In particular, the NMH mobile clinic and home program rely upon the availability of transportation for home visits. Staff there are thus more sensitive to the need for transportation availability.

Presumably, if professionals felt frustrated in their efforts to provide an adequate structure for intervention due to the limitations of resources, it would be reflected in their judgments of a low success rate. In the case of the Philippines, unlike that of Taiwan, fewer than 20 percent viewed low success rate as more than a slight problem; 27 percent saw it as no problem at all. Understandably, several NMH staff identified this as a problem for their facility. Yet, PGH and PMHA personnel also responded in this manner. It may well be that these latter two cases are a function of heightened sensitivity on the part of respondents to what an idealized therapeutic outcome should entail, at least according to the standards of contemporary psychiatry.

COMMUNITY INTEGRATION AND ACCEPTANCE OF THE
MENTAL HEALTH SYSTEM

Institutional ties to the community are strengthened through involvement of community agents, particularly family members, in such intervention tasks as goal setting, treatment selection, service delivery, and rehabilitation. Encouraging participation of persons from the patient's social network simultaneously provides enhanced continuity of care, integration, and community acceptance of agency programs.

A distinct pattern of community involvement in agency therapeutics is evident in table 4.8. Nonrelatives from the patient's immediate social environment are seldom brought into case management. On the other hand, agencies do apply a host of methods for getting family members to take some form of responsibility for helping in the patient's recovery. Family therapy, counseling with spouses, weekly family education sessions, and reliance on relatives to report problems and improvement at home are frequent methods used. However, the family "watcher" system, involving the overnight stay of a member who has a positive relationship with the patient, is perhaps the most dramatic penetration of the community into residential treatment.

At PGH in particular, the watcher has been recognized as a vital force for assistance. Staff take time to train, educate, and offer professional support to those accompanying an admitted relative. Visitation is encouraged in all settings; staff sometimes take advantage of family presence to gather information, offer suggestions, or encourage activities such as picnics or outings.

However, for the most part, family input into the selection of therapeutics and specific goals of treatment is seldom sought out. The power to make these decisions—as in the case of Taiwan—rests almost exclusively with the psychiatrists. In some instances, other professionals are called upon to make team judgments. Yet, it is the physician in the standard medical tradition who is the final decision maker and authority. This is not the case in only one instance: PMHA's nonresidential programs. There, the social workers and rehabilitation specialists carry the burden of client contact and consultation. Not surprisingly, PMHA is noted for its emphasis on the family unit in therapy, education, and research.

A second measure of integration entails agency openness to community input at the level of program policies and goals. The conception of community consultants or an advisory board empowered to assist in program development was alien to the Philippines as it was to those in Taiwan.

The one exception was PMHA. Its basic policies and orientation are guided by a national board made up of well-known professionals—lawyers, physicians, psychiatrists—and representatives of the business world and government. The recent president of PMHA was a former chief justice of the Supreme Court. PMHA chapter offices are also directed by local boards composed of community volunteers, both professionals and members of higher social classes. Although neighborhood or *barangay* political leadership is not formally represented in PMHA administration, certain PMHA programs are directed toward cooperation with these local units.

Perhaps of more direct consequence, however, is the voice of higher political authority, especially Imelda Marcos. She recently began a campaign to assist out-of-school youth which was taken up by PMHA. In short, PMHA is substantially tied to local interests in its orientation, although those interests are perhaps most closely associated with the values, attitudes, and beliefs of the educated elite of the country and its current political leadership.

A survey of staff opinion regarding the agencies' integration with their consumer communities firmly hints of agency alienation (table 4.10).

TABLE 4.10 Staff Perceptions of Agency Acceptability in the Philippines (*N*=22)

	Seriousness of problem			
Questionnaire item	Very serious	Moderately serious	Slightly serious	Not a problem
1. Community people don't know about or understand the treatment program.	23%	32%	41%	4.5%
2. Community people have a bad opinion of the treatment program and use it as a last chance.	18%	27%	41%	14%
3. Patients and their families don't believe the treatment will help.	4.5%	4.5%	50%	41%
4. Patients returning home have problems because people know they were in a mental hospital.	32%	32%	32%	4.5%
5. People with traditional beliefs about mental problems won't use the treatment program.	14%	14%	64%	9%
6. People go to "folk doctors" instead of using the treatment program.	14%	32%	50%	4.5%

Less than 5 percent of the respondents found no problem in the community's knowledge or understanding of their program. The sense of alienation is reinforced to a moderate degree by the view of just under half of those sampled that people hold negative opinions of psychiatric facilities and use them only when forced to. None of the sites reported being completely free of this problem, although VMH, UERM, and UST saw it as a minor issue.

Concern for the stigmatizing effects of psychiatric contact has the most agreement among respondents. Only one staff member (at PGH) did not see stigmatization as a problem; a clear majority saw it as moderately serious or worse. In fact, staff firmly believe that their treatment carries the burden of social ostracism for patients. Those who come do so only as a last resort when other alternatives have failed. Yet, personnel feel quite certain that those who arrive bring with them a certain amount of faith in the treatment itself. The act of seeking help may require faith by those participating, a faith not shared by nonparticipating observers. Faith in psychiatry is evoked at the point when other intervention avenues such as general practitioners or folk methods have failed.

An interesting difference emerged when personnel were asked to rate problems associated with tradition-minded persons (those whose beliefs about disorder might be incongruent with modern psychiatry's) and those who prefer to use folk doctors instead of clinic services. More staff rated folk doctor visitation as more of a problem than the simple reluctance of people with traditional values to attend their clinics. It may be that staying away because of traditional-mindedness is only a minor difficulty, at least in regard to urban Manila. It may also be that the highly visible, dramatic, and well-publicized spiritualists and faith healers of the country—including the internationally known psychic surgeons who practice in Manila—are perceived as threatening by certified personnel. This could explain the finding that only one respondent did not label folk doctors' attractiveness to patients as problematic.

Taken as a whole, these three sources of evidence regarding integration suggest that a community penetration of agency functioning is limited to a few key points of contact involving the family. Furthermore, staff do recognize a modicum of alienation. But this is by no means thought of as overwhelming or severely isolating of extant programs.

CULTURAL CONTINUITY AND ACCOMMODATION OF MENTAL HEALTH SERVICES

The pursuit of cultural continuity in the delivery of psychiatric services is the third attribute of a mental health system investigated. Instances were sought depicting accommodation of psychiatric practice and procedure with patterns of recipient culture. Five dimensions of Philippine culture accommodation, similar to those of Taiwan, were observed and interpreted in the light of ethnographic reports.

Prominence of Philippine Kinship Ties

A force requiring recognition in any designated therapeutic encounter is the Philippine family structure within which each patient lives. First, a Filipino's sense of personal identity is almost exclusively defined through kinship ties (Shakman 1969). The eminent Filipino anthropologist, F. L. Jocano, emphasizes the cultural ideal that an individual's most important duty and responsibility are to his close kin, doing nothing to bring disgrace to the family (Jocano 1973: 34). Extreme loyalty demands by the family are presumably compensated for by its extensive support of each member and its function as satisfying emotional and dependency needs (Sechrest 1969; Shakman 1969). Helping professionals must consider that the patient's source of emotional well-being and reassurance is derived through successful negotiation of interpersonal affairs with family and friends (Lapuz 1972). In Bulatao's (1969) analysis, only family members are to be trusted and no one else.

A second aspect of family influence is the family's role in recognizing "illness" and deciding upon treatment action. A host of etiologies are held regarding perceived illness (Jocano 1973) and determine family reaction to it (see discussion below). What is significant to the agencies, however, are those behaviors that lead to a psychiatric referral by relatives. It appears that as long as the behavior dysfunction is passive in nature—the person quiet and manageable even though actively hallucinating—she will be maintained in the home.

Professionals complain of a general inability among relatives to recognize the cues of an impending disorder (Sena 1974) or simply a high tolerance of mild psychotic symptoms (Santiago, personal communication). Supporting this latter point, Maguigad (1964) reports that family and friends may not actually consider visual hallucinations as unnatural. Jocano (1971) recorded in his visit to Panay that hallucinations are one method of social control used by the people and are an established part of the peasants' "idiom of cognition."

On the other hand, violence or threat of violence to family members and neighbors is definitely intolerable. In a culture where modesty in speech and actions is highly valued, where public display of feelings is discouraged (Jocano 1973), and where hostility toward parents is never legitimately expressed, severe social sanction is likely to befall the member who acts violently toward his kinship group. It is often under these conditions of extreme alienation that a person is finally brought to the attention of a psychiatrist and hospitalized. It becomes the challenge of the agency worker to recognize the severance in the relationship and set in motion ways to begin a rapprochement. Without family support and cooperation, the agency will end up being a long-term caretaker for the patient.

The point of initial institutional contact is critical for establishing a cooperative link between the staff and family of the patient. Relatives' initial expectations of treatment function are dominant and must be considered. Frequently, they expect a quick, complete cure, regardless of the patient's condition. They look around for the "best" healer—someone who can demonstrate quick results. The family may demand to have the patient released by a certain time, tell the staff how to handle the case, or remove their patient against the physician's advice when these expectations are unmet.

In response to this situation, facilities work to get the family's commitment for a full treatment program. For example, at UST the patient is admitted with perhaps the whole family in attendance. They are interviewed and the program is described to them; ECT is explained and consent for its use is sought. Personnel feel that if the physician explains the significance of the treatment modalities the family is easily convinced of its value and is satisfied with the treatment program. At PGH, it was stressed that it is important to deal immediately with reduction of overt symptoms that the family fears. Rehabilitation involving broader treatment activities and family participation is discussed later.

The tendency to abandon the patient to residential care, especially those alienated from kin through acts of violence, is the greatest challenge to agency professionals. Its counteraction requires culturally appropriate procedures. Families often eschew responsibility for rehabilitation. They prefer to have their aggressive patients remain in the hospital forever, even those cases the psychiatrist advises can be treated on an outpatient basis (Manapsal 1974). This may be related to fear of being harmed again, a sense of hopelessness, or to notions of incurability and a desire to avoid dealing with the stigmatization and shame that a discharged mental patient may bring to the family. At NMH it was remarked that if a patient is not completely recovered, although functionally improved, the family still wants him to remain in the hospital employed in menial labor rather than returned home.

Hospitals adopted a variety of measures to keep the family engaged with the patient, avoid abandonment, and facilitate recovery. These measures all entail encouraging different levels of family participation in treatment. NMH staff wait for the hostility to die down before asking the family to make regular visits to their relative. They are allowed to bring a supplementary diet to the patient. This not only promotes health but is a concrete expression of affection between family members (Jocano 1973).

Of course, the watcher system is another example of how agencies can rely upon existing ties of emotional dependency and support to provide intensive treatment for a case. This is especially true at PGH and UERM, where the watchers are instructed on how to be maximally useful to the patient. Parent and spouse groups and family education sessions with treatment staff at VMH are examples of responsive efforts to exploit kinship structure for rehabilitation goals. These methods aim to insure that the patient maintains her position safe within the family.

Accommodation to Popular Indigenous Conceptions of Disorder

Filipino mental health workers in contact with less-educated and barrio populations revealed a certain awareness of folk conceptions of disorder. Professionals recognize that it is those patients whose distress proves refractory to the healing power of local folk specialists who are referred finally to the hospital. In the course of this referral process, illness interpretation may change for those experiencing treatment failure. This in turn dictates selection of a different type of specialist by the family. In general, however, the decision between folk and modern doctor is based on recognition of natural or supernatural causes (Lieban 1967; Manapsal 1974). A scientific doctor is assumed to be inadequate if an illness is said to result from malign magic (sorcery) or an encounter with a malevolent spirit. The shaman or sorcerer is the correct expert, in the logic of barrio people, to resolve illness induced by man-eating spirit possession *(answang),* loss of soul, and taboo violation.

Psychiatrists have little sympathy with indigenous explanations involving "devil possession." It is diagnostically termed "Follie a Familia"— delusional ideation shared among an entire family—and associated with lethal consequences. An NMH psychiatrist reported a case in which a husband and wife thought that their child was changing into a monster. They put a cross into the child's mouth, causing death by asphyxiation. All too often, professionals' knowledge and judgment of cultural interpretations are determined by these extreme, although rare, examples. Similarly, psychiatrists complain that local healers called in to exorcise spirits employ sadistic procedures, such as burning the flesh of disturbed people with cigarettes, and delay "proper" medical attention (Sena 1974). These accusations fail to consider the substantial health contribution of community-sanctioned folk specialists (Lieban 1967; Shakman 1969) and, of course, the fact that barrio populations are out of contact with primary health care, let alone psychiatry. Yet a disturbing report by Sechrest (1967) cannot be dismissed. He found in Negros Oriental that there was an *intentional* lack of treatment given certain cases; even contact with native healers was denied as it was deemed futile and thought unnecessary.

In contrast, maladies popularly attributed to physical or psychological causes not associated with sorcery or witchcraft raise less professional ire. This category contains illnesses treatable by physicians and includes sickness brought on by incorrect personal habits such as taking a nap after a bath, bathing during the menstrual period, getting caught in the rain, or neglecting to eat meals on time (Sena 1974). Common ailments like colds and stomachaches are attributed to an unbalanced relationship of elements inside the body due to overconsumption of "cold" or "hot" food (Woolley et al. 1972). Injury, infection, vulnerability arising from previous sickness, and hereditary transmitted ailments are also viewed as "natural" in etiology (Lieban 1967; Sechrest 1967). Interpersonal conflicts are frequently cited by respondents as disorder producing—abandonment by loved ones, quarrels in the family or with employers—as are unbearable frustrations like death of a close relative, inability to find work, overstudying for or failure of an exam, and financial problems.

Psychiatrists at PMHA and PGH were most articulate on how the institution responds to indigenous notions of psychopathology. The first strategy is to teach the family to view the problem in psychiatric terms, "educating" them to psychiatric methods. PGH staff found analogies useful in communicating concepts of disorder, such as the image of an overflowing or cracked clay pot when describing emotional repression.

Second, veteran professionals agreed that direct confrontation of superstitious beliefs and use of local healers were ineffectual. For example, saying that consulting a herbalist was a waste of time only leads to resistance. Often, herbalists enjoy patient trust, which remains to be won by psychiatrists. It was thought best to try to remain nonjudgmental, although professionals usually asked their patients to try their therapy as an alternative and avoid seeing a herbalist while under treatment.

Generally, staff attitudes toward folk healers were that they interfere with proper care, confuse patients, and may cause more anxiety than they dispel. One PMHA staff member, however, felt that it was best to try to make herbalists more scientific in their approach: to invite them as allies rather than antagonize them. This approach has been used for twenty years with *hilots* by public health administrators with established success (Del Mundo, Morisky, and Lopez 1976; Mangay-Angara 1977).

In essence, the accommodation strategy for handling clients with "unscientific" ideas is either to gently ignore them or to persuade them to acquire an alternative conception—one that is more "psychological minded." At least one staff member at PGH, however, expresses frustration that the Western theories studied so diligently are inapplicable with many patients who hold folk conceptions. Thus, therapists are forced simply to look at the individual's life situation and give small, realistic assignments that are aimed at helping them secure a better adjustment.

Providing Expected Therapeutics

As was the situation in Taiwan, staff believe that physical forms of treatment have the highest credence since more presenting problems are expressed in somatic terms. Lapuz (1972) listed the most frequent complaints from her clients: males generally reported poor balance, eye pain, low back and groin pain, and urinary disturbance; women complained of numb feelings, tremors, tingling hot and cold sensations, and body weakness. The most often reported symptom mentioned by agency respondents was disturbed sleeping patterns and loss of appetite. Lapuz (1972) also notes that for Filipinos, such physical ailments are readily given credence and are greatly effective in eliciting concern from others.

In correspondence with bodily complaints are expectations from the patient and his social group for the physician's biomedical armamentarium to alleviate these symptoms. Those with undifferentiated perceptions simply want the person hospitalized with a physician to care for him. However, many others specify that drug injections should be given. Remarkably, many staff report that families specifically asked that electric shock be administered as preferred treatment. Shock was seen by some as an immediate curing device preferable even to drugs. Some families insisted on taking their member elsewhere if shock wasn't provided. Except among the educated elite, talk therapy is disregarded as anything of curative value. Nevertheless, several therapists at PMHA and elsewhere expressed their faith in the use of group dynamic approaches. They felt that group interaction has more impact and a deeper effect on Filipino patients than do one-to-one therapies.

Ethnographies of Filipino folk medicine enrich our understanding of these staff observations and underscore psychiatry's failure to fulfill cultural expectations as well as its isolation from the popular health sector. At the core of the Philippine belief system, Jocano (1973) notes, is an understanding of human existence as a configuration of harmonic relations between the physical body and spiritual well-being. Illness and misfortune are brought about by the disruption in the relationship between a person's organic and spiritual duality. Hence, curing involves attention to both pharmacological techniques and ritual symbols—such as prayers —directed at the metaphysical aspects of disease. Prayer is the most important part of healing as it serves as the link between a practitioner and the supernatural power which does the healing. This aspect is hardly attended to by scientifically trained doctors. Furthermore, both the healer and the patient must have faith in the healer's prayers or they will not work. In essence,

> it is this reciprocal faith that healers and patients have that folk medicine finds appropriateness, strength, and continuity in the lives of the peasants . . . It may be lacking in all that scientific medicine has to offer, but certainly it is the unquestionable source of assurance—assurance that a sympathetic hand is zealously doing something to relieve the pain and the anxiety that accompanies it. Thus, even if the patient suffers more because of the procedure intended for his relief, the folk healer is still looked up to with respect, hope, and gratitude (Jocano 1973: 195).

Secular psychiatry could profit immeasurably from fully grasping these therapeutic principles guiding patient-therapist transactions in sacred healing. Yet, except for legal opposition, professionals afford little regard for the shamans *(arbularyos),* diviners, folk doctors *(medicos),* and faith healers *(spiritistas)* whose ritual base and pharmacopoeia engender such profound faith of curing in nearly every Filipino community.

Accommodation through Staff Qualities and Mannerisms

Agency personnel delineated three personal and interpersonal qualities thought to be prerequisites for securing a therapeutic relationship with Filipino patients. The major attribute expected of a therapist is authoritative stature: he or she should have an air of almost godlike authority and fit a parental image. As an omnipotent expert in command of the situation, the physician should give assurances that the treatment will help. Lesser-educated persons simply turn over responsibility to the physician with complete trust and may find it difficult to question the high-status authority. More-educated clientele at the private clinics usually request some sort of explanation of what therapeutics entail.

Along with the parental quality, there is an expectation of allowance of dependency and emotional closeness between patient and staff. They look for the physician's human side and ask about her personal life in order to feel comfortable in the relationship. Patients seek security in physician acceptance, patience, and understanding. They hope for a supportive and familylike emotional relationship with the nursing staff. Besides an emphasis on tender loving care, staff also recognize that delicacy with individual feelings is essential. To avoid shaming the patient or violating his self-respect, it may be necessary not to go directly to the

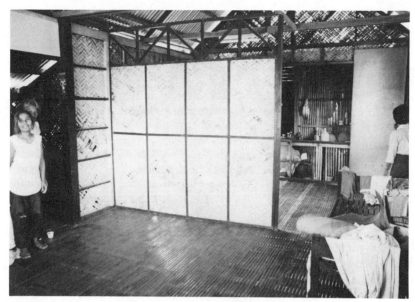

Patients' quarters at the rural-oriented rehabilitation center in Cavite.

point in problem solving. Rather, therapists should send out "feelers" and use gentle suggestion. In short, a parental and warm emotional approach is generally recognized by therapeutic staff as the basic approach to developing a good working relationship with patients and their families.

While hospital staff may seek patient cooperation through creation of pseudokinship ties, folk specialists are able to accumulate high esteem in the community by adhering closely to expected role obligations. Certain healers carry out their work without asking for payment. They are thus respected for their convictions and high sense of civic duty to community and fellowmen (Jocano 1973: 126). Reputable shamans, in fact, frequently have quite lively and demanding caseloads and may have a greater proportion of clients visiting them from outside the district than do nearby licensed physicians (Jocano 1973; Lieban 1967). Incompetent or unethical healers are socially censured by withdrawal of patronage and repudiation of confidence, community sanctions from which hospital staff are immune. Moreover, the *arbularyo* or *mananambal* (shaman) is prominent among folk practitioners because her supernatural power— God-given gift of diagnosis and cure—is not restricted in the types of illnesses that it affects. The socially sanctioned preconditions for *arbularyo* stature involve visitation by a supernatural being; long training under the direction of an experienced *arbularyo;* mastery of prayers, ritual procedures, and pulse taking; and, especially, expertise in the use of available pharmacopoeia (medicinal plants). Unlike the sorcerer, *arbularyos* are believed to follow strictly the will of God in using their "gift" of curing and cannot subvert their power for evil purposes such as causing sickness.

Accommodation in Ward Activities

Elements of accommodation in ward organization and events were observed in many institutions. A common practice was linguistic matching. Having so many major dialects and serving patients from throughout the islands necessitated assigning patients to treatment personnel or aides who could understand their dialects. Attending to sex role differences was recorded at NMH. Efforts were made there to simulate a homelike atmosphere for certain female wards. Male programs involved a strong work orientation—learning work skills and even being sent out on weekends for part-time jobs. PMHA's rehabilitation program catered to cultural background in the employment domain: patients could be referred either to an industrial or farming training center. Another procedure to reinforce the patient's sense of community was the establishment of ward self-government organizations by PGH and VMH. The VMH patient government met several times weekly, elected its own officers, discussed problems, and had a definite impact on ward policies such as food choice, TV usage, and resolving peer conflicts. Ethnic minorities were given some attention within these institutions. At NMH there are two pavilions set aside for Chinese-Filipinos. The buildings were donated by the Chinese Chamber of Commerce. The unique needs of Muslim patients at VL were somewhat addressed by recognition of food restrictions, acceptance of certain religious rituals, and permission to wear necklace charms *(anting-anting)* believed to protect the person against evil.

Perhaps the most concrete institutional recognition of the need for culture accommodation was found at UST and VMH. UST has sought to remove the stigma of psychiatry by calling its unit a "Community Center." The hope is to create the image of a community-based service like a boarding house or general ward. Pleasant eating quarters and the absence of uniforms are intended to add to the atmosphere. Similarly, VMH is hoping to remove its outpatient clinic from the ward to reduce the stigma and apprehension evoked by clients visiting the hospital for consultations. Finally, it can be noted that MC seeks to keep a lively and "normal" atmosphere by including such events as bingo socials, cookouts, parties, films, marketing, and garden strolling as essential components of its therapeutic regimen.

STAFF PERCEPTIONS OF CULTURE ACCOMMODATION

Agency respondents were also asked to state their perceptions of the availability of certain accommodation practices and their attitudes toward various accommodation dimensions (table 4.11). Only two practices—"Staff adjustment of personal manner to fit patient expectations" and "Patient's family helps with hospital care"—are clearly seen to be part of clinic routine. That staff indeed do adjust their personal manner in relation to patient expectations is suggested by very strong agreement with item 6, table 4.12. This is further supported by the examples of staff offering physical treatments and explicitly desired emotional closeness or parental relationships mentioned earlier. Endorsement of the family participation item (table 4.11, item 8) reinforces the examples we gave describing the prominence of Philippine kinship ties.

Staff were more reluctant to describe their agencies as creating living environments that approximate the "real" outside world. This is some-

TABLE 4.11 Perceptions of Institutional Accommodation
Practices in the Philippines (*N*=20)

	Percentage of staff endorsing accommodation item	
Accommodation practice	Always/ sometimes	Seldom/ never
1. Native healer involvement in patient care	5	95
2. Staff seek to reeducate those with traditional beliefs about mental problems	100	
3. Staff adjust their personal manner to fit patient expectations	95	5
4. A policy exists to find staff whose backgrounds are similar to those of the patients	40	60
5. Inpatient activities are similar to their activities outside the hospital	57	43
6. Patients make choices about their daily activities	63	37
7. Patients are encouraged to participate in community activities outside the hospital— work and recreation	68	32
8. Patient's family helps with hospital care	89	11
9. Problems occur because patients and staff have different social backgrounds	5	95

TABLE 4.12 Staff Endorsement of Culture Accommodation Dimensions in the Philippines (N=49)

Accommodation statement	Percentage of staff endorsing statement
1. While in the hospital, patients should remain isolated from activities in the community.	98% disagree
2. Staff should know the traditional names for mental disorder.	96
3. Community leaders should help in planning and directing facility activities.	96
4. Patient activities in the hospital should be as similar as possible to their activities in the community.	96
5. It is useless for staff to know the traditional beliefs about the causes of mental disorder.	90% disagree
6. Staff should adjust their professional manner to fit the expectations of patients from different social backgrounds.	90
7. What is considered as "normality" or "good personal adjustment" is the same for all cultures.	86
8. Patients should go to large central hospitals for their treatment.	85% disagree
9. Staff should know the traditional healing practices for mental disorder.	83
10. The doctor alone should decide what the appropriate treatment outcome will be.	83% disagree
11. What is considered the appropriate outcome of treatment should be different for different cultures.	83
12. Only those trained in scientific treatment techniques are qualified to help people with mental problems.	63% disagree
13. It is best to hire staff whose social backgrounds are similar to those of the patients.	52
14. The patient and his family should help choose the type of treatment given.	51
15. It is useless to consult with native healers since most of them cannot really help patients with mental problems.	43% disagree
16. Staff should try to correct or reeducate patients who maintain their traditional beliefs and customs about mental disorder.	4% disagree

what surprising as it is at variance with the unanimous attitude that patients should not remain isolated from activities in the community when hospitalized. The accommodation component regarding hiring staff whose backgrounds are similar to those of the patients appears to have meaning in the Philippines only in regard to linguistic matching. Otherwise, social background differences will not be thought of as a problem.

It was brought out earlier that staff accommodate patients with folk beliefs only to the extent that they gently reeducate them to alternatives and avoid direct confrontation of traditional idioms. Two items (item 2, table 4.11 and item 16, table 4.12) show unvaried intention among all respondents toward correction and reeducation of folk beliefs when they intrude upon the treatment setting. Lastly, there is neither perception of native healer participation in these clinics nor more than minimal endorsement of the statement that such healers should be consulted in some aspect of treatment.

As with the responses of Taiwanese professionals, 80 percent or more of those interviewed endorsed almost three-fourths of the sixteen accommodation statements shown in table 4.12. There is almost unanimous agreement among these diverse personnel on three issues: (1) the folk names and causes of disorder should be known by staff; (2) professional manner should be flexible; and (3) the barriers between the hospital and community should be minimal, both in terms of making the hospital environment similar to what is outside and in allowing community input into agency programs. This last point is worth commenting upon. Although 96 percent agreed that community leaders should help in planning and directing facility activities, in only one instance—the board of directors for PMHA—was such community involvement noticed. Cultural relativism received over 80 percent approval (items 7 and 11), as did the opinion that others besides the doctor should help decide treatment outcome.

However, only about half of those sampled thought the patient or his family should be involved in decision making in terms of treatment per se. Finally, although most would agree that it is important for staff to know about traditional healing practices, far fewer were comfortable with the notion that nonscientifically trained people are qualified to help those with mental problems. Fifty-seven percent agreed that it is useless to consult with native healers as most of them cannot really help patients with such problems. Apparently, it is thought good for mental health workers to have knowledge of what indigenous healing entails, but actual involvement of folk healers is not endorsed. This confirms the antagonistic attitude toward nonprofessional therapists we described earlier.

In conclusion, accommodation to distinctly Filipino cultural patterns by the mental health system appears to move along several lines simultaneously. Broadly speaking, these efforts are threefold: engage the patient's family in a cooperative relationship with the clinic (to avoid patient abandonment); gently orient them to the merits of a psychiatric approach (dispelling myths); and make the institution more attractive (lowering stigmatization) to the community as a whole. Accommodation practices intended to carry this out included the twenty-four-hour watcher system; involvement of the whole family during the intake interview; NMH encouragement of families to bring in food; family therapy sessions at some sites; staff willingness to provide the close, emotional, and dependent relationships expected by patients; and a few attempts to create the image of community-oriented services casting off the trappings of highly stigmatized and isolated psychiatric treatment.

Culture accommodation within Philippine agencies is primarily an initial effort to gain confidence and cooperation until education and persuasion can coax the uninitiated into accepting an established psychiatric regimen. Families are invited to visit and get involved in inpatient care, but in a circumscribed manner, under the supervision of treatment staff. Their input into decisions about therapy or outcome goals is restricted. Such decisions remain the medical staff's prerogative, specifically the attending physician's—a practice fundamental to Western biomedicine. Nowhere did we discover a deep appreciation of the sacred healing principles so prominently expressed within the popular health sector. Given that illness in the Philippines is interpreted predominantly through a religious idiom, it is unfortunate that the profound faith engendered in divine cure is untapped by the scientific bias of secularized professional intervention.

NOTES

1. See *Fookien Times,* 1980, 1981/82; *Quarterly Economic Review of the Philippines,* annual supplement, 1982.

2. These figures are a far cry from Sechrest's (1969) estimate of 1:1,000 based on his own observations of rural areas. Diagnostically, the following incidence rates were reported per 1,000 population: psychoneurosis, 15.2; psychosomatic disorders, 6.8; mental retardation, 5.9; psychosis, 3.9; personality disorders, 2.5; and epilepsy, 1.8 (Escudero 1972).

3. For a list of psychological investigations done on topics concerned with mental health in the Philippines, see Virgilio Enriques, *An annotated bibliography of mental health works in the Philippines* (Manila: Philippine Mental Health Association, 1976), and Shiro Saito, *Philippine ethnography: A critically annotated and selected bibliography* (Honolulu: University Press of Hawaii, 1972).

4. Five private agencies dealing with mentally retarded children were found in

Bonificio Amor, ed., *Focus on mental health resources* (Manila: Philippine Mental Health Association, 1975, 1981).

5. PMHA reports giving consultation to the Department of Local Government and Community Development; the Institute of Labor Relations, Education, and Manpower; the Division of Mental Hygiene; the Department of Education and Culture; and the Juvenile and Domestic Relations Court. Relationships are also maintained with the Philippine Guidance and Personnel Association, Public Schools Guidance Service, and various private schools.

6. See *Philippine Journal of Mental Health,* 7, no. 1 (1976).

chapter 5

The Mental Health System
of Thailand

Psychiatry has a long and rich history in Thailand. In his chronicle of the discipline's evolution, one of its principal developers, Dr. Phon Sang-singkeo (1965, 1975), traces three threads: the development of physical facilities, the development of educational curricula and manpower training, and the involvement of the World Health Organization.

The development of facilities began in 1889, during the reign of King Chulalongkorn, when a small (thirty-patient) mental hospital was opened at Klong Sarn, Dhonburi, across the river from Bangkok. The original purpose was to confine (via imprisonment and chains) prisoners who were unable to live together with regular medical patients. British medical influence began in 1905, when Dr. H. Campbell Hyde took charge of Klong Sarn Mental Hospital *inter alia* as head of the Bangkok Health Ministry. Unfortunately, Hyde had little time to supervise this expanding unit and conditions deteriorated to such a point that he was forced to report, "This hospital is shamefully falling apart. It is quite apparent that the government should do something to improve it. I myself cannot find stronger words to show how humiliated and disgusted I am" (Hyde, quoted by Sangsingkeo 1975: 652).

That plea was answered two years later with the construction of hospital buildings on seventeen acres of land close to the original asylum. From its inception, Somdej Chaopraya Mental Hospital (presently Thailand's premiere teaching facility) was administered according to the strictures of modern medicine. The Department of Public Health took over Somdej Chaopraya in 1918, and seven years later all European supervisors and doctors were discharged and their positions filled by Thai.

The second phase of facility development, 1930 to 1950, is characterized by construction of four new regional mental hospitals, the expansion and modernization of Somdej Chaopraya under Dr. Sangsingkeo, and establishment of a division within the Ministry of Public Health to oversee psychiatric facilities. Subsequently, specialized services were added, often at the suggestion of WHO experts, to form a more comprehensive mental health system. For example, the Child Guidance Mental Hygiene Clinic was begun in 1953 with help from WHO consultant Margaret Stepan. Intended for neurotic and neurological complaints, its success led to the founding a few years later of Prasart Hospital and Research Institute in Neurology. In 1960, a special hospital for mentally handicapped children and adults opened on Samsaen Road, Bangkok. Specialty units for other childhood disorders, drug addiction, and the criminally insane were built in the metropolitan area between 1965 and 1971. Meanwhile, community-oriented care had come early to the system. Dr. Sangsingkeo reported that by 1946 a general effort was made at Dhonburi to organize outside housing for patients so they could live and work in the community. It wasn't until 1958, however, that the first farm village-style halfway house opened, operated by Nondhaburi's Srithunya Hospital.

The pioneers of psychiatric education in Thailand were forced to acquire their expertise at foreign universities. Dr. Luang Vichien Bhatayakom, Somdej Chaopraya's first director, initiated the Thai-American connection for acquiring mental health technology in 1927. Upon his return from postgraduate studies in 1931, Bhatayakom began the first lectures on this subject. Two years later, psychiatry was included in the curriculum of last-year medical students at Siriraj Hospital.

In the late 1930s, three other Thai physicians, including Phon Sangsingkeo, were sent also to the United States. Dr. Sangsingkeo made his way to the University of Colorado and then to Johns Hopkins University. After the war, returnees from another group of seven doctors educated in America became powerful figures in teaching and administration. For example, Dr. Prasop Ratanakorn founded Prasart Neurological Hospital; Dr. Subha Malakul began the first child guidance clinic; services and training for the mentally retarded were started by Dr. Rosjong Dasnanjali; Dr. Arun Bhaksuvan directed Somdej Chaopraya and transformed it into the nation's major teaching center; and Dr. Chantana Sukavajana became the director for mental health services within the Ministry of Public Health.

A major conference to revise medical education in Thailand was held in 1956 under the auspices of the United States Agency for International Development and WHO. It proved to be a major turning point for psychiatry: recommendations were made to elevate its status to a separate area of study, worthy of its own teaching track and department. Yet, it was a struggle to get curricula included in the four-year medical coursework, and it wasn't until 1969 that Siriraj Medical School opened a separate department of psychiatry. In subsequent years, the other three medical schools—Chulalongkorn, Mahidol, and Chiangmai—followed suit.

The World Health Organization became more directly involved in Thai mental health service development than in any other Asian country except India. Thai physicians have participated in WHO programs since its inception in 1948. Dr. Sangsingkeo, for instance, served on the Committee of Mental Health Experts in 1952. The scope and depth of more than ten expert surveys in the ensuing thirty years, and their acceptance by Thai officials, have enabled WHO advisors to make significant contributions to the status and direction of Thai mental health care.

THE PUBLIC HEALTH SYSTEM AS THE CONTEXT FOR MENTAL HEALTH SERVICES

The Ministry of Public Health (MOPH) is the national agency responsible for administering all public and most governmental health services (MOPH 1977). The Office of the Under Secretary of State for Public Health coordinates five major departments (e.g., Medical Service, Communicable Disease Control, etc.) and the health program carried out by the seventy-one provincial health officers. Significantly, separate administrative structures govern health services provided by the Provincial Health Offices and the Bangkok Metropolis Administration. For example, provincial and district health officers—operating provincial hospitals, health centers, and midwifery clinics—receive assistance from an office within MOPH. However, they answer directly to the governors of their provinces, who are under the authority of the Ministry of the Interior. Thus, administrative control of primary services is actually more diffuse than figure 5.1 indicates.

Mental health concerns are dealt with exclusively by MOPH's Department of Medical Services. It is responsible for psychiatric services for the entire country and also handles a part of metropolitan Bangkok's medical care. Currently, five psychiatric agencies of equal status exist within this department. Four are individual hospitals—Srithunya, Pan Ya On, Prasart, and Somdej Chaopraya—and the fifth is the Division of Mental Health. It supervises twelve facilities, including all provincial mental hospitals and various units within the metropolitan area. This administrative configuration is under pressure for revision to make it more equitable and efficient (Kiernan 1976).

Public Health Resources

Public health resources are moderately well developed in Thailand, but not equitably distributed. Clearly, Bangkok Metropolis maintains an unequal proportion. For its estimated 4.3 million population, Bangkok has thirty-four government hospitals with 13,000 beds, thirty-nine private hospitals of more than 25 beds, four of the five university medical

Figure 5.1
Organization of the Thai Ministry of Public Health

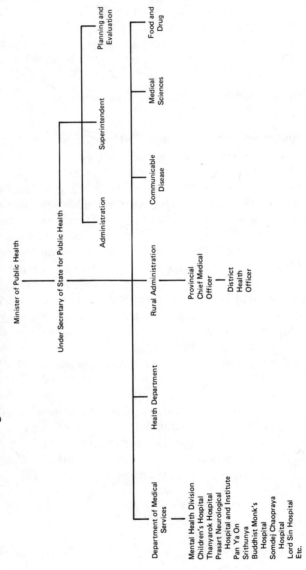

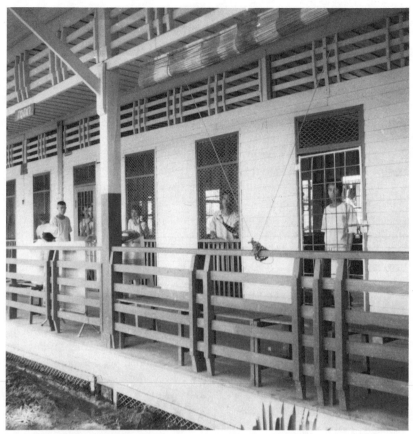

Patients peer through the windows of a maximum-security ward for men at a facility in northern Thailand.

centers, and approximately 75 percent of the health manpower (MOPH 1976). The private sector, with an average per capita health expenditure several times greater than the government's, concentrates on curative medicine in Bangkok and other municipal locations. In the remaining seventy provinces of thirty-six million Thai, the public sector dominates health delivery. The provinces have ninety-seven government hospitals— about 22,000 beds—and only twenty-four private facilities.

Besides local hospitals, there are three components to rural health delivery. The country's 570 districts (catchment areas of 50,000) have 288 District Health Centers. Each center is supposed to have at least one doctor, one qualified nurse-midwife, two junior health workers, one auxiliary midwife, and ten to twenty-five beds for emergency use. Yet, over ten percent of these have M.D. vacancies.

There are 3,720 *tambon* (commune) health centers covering about 70 percent of Thailand's designated *tambons* (population catchment of 5,000). *Tambon* health subcenters employ one junior health worker and one nurse-midwife. Their objectives are limited to maternal and child welfare, environmental sanitation, control of communicable disease, health education, and attention to minor physical ailments.

There are 1,456 midwifery clinics serving 48,847 villages and hamlets throughout the country (approximately 2,000 persons each). In addition, four regional Maternal and Child Health Centers were set up, each with 200 maternity beds. These provide complete services, training, and public information (see table 5.1).

Other indicators of medical resource strength are found in manpower numbers, budgeting, and the guidelines for the 1977–1981 five-year plan. In terms of distribution, statistics for manpower and facilities are very similar. There is a physician to population ratio of 1:1,000 in Bangkok. In smaller municipalities, the ratio is 1:30,000, while in the far-flung provinces it is up to 1:150,000 (MOPH 1976). Of the approximately 5,000 physicians in Thailand (1 per 8,455), 400 are in private practice exclusively; 1,800 are employed by the MOPH; universities and the Ministry of Defense have 2,200; and another 600 work for city and province enterprises. There are also 12,653 qualified nurses (one per 3,342 population), approximately seventy psychologists (B.A. level) working in clinical settings, and an overall ratio of one hospital bed per 823 population.

Budgetary allocations for health have been quite modest in the past, but have edged higher in recent years. In 1975, MOPH received $7.5 million for operating expenses, 3.2 percent of the total government bud-

TABLE 5.1 Private and Public Medical Facilities in Thailand

Type of facility	Number	Number of beds
General hospitals	50	10,322
Local/rural hospitals	178	27,210
Medical centers	53	977
Maternity hospitals	2 (private)	423
Pediatric hospital	1 (public)	450
Infectious disease hospital	1 (public)	230
Mental hospitals	14 (public)	7,483
Mental deficiency hospitals	2 (public)	520
Drug addicts hospital	1 (public)	500

Source: World Health Organization. *Annual Statistics.* Geneva: World Health Organization, 1977.

get. This sum increased to almost $18 million in 1977, or 5.1 percent of the national expenditure. Seventy percent was earmarked for provincial health needs (free medical care, maternal and child health, etc.). Even so, the government per capita spends a little over two dollars for citizens; private expenditures are three times this amount. Yet MOPH planners are optimistic that 8 percent of the national budget will be spent on health by 1981.

Health development is also progressing with financial and technical assistance from various international agencies. Through several projects such as the Population Planning and Health Project and the Lampang Project, USAID alone budgeted close to $15 million during 1977–1981. MOPH publications do not detail future allocations for mental health care. At present, psychiatric facilities (excluding Pan Ya On) spend only $7 million annually, half of which is generated by hospital revenues (MOPH 1977).

Health Needs and Problems

Constraints of the public health system are especially pertinent to note. Woolley's (1974) analysis revealed fundamental impediments in the areas of personnel, administrative planning, and receptiveness of users. Besides the shortage of personnel at the middle management and supervisory levels, problems involve inadequate training, insufficient specialization, and the familiar dilemma of brain drain. During a five-year period in the 1960s, the number of physicians training abroad was equal to seven years of output from Thai medical schools.

The lack of a dynamic national health plan means that MOPH only trains special health workers for projects when needed. Furthermore, there is no coordination between the universities producing the manpower and the government agencies employing them. The conflict arises when curricula aim at one-to-one office practices and specialist work. Yet, the health system actually needs providers capable of addressing curative and preventive services at the community level.

The problem of user receptiveness is dramatized by MOPH (1976) statistics. In 1970, only 17 percent of the people in rural areas were using public services to handle illness in spite of the fact that most of the population average biannual illnesses. In fact, the only people who actually use health centers are those living close to the facilities. Health center personnel exacerbate this by failing to venture beyond 5.5 kilometers from their institutional base into outlying areas. Besides inconvenience of location, dissatisfied users surveyed by MOPH mentioned that center services were slow and wasted much of the client's time, that the staff spoke rudely and seemed uninterested, and that the illness was not cured.

User resistance is further accentuated by social class divergence, inhib-

iting a positive working relationship between physician and rural peasant. On the one side are upper- and middle-class, urban-educated doctors. On the other side are Thai farming people who by cultural norm
(patron-client) are inhibited from expressing their complaints, mistrust,
lack of understanding, or disagreement with the treatment. The result is
insufficient information to guide medical decisions and unexpressed dissatisfaction. Still, as Woolley (1974) sadly concludes, even if health centers were better received, their impact would continue to be insignificant
as long as the absence of potable water contributes to the spread of infectious diseases.

NATIONAL ORGANIZATION OF PSYCHIATRIC RESOURCES: INSTITUTIONS AND PERSONNEL

Reviewing Thailand's health picture gave a realistic context for describing psychiatric services in three important ways. First, it pointed up the
position of mental health in the Ministry of Public Health as an uncoor-
dinated collection of units within the Department of Medical Services.
Secondly, knowing the components and structure of public medical care
establishes a standard against which to contrast the availability of psychiatric services and reflects the extent to which psychiatry could be
extended if it were incorporated into the existing network. Lastly, assessing general medical care delivery problems anticipates the difficulties
mental health workers face. Examples include restricted funding, poor
national planning, maldistribution, inappropriate medical curriculum,
manpower shortages, undertrained workers, and poor reception by rural
peoples due to staff-user cultural differences.

A field visit by W. E. S. Kiernan (1976), WHO regional advisor for
mental health, offers a current analysis of the Thai mental health picture.
According to Kiernan, an MOPH reorganization in 1972 resulted in a
two-tiered administrative scheme (fig. 5.2). Prior to this date, the Division of Mental Health (DMH) was responsible for nearly all psychiatric
facilities.

At present, the DMH has no direct role in determining the operations
of the four major Bangkok institutions on the same administrative level.
Rather, the Division is restricted to overseeing the smaller psychiatric
centers in the metropolitan area and the mental hospitals in the outer
provinces. Moreover, DMH's advisory role within the Ministry is at best
perfunctory; a coordinating committee made up of representatives from
DMH and the Bangkok institutions exists without a clear mandate (Kiernan 1976). Under these conditions, it is nearly impossible for DMH to
discharge its principal functions: "The planning, policy making, re-

Figure 5.2
Organization of Mental Health Services in Thailand

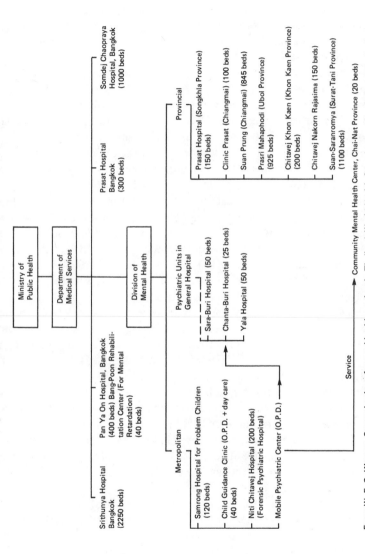

From W. E. S. Kiernan, Strengthening of mental health services in Thailand. World Health Organization, South-East Asia Region, Mental Health Division, Report No. 34, August 20, 1976.

source mobilization, training, evaluation, and supervision of the total mental health service" (Kiernan 1976: 9).

The public sector accounts for all mental health resources except for a few psychiatrists working full-time in Bangkok's private general hospitals (e.g., Paolo Memorial Hospital) and those government psychiatrists carrying on part-time private practices (fig. 5.2). The vast majority of resources are under the Department of Medical Services (DMS). However, five independent units are run by university psychiatry programs, the Army Hospital has forty-five beds, and the Social Welfare Department operates a halfway house.

In terms of geographical coverage, the problem of rural-urban maldistribution seen with public health centers also holds true for psychiatric agencies. For the nine health regions outside of Bangkok there are 3,465 beds, or 0.096 per 1,000 population. In marked contrast, Bangkok figures show 1.06 beds per 1,000 population based on 4,400 available beds (most are located at Srithunya and Somdej Chaopraya).

The rural-urban gap is further widened by the limited availability of programs for special needs (e.g., mental retardation). Alternatives to inpatient care such as day care, after care, sheltered workshops, walk-in clinics, and so forth exist only to a limited extent in Bangkok itself and not at all in the provinces (Kiernan 1976). The Mobile Mental Health Center, an active unit giving consultation to outlying general hospitals, was forced in 1976 to restrict its operations due to funding cutbacks.

The distribution of psychiatric manpower follows the same pattern. The seven provincial area hospitals together have twenty-two physicians, 165 staff nurses, 213 practical nurses, seventeen psychologists, and twenty-one social workers. The doctor-to-bed ratio is 1:157, and there are twenty-one beds for each nurse.

Bangkok, on the other hand, has the services of eighty-one doctors, 276 nurses, thirty-two psychologists, and thirty-seven social workers within its collection of eight MOPH agencies. With these personnel, the physician-to-bed ratio is three times lower than that of the provinces (Kiernan 1976). The five medical school psychiatry programs, two of which have small inpatient wards, employ about thirty-five faculty to teach psychiatry.

Further aggravating this uneven user access, Kiernan (1976) found, 50 percent of the psychologists and social workers in Bangkok held positions in 10 percent of the agencies—those handling children with emotional and developmental disorders. Kiernan also noted that staff were poorly utilized: nurses were employed as technicians, record clerks, and secretaries, while practical nurses were left to handle ward operations. What was especially startling, however, was that provincial units, like their health center counterparts, were not overwhelmed with demand. This question of acceptability and what it implies about nonmedical healing will be taken up later.

OTHER FACTORS INFLUENCING THE DELIVERY OF PSYCHIATRY IN THAILAND

Manpower Training

Psychiatric education for physicians began in the early 1930s with Luang Vichien's return from the United States. Postgraduate residency instruction started twenty years later, in 1954, at the Dhonburi site. Carl Bowman, an American consultant at the 1956 conference on medical curriculum, pushed for a four-year program of instruction. Today, thirty-two faculty in Thailand's five medical colleges teach undergraduate and postgraduate psychiatry.

A WHO progress report on the place of psychiatry in Southeast Asia indicated that Thai undergraduate curricula range from thirty-three to ninety-four hours, with an average of fifty-seven hours of instruction, excluding clerkship (WHO 1975c). Behavioral sciences are taught in the premedicine courses by academic psychologists, although these professors have no formal links with the department of psychiatry. In contrast, teaching resources are gravely lacking for developing allied professions— clinical psychology, social work, psychiatric nursing. Universities select the candidates and determine curriculum and teaching methods for these professions, but do not coordinate with the needs of the mental health delivery system. Although a six-month Somdej Chaopraya training program prepares practical nurses, psychologists, and social workers for service in mental health agencies, postgraduate studies in these fields are unavailable.

In short, the last twenty years has seen a gearing-up of educational curricula to train allied workers. Still there is not yet a critical mass of qualified instructors and students to give the field momentum, identity, and a position of strength from which to deal with the problem it seeks to solve.

World Health Organization Influence

Contact with WHO experts has had a significant influence on the direction of mental health development at the national level and continues to guide innovation and the elaboration of existing institutions. Each advisor in the series of consultations made a unique contribution.

Charles Gundry in 1952 recommended the establishment of a Child Guidance Clinic. A year later, psychologist Margaret Stepan was sent to help actualize this concept. Alan Stoller followed Stepan in 1958 to push for the regionalization of facilities and the creation of a Division of Mental Health. He also urged a follow-up visit by an expert in epidemiological research. Tsung-yi Lin, an international leader in field survey methods and epidemiology, arrived in 1964 to promote Thai psychiatric research and manpower expansion. In 1968, a specialist in psychiatric nursing, L. M. Harwood, was assigned by WHO at the government's request to help initiate post-basic training for psychiatric nurses. Lin, who returned in 1972, and Milton Miller, an American psychiatrist who arrived in 1975, focused their consultations on boosting educational curricula and upgrading training.

The latest WHO survey was carried out by W. E. S. Kiernan in the summer of 1976. Kiernan gave special attention to strategies for operational research, integration of services, development of community-based prevention and after-care programs, and the reorganization of national administration. Moreover, Thai educators have actively participated in the WHO South-East Asia Region (SEAR) seminar series on the teaching of psychiatry. Thailand hosted the fifth seminar in 1974 which dealt with "education and training of personnel for mental health work in the community" (Harper, Shapiro, and Zusman 1975). In addition, four projects in the WHO Medium-Term Mental Health Programme (1975–1982) involve Thailand.

In the course of their site visits, WHO consultants pinpointed ten critical issues that we should bear in mind for comparison with data gathered in October 1977. First and most prominent are the acute shortages of qualified personnel and mental health educators in all disciplines and the nonindependence of psychiatry departments. Integral to this concern is the failure to coordinate between programs providing basic training and the government-administered delivery system. The third problem involves unequal distribution based on geography and the dilemma of lower socioeconomic segments of the urban cityscape who are completely out of touch with these services even though they are close at hand. Fourth, even the large service institutions of Bangkok lack effective after-care programs aimed at preventive mental health.

The strong need for a Mental Health Division with administrative sanction to create and guide national programing is the fifth issue. A sixth problem spotlighted is the indifference and negative attitudes toward psychiatry, limiting both client and staff recruitment efforts. Similarly, adverse public sentiment was implicated as responsible for the refusal of families to accept returning patients, an action that would cut hospital caseloads by one-third. Two further problems pinpointed were lack of interest in epidemiological research and low patient turnover rate, resulting in a buildup of chronic inpatients. Stoller urged screening out the profoundly disturbed and aggressive male "schizophrenics" who had become the bulk of these chronic cases. Last is the issue of legislative provisions for admission and treatment. Curran and Harding's (1977) survey found that Thailand had no mental health legislation, functioning instead on an informal system of admissions.

Input from Mental Health Research

Mental health research has the potential to play a vital role in guiding clinicians and planners alike. In Thailand, a good start has been made in studies concerned with operational research, symptom expression, and culture change, although the potential has not been fully exploited due to the lack of applied researchers and the absence of pressure for program evaluation from the Division of Mental Health.

One type of Thai operational research involves measuring the incidence and prevalence of psychiatric problems. Stoller's 1959 visit initiated concern for estimating the prevalence of untreated cases. Since no epidemiological data were available on psychosis, a village survey was undertaken and found a 3/500 rate for schizophrenia. This figure closely matches the only other prevalence study of psychosis, done by Dr. Sangsingkeo with a Hill Tribe village (Visuthikosol and Suwanlert 1977).

Stoller went on to discover in 1959 that there were 40,000 registered opium smokers in Bangkok alone and 1,041 opium dens throughout the country. He then estimated there were 100,000 addicts in Thailand. Subsequently, research intensified in the area of substance abuse. Ratanakorn (1975) noted the steady increase of admissions for alcoholism and was instrumental in founding a research unit for its treatment.

Other investigators reported drug addiction at epidemic proportions— 30,000 addicts in 1973 with half of the 43,000 prison inmates addicted (Sangsingkeo, Punahitanont, and Schneider 1974). Later, surveys of drug use among school students found that between 10 and 23 percent had experimented with illegal drugs, most often choosing marijuana and a mildly narcotic plant called *kratom* leaf (Otrakul et al. 1975; Sangsingkeo et al. 1974). Suwanlert (1975) then gathered case studies on *kratom* eaters and found them to be almost exclusively middle-aged, ethnic Thai males from the lower and middle classes. *Kratom* addiction is primarily a rural phenomenon; it is taken to stimulate a strong desire to do manual labor in the user's field, but may induce psychotic symptoms among chronic users.

The second type of operational research focuses on the description of current institutions and especially the make-up of inpatient populations. Visuthikosol and Suwanlert's (1977) report that Srithunya had 84 percent chronic schizophrenics in 1974 matched Ratanakorn's observation made twenty years before. Ionescu-Tongyonk (1978) is disturbed by the overuse of this one category. He posits that a greater number of endogenous depressives, masked by somatic symptoms, go unnoticed or are diagnosed inappropriately.

Malakul in 1964 noted that one-third of the 296 children seen at her child guidance clinic were brought in for academic difficulties. The ratio of aggressive, hyperactive, and antisocial children to passive, withdrawn, and asocial ones was 2 to 1 (Sangkingkeo 1969). This points to a lower tolerance threshold for active as opposed to passive behavioral problems among Thai children, meshing with broader cultural expectations regarding behavioral norms.

Descriptions of institutional practices are also available, but to a lesser degree. Visuthikosol and Suwanlert (1976, 1977) have written about the therapeutic community groups operating at Srithunya and commented on the lack of individual therapy and overreliance on long-acting phenothiazine and ECT. They have also rank-ordered referral sources for Srithunya: relatives and siblings were the highest, followed by police and social agencies. Surprisingly, no systematic studies evaluating program effectiveness or treatment outcome were encountered apart from the yearly discharge figures gathered by the Division of Mental Health (MOPH 1977). Nor were links discerned between surveys of psychopathology and proposals for new programs, a responsibility of DMH. Quite often, the impetus for program development came from outside consultants and the interests of returning professionals trained overseas.

In contrast to Ionescu-Tongyonk's (1977) attempt to penetrate Thai somatic symptoms to locate Western syndromes, Sangun Suwanlert has sought to document the culturally unique aspects of Thai psychopathology. In doing so, he has gathered clinical as well as ethnomedical data on psychotic states attributed to *phii pob,* or spirit possession, *latah* and *koro,* both culture-bound syndromes, and treatment approaches for spirit possession cases (Suwanlert 1972, 1976a, 1976b, 1977; Suwanlert and Coates 1977). Suwanlert's findings on indigenous beliefs and cures of psychopathology will be examined in our discussion of indigenous conceptions of psychiatric care.

The pathogenic effects of cultural transformation is another topic receiving intense attention. Several authors argue that the cultural basis of Thai society has weakened of late and cannot be compensated for by imported Western institutions. According to Meesook (1975), industrialization and urbanization are incompatible with the perpetuation of traditional Thai values built around Buddhism and the socioeconomic structure of the agricultural village. Bureaucracy now regulates citizen relationships and handles conflicts that before were directly dealt with by those involved. It thus usurps the authority of senior members of extended families.

As children come to have more education than their parents, they desire independence from restrictive customs and choose their own occupation and marriage partners. Besides generational conflict and stress on kinship ties, the omnipotence of Buddhism itself may be on the wane among youth. Kamratana (1972) surveyed 500 secondary school students fourteen to eighteen years old and found that most of them practiced no religion and considered it to be outmoded.

Women's roles, too, are dramatically shifting. Instead of being limited to home activities, women are securing more education and employment to enhance the economic status of the family (Suwana 1969). Along with rising expectations, Suwana found increased anxiety among women, the result of unchanging legal discrimination and traditional male attitudes.

Kiernan (1976) noted two sequelae of these shifting cultural patterns which summarize the concerns of many Thai psychiatrists: (1) declining family care of psychologically impaired members due to the pressures of economic survival in urban areas and (2) rising prevalence of disorder due to continued incidence of traditional forms of illness and the appearance of newer patterns of dysfunction related to stress, growing numbers of old people, and iatrogenesis.

PSYCHIATRIC RESOURCES AVAILABLE: SELECTED EXAMPLES

As with Taiwan and the Philippines, a framework of seven variables is applied to judge the resource potential of Thailand's mental health network, the major centers of which are summarized in table 5.2. At eight centers, staff were interviewed for this survey. Elsewhere, unstructured interviews were held with key figures in Thai psychiatry and psychology.[1] Also, Dr. Suwanlert arranged a visit to the shrine of a Thai shaman to view the healing ceremony of a popular Nondhaburi medium (Khon Chung). In all, the Thai case study data were derived from twenty psychiatrists, seven psychologists, and one social worker responding to the questionnaire on institutional practices and from twenty-three staff members completing the instrument measuring accommodation attitudes. Interviews were recorded in twelve settings—nine in metropolitan Bangkok, three in Chiangmai—and thirteen informants were sampled through open-ended discussions (table 5.3). Thus, the information comes from about thirty-five professionals, almost entirely psychiatrists and psychologists, three-fourths of whom work in Bangkok agencies. This

TABLE 5.2 Residential and Outpatient Treatment Centers in Thailand

	Number of beds
Bangkok inpatient facilities	
*Srithunya Hospital	2,250
*Somdej Chaopraya Hospital (teaching)	1,000
*Pan Ya On Hospital	400
*Prasart Neurologic Hospital (including neuroscience research center; teaching)	360
Niti Chitavej Forensic Hospital	200
Samrong Hospital for Problem Children	120
Bang-Poon Rehabilitation Center for Mental Retardation	40
Srithunya Hospital Quarterway House and Rehabilitation Village	150
Social Welfare Department Welfare Home	(1,200)
Army Hospital	45
Chulalongkorn University Hospital Department of Psychiatry (teaching)	20
Total	4,585
Provincial inpatient facilities	
Suan-Saranromya, Surat-Tani Province	1,100
Prasri Mahaphodi, Ubol Province	925
*Suan Prung, Chiangmai (including Clinic Prasart)	1,000
Chitavej Khon Kaen, Khon Kaen Province	200
Chitavej Nakorn Rajasima, Nakorn Rajasima Province	150
Prathumthani Provincial Halfway House	250
Prasart Hospital, Songkhla Province	150
Sara-Buri Hospital Psychiatric Unit	50
Chanta-Buri Hospital Psychiatric Unit	25
Yala Hospital Psychiatric Unit	50
*Chiangmai University Department of Psychiatry (teaching)	25
Total	3,925

Bangkok outpatient clinics
    Chulalongkorn University Department of Psychiatry (teaching)
   *Ramathibodi Hospital Department of Psychiatry (teaching)
    Siriraj University Department of Psychiatry (teaching)
   *Child Guidance Clinic (day care 40 beds)

Provincial outpatient clinics
    Chai-Nat Province Community Mental Health Center

*Interview site

TABLE 5.3 Personnel Administered Questionnaires 1, 2, and 3 (Thailand)

Facility and staff	Questionnaire 1	2	3	Open-ended interviews
Srithunya (SH)				
Psychiatrist (hospital director)				1
Psychiatrist (medical director)	1	1	1	
Psychiatrist (consultants)		1	1	
Chief psychologist		1	1	
Chief social worker			1	
Somdej Chaopraya (SCP)				
Psychiatrist (hospital director)	1	1		1
Psychiatrist (consultants)		2	3	
Psychologist		1	2	
Social worker		1	2	
Pan Ya On (PYO)				
Psychiatrist director	1	1	0	1
Child Guidance Center (CGC)				
Chief psychologist	1	1	1	1
Staff psychologist		1	1	
Ramathibodi Hospital (RH)				
Chief psychologist	1			1
Prasart Neurological Hospital (PN)				
Psychiatrist (director)	1	1	1	1
University of Chiangmai, Department of Psychiatry (CU)				
Psychiatrist (director)	1	1	1	1
Chief psychologist		1	1	
Chief nurse			1	
Suan Prung Hospital (SP)				
Psychiatrist (director)	1	1	1	1
Psychiatrist		2	1	
Psychologist			3	
Dr. Phon Sangsingkeo (psychiatrist)			1	1
Division of Mental Health (DMH)				1
University of Chiangmai Hospital				1
Drug Research and Prevention Center				1
U.N. Asian Development Institute				1
Totals	8	17	23	13

suggests that the study may be biased toward the perceptions of these two groups and may not present a picture of the conditions beyond Thailand's capital and its second-largest city, Chiangmai.

FRAMEWORK FOR MENTAL HEALTH RESOURCES

Comprehensive Services

The basic treatment functions and modalities that constitute a comprehensive service system are available among the Thai sites sampled (see tables 5.4 and 5.5).

At almost every agency, an adult psychiatric case would receive the core elements of "modern" services—inpatient, outpatient and follow-up care, diagnostic, and neurological assessment. If easy access to alternative agencies is possible in Bangkok, more specialized units such as emergency care, partial hospitalization, childhood and geriatric services, and treatment for drug abuse are within grasp.

In essence, the actual therapeutics administered are indistinguishable from those of Taiwan or the Philippines either in substance or emphasis. Chemotherapy, individual, group, family, and occupational therapy are all given "often" or "sometimes." ECT is evident but less frequent than drug regimens. Supportive psychotherapy is the most popular mode of talk therapy; selected patients are exposed to psychoanalytic, eclectic, client-centered, and behavioral orientations. These choices reflect the American and British training of many professionals.

Group work is done to remotivate chronic patients. Therapeutic community groups, an integral part of Srithunya wards since the early 1960s, have spread to several other hospitals. Work therapy is carried out at two vocational rehabilitation units set up by Srithunya and Pan Ya On. Public education activities and consultation to gatekeeper agencies in the community—high schools, police, professional associations—were reported at all but one site.

The attributes of these institutions can be compared for perspective. Somdej Chaopraya (SCP), Srithunya (SH), and Suan Prung (SP), Thailand's three largest mental hospitals, differ in several important respects. SCP is the premiere training facility. It has almost three times as many physicians as the other two hospitals combined and has more specialized departments, including a Department of Public Relations and Education. Srithunya, with twice as many patients as any other hospital, has pioneered in creating partial-hospitalization and halfway house programs and has several prolific researchers. SP, Chiangmai's nonteaching regional mental hospital, has almost a skeleton crew of professionals. But it still manages to operate one of the country's three halfway houses and undertake research.

TABLE 5.4 Availability of Comprehensive Services in Thailand

Service function	SCP	SH	PN	PYO	CGC	RH	SP	CU
Inpatient	+	+	+	+	−	2 beds	+	+
Outpatient	+	+	+	+	+	+	+	+
Emergency	+	+	−	−	−	−	+	−
Partial hospitalization	+	−	−	+	+	−	−	−
Transitional living	−	+	−	+	−	−	+	−
Follow-up	+	planned	+	+	+	+	+	+
Children's services	+	+	−	+	+	+	−	+
Geriatric care	−	+	+	−	−	−	−	−
Drug abuse	−	−	+	−	−	−	−	+
Diagnostic	+	+	+	+	+	+	+	+
Neurological	+	+	+	+	−	−	+	+
Suicide prevention	−	−	planned	−	−	−	−	−
Educational	+	−	+	+	+	+	+	+
Mental health research	−	+	+	+	+	+	+	+
Program evaluation	−	−	−	−	−	−	−	−
Teaching/training	+	−	+	−	+	+	−	+

+ indicates available
− indicates unavailable

TABLE 5.5 Treatment Modalities Available in Thailand

Modality	SCP	SH	PN	PYO	CGC	RH	SP	CU
Electroconvulsive therapy	++	+++	+	+	–		+++	++
Physiotherapy	++	–	++	+++	+		+	–
Drug	+++	+++	+++	+++	+++	+++	+++	+++
Psychotherapy	++	+++	+++	+++	+++	+++	++	++
Behavior modification	planned	–	–	++	+	+++	–	++
Group therapy	+++	+++	+++	+++	–		++	+++
Family therapy	++	+	++	++	++	++	–	++
Occupational therapy	+++	+++	+++	+++	+++		+++	+++
Work therapy	–	+++	–	+++	–		–	–
Other	milieu, recreation	therapeutic community groups		rehab. schooling	yoga exercises		therapeutic community groups	recreation

+++ often
++ sometimes
+ seldom
– never

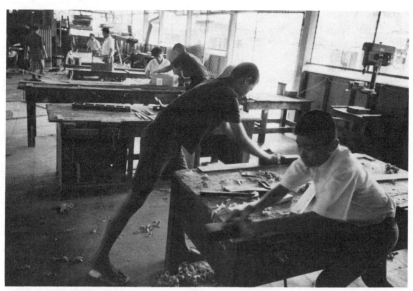

Young patients train for a craft occupation at Pan Ya On Hospital in Bangkok.

Pan Ya On (PYO) is the other large residential program visited. As a treatment facility for some 450 mentally deficient children and young adults, it makes no pretext of being comprehensive except in reference to its mandated group. In this regard, it offers a spectrum of clinical modalities: individual and group therapy to remotivate children and deal with their emotional problems; special educational curricula; family therapy; and twice-weekly well-baby clinics to screen for mental retardation and phenylketonuria (PKU).

The remaining four sites concentrate on outpatients but maintain some bedspace for acute patients. Within the Prasart Neurological Hospital (PN) is the forty-bed psychiatric unit, the country's Research Institute for Drug Addiction, and an alcoholism treatment ward. The Bangkok Child Guidance Clinic (CGC), the first center of its kind, has now expanded its capacity to include adult outpatients and operates as a community mental health center. Its foci remain with day-care services for children (providing a forty-bed partial hospitalization unit), training in child psychology, and community/professional education projects. The least comprehensive of the hospital-based programs were recently established at Mahidol University's Ramathibodi Hospital (RH) and Chiangmai University Hospital (CU) respectively. When surveyed, RH had two and CU twelve beds for short-term admissions. Teaching and research were the primary roles within these settings, although both carried demanding outpatient loads based on their staffing capacities.

Gaps in the system's ability to provide comprehensive services are also apparent from tables 5.4 and 5.5. Most obvious is the absence of a suicide or crisis center in Bangkok. Without figures on self-injury, it is hard to determine whether this dysfunction is prevalent or simply not a concern. PN operates the only alcoholism treatment ward in the system. Drug dependence is a major government concern, as shown by the amount of research on this topic and the founding of the Drug Dependence Research and Prevention Center. Drug cases amount to 50 percent of the prison population (Sangsingkeo et al. 1974) and are most probably handled at the Niti Chitavej Hospital (forensic). But how many are treated and by what means are unknown. Programs for geriatric cases were just introduced at SH and PN. Provisions for childhood disorders outside of PYO and CGC tend to be makeshift. As an example, childhood schizophrenics were admitted to the convalescent ward at SH. Child inpatients are best served by referral to the Samrong Hospital for Problem Children.

Except for gaps in application of behavior modification and work therapy, the Thai sites afforded the full complement of therapeutic modalities. The lone psychologist at RH and the chief psychologist at SCP were both experts in behavior therapy, having been exposed to his approach at English universities. Still, Kiernan's (1976) earlier comments on the dearth of special programs and alternatives to inpatient care are confirmed by our findings. Units for inpatient child care, substance abuse research and intervention, mental retardation, geriatric care, and neurology are all concentrated in the capital. Suicide prevention and program evaluation components remain unfounded.

Preventive Orientation

Surprisingly, public consultation is by far the most active prevention service at the Thai sites surveyed (table 5.6). It involves extending technical assistance and advice to other social agencies handling various client populations. Each site except CU has ongoing consultative relationships with professional groups and other institutions. Looking at the three large mental hospitals: SP sends psychologists to surrounding vocational and high schools to handle behavioral and learning problems; SH renders assistance to staff operating nearby institutions for welfare cases and prostitutes; and SCP has a formal program of consultation to the police academy, Bangkok schools, and lawyer groups.

However, PYO and CGC are the most deliberate in their efforts to extend support services to allied agencies. Besides continuing-education seminars for helping professionals, CGC cooperates with the Ministry of Education in early detection of children with emotional problems and has three mobile mental health teams visiting more than a dozen Bang-

TABLE 5.6 Availability of Preventive Programs in Thailand

Prevention type	SCP	SH	PN	PYO	CGC	RH	SP	CU
Public information	+++	–	+	++	+++		–	–
Public education	+	–	+	+++	+++		–	–
Public consultation	++	++	+	+++	+++	++	++	–
Ecological change	–	–	–	–	+		–	–

+++ often
++ sometimes
+ seldom
– never

kok universities and demonstration schools. Physicians from PYO sometimes attend normal schools, teacher training centers, prenatal care
clinics, and a facility for profoundly retarded children to advise on matters dealing with developmental disabilities.

Efforts to generate heightened public awareness of mental health issues are evident in only three institutions. Public information at SCP is
the purview of the Department of Public Relations/Education, which
promotes public tours of the hospital to acquaint citizens with the facility
and coordinates information dissemination through the mass media,
including television appearances by SCP psychiatrists. Public lectures in
conjunction with the Thai Mental Health Association, newspaper arti-
cles, and a pamphlet on mental health are avenues CGC uses to affect
public attitudes. The CGC day-care unit is a response to an emerging
urban problem—working parents who cannot care for their preschool
children. CGC holds lectures and discussion groups for these parents
regarding normal child development and appropriate child-rearing techniques. Furthermore, PYO undertakes two "high risk" prevention projects: first, it organized and holds monthly meetings for the Association
of the Parents of Mentally Retarded Children to teach problem-solving
skills. Secondly, a well-baby clinic is conducted to screen for undetected
metabolic disorders requiring early care.

As in the Philippines, there was little evidence that these agencies saw
their roles as ecological change-agents for sociopolitical institutions.
Programs were not devised to reach out to people living in the slum areas
of Bangkok, nor to tackle the psychosocial stress resulting from high-
density urban living, poverty, and rapid social change. CGC's efforts to
make educational institutions more responsive to the needs of students—
through the creation of counseling services—came closest to the concept
of ecological change.

Other than public consultation, only two or three of the eight institutions follow a clear mandate to organize prevention programs. Yet, it is
clear that MOPH sees prevention of drug abuse as a major mental health
thrust for the 1977–1981 five-year plan. Even though previous research
cited showed insignificant "hard drug" use among youth, the presumed
population at risk is students: MOPH has planned 111 guidance units
manned by school teachers and serving 4,225 schools to prevent the rise
in the present addiction rate.

Continuity of Care within the Facility: Manpower

The manpower situation among the eight institutions is almost identical
to that of the Philippines (table 5.7).[2] There are nine times as many psychiatric nurses as physicians; psychologists, occupational therapists, and
social workers are least available. The parity in representation among

TABLE 5.7 Multidisciplinary Teams and Manpower Availability in Thailand: Staff Numbers and Staff-to-Patient Ratios

Profession	SCP	SH	PN	PYO	CGC	PM	SP	CU	Total
Psychiatrist (including residents)	32	11	4	6	3	3	2	1	62
Psychologist	8	4	4	3	8	3	4	1	35
Nurse (including assistant)	137	125	24	65	15	73	85	8	532
Social worker	10	8	3	5	6	2	5	—	39
Occupational therapist	12	10	2	5 / 15 teachers	2 teachers	—	4	—	33
Beds	1,000	2,250	40	450	40	925	900	12	
1976 average monthly outpatient visits	4,958*	2,611*	3,750*		1,450	2,307*	862*	108*	
1976 total new outpatients	10,189	4,116			1,657	5,345	2,252	500*	
1976 total outpatient visits	59,449	31,333	50,564*	150 day students	17,397 total clients	27,688	10,342	1,300*	
1976 total inpatient admissions	2,255	4,609		60	72	1,087	1,682	250	
Inpatients per therapeutic staff	5.025	14.25	1.08	4.54	511.67 (outpatients)	11.41	9.0	1.2	

*Estimate

these last three types of workers and the fact that in most instances they are not numerically inferior to psychiatrists is significant. It suggests that the Thai psychiatric system permits a more active involvement of non-medical disciplines than observed in the other two countries.

The optimism stimulated by apparent equality in professional ranks quickly gives way to dismay upon inspection of the patient/staff ratios. The overall ratios are adequate, ranging from 1.08 and 1.2 inpatients per therapeutic staff at PN and CU to 9, 11, and 14.24 inpatients per professional at SP, PM, and SH respectively. These figures are lowered by the high numbers of psychiatric nurses and their trained assistants.

However, in the large residential institutions, the scarcity of professionals becomes distinct. At SP and Prasri Mahaphodi (PM), each with almost 1,000 residents, there are only two or three psychiatrists. SH in Bangkok has a ratio of 204 patients per psychiatrist, while nearby SCP enjoys a ratio of thirty-two residents per physician. Allied therapists fare little better. In fact, SH's four psychologists are theoretically responsible for 562 patients each. Similarly, PM's two social workers confront 462 needy persons.

The pressures on professional time are felt even more profoundly when outpatient figures are brought into account. SCP had a total of 59,449 contacts in 1976, while PN had 50,564 visits. Likewise, SH, PM, SP, and CU gave consultations on 31,333, 27,688, 10,342, and 1,300 occasions respectively. In the same year, CGC's total program, including outreach work, brought their thirty-four staff into contact with 17,397 cases—approximately 511 clients per staff member. In contrast, smaller inpatient settings, PN and CU, have excellent ratios for all types of workers.

The team concept, with close collaboration among medical and allied workers, is evident, but not uniformly practiced. Physicians covet their position as primary decision makers at PN and SCP. Recently, SCP administrators sought to foster teamwork among the separate disciplines but were without success due to the hesitancy of some status quo-minded staff.

Integrated team approaches and flexible use of staffing appear strongest at sites following contemporary philosophies of treatment. At SH, where group therapy and the therapeutic community were introduced in 1963, psychiatric teams are assigned to each section. Moreover, each team member serves as leader for her own therapeutic group (Visuthikosol and Suwanlert 1976). CGC has several mobile teams of mixed professions carrying on training and evaluation at Bangkok schools. CU also endorses the therapeutic community philosophy for organizing group discussions. Nurses there handle recreational, occupational, and individ-

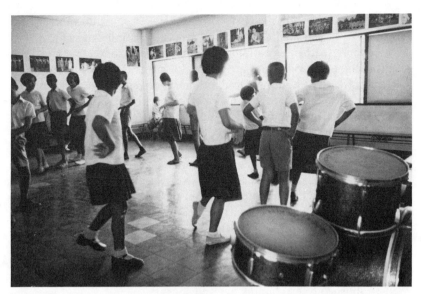

Thai youngsters participate in music therapy at Bangkok's Pan Ya On Hospital.

ual group therapy sessions, and all disciplines contribute to discharge planning. PYO's program is built around close cooperation among teachers, physicians, occupational therapists, and social workers. Retarded children are provided with three training phases—daily living, social adaptation, and vocational.

Duties assigned to different personnel vary from traditional assignments to those offering new responsibilities. Staff psychologists are primarily active with test batteries, giving Thai versions of standardized intelligence tests (WAIS, WISC), personality inventories, and projectives. The few psychologists allowed to do psychotherapy choose either supportive talk therapy or psychoanalytic techniques. Behavior therapy may grow in popularity, though, now that the chief psychologists at RH and SCP have begun to teach and practice it. RH's behavior therapist is frequently referred patients with phobic complaints and sexual dysfunctions. As an agency dominated by nonmedical practitioners, CGC psychologists occupy their time in community consultation, research, and individual work. The four psychologists at SP have introduced dance and music therapy on several wards and hold last-minute sessions with all patients prior to discharge.

Social workers at certain sites have been able to define their role more broadly. SCP social workers, whose chief was trained overseas, handle group therapy sessions, intake interviews, and home visits and coordinate referrals with other agencies. PYO social workers do therapy with the families of retarded children and help the institute's graduates find jobs suitable to their vocational training. Social workers at CGC and their psychologist colleagues are the backbone of the center's outpatient and outreach consultations. Occupational therapists at SH's quarterway house rehabilitation unit enhance chronic schizophrenics' chances of making the transition back into the community.

In conclusion, intrainstitutional continuity of care is probable within those Bangkok programs that have an adequate complement of specialists and organize them into integrated psychiatric teams. PM and SP, typical of provincial mental hospitals, have frightfully small numbers of therapeutic staff. Each professional (except for nurses) in principle is responsible for literally hundreds of inpatients. Other facilities' capacity to provide sufficient intrainstitutional referral and follow-up is brought into question when the figures for outpatients are considered.

Continuity of Care: Interinstitutional

Well-established referral pathways and consultation relationships among mental health resources enable a system to function as an integrated unit for diverse needs. The most significant sources of referrals into the Bangkok and Chiangmai institutions are family and friends, schools, and physicians (fig. 5.3). Traditional healers, priests, and employers play lesser roles as "gatekeepers," according to informants. The strong endorsement of schools, social welfare agencies, and physicians as referral agents implies good links among professionals in allied fields and viable referral pathways among government mental health programs. Interestingly, the least stigmatized agencies—those with the easiest patient access —are the community clinic (CGC) and neurological unit (PN).

Well-defined links appear among several of the Bangkok programs. Yet, the sense of unity and coordination among these elements is less than would be expected, given that they all fall under the Department of Medical Services. This opportunity for centralized leadership in mental health service, a luxury not found in Taiwan or the Philippines, is not fully exploited, as Kiernan's (1976) report suggested. Nevertheless, positive examples may be cited.

CGC is clearly well-integrated both with other community groups (schools, police, public welfare agencies) and with other service providers. CGC clients needing more intensive care than is offered there— including those requiring hospitalization and those diagnosed as mentally deficient—are readily passed along to either PYO, PN, RH, SCP, or the Children's Hospital. University psychiatry departments in Bangkok have similar relationships with SCP, PN, and SH. PYO, with its resi-

Figure 5.3
Referral and Consultation Relationships among Bangkok and Chiangmai Psychiatric Centers

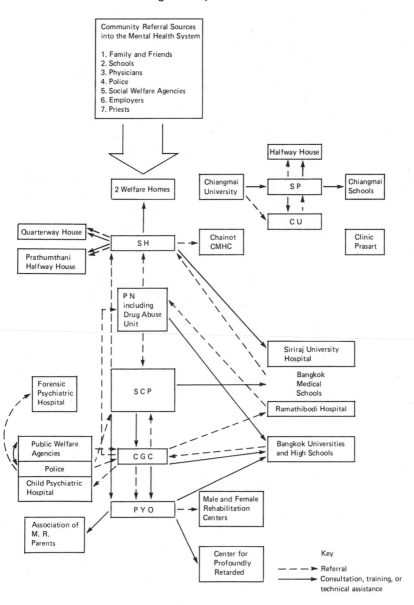

dential rehabilitation centers, and SH and SP with their own halfway houses, are able to transfer patients smoothly along to less-restrictive environments. SCP is the prime focus of communication and consultation in the network because of its historical significance, large multidisciplinary staff, and role as the training center for all categories of workers sent by other institutions. Further underscoring its prominence in the information flow, SCP organizes scientific meetings and case conferences and houses the best psychiatry library in Thailand. The strongest evidence of coordination among these sites is the mutual consultation between SCP and PYO and between CGC and PYO and the fact that all facilities either gave to or received from another agency some sort of technical assistance. That each hospital may in actuality operate as a separate entity is suggested by the fact that there is only one meeting per year of mental institutions.

In Chiangmai, the relationships are less complex since there are only three official programs serving psychiatric populations. Chiangmai University Hospital, SP, and CU have mutual ties. The form and extent of their relationships are still developing due to the recent inauguration of Chiangmai University's Department of Psychiatry. SP relies primarily upon family and friends and police for its admissions. CU does occasionally refer long-term patients to SP, given its own limited dormitory space. SP's consultative activities include its contacts with Chiangmai schools, the province's halfway house, and the supervision of CU's medical students in practica work. Chiangmai University Education Department sends instructors to SP to provide counselors in-service training.

In contrast, CU gets most of its admissions from the University Hospital medical departments. At the time of the survey, CU did not have enough manpower to provide consultation outside of the clinic. Clinic Prasart with its 100 beds for neurological cases handles a fair number of psychiatric intakes based on the pattern found at PN.

Continuity with Community Care-Giving

In line with Kiernan's observation of the failure to provide alternatives to inpatient care (Kiernan 1976: 3), there does not appear to be an easy flow of patients from highly restrictive into minimal supervision settings or into the hands of responsible community agents. Moreover, the residential programs seldom encourage or make use of family member participation in hospital treatment. Rather, it is at the moment of discharge that relatives are brought into the picture and given instructions for home care.

Home or village-level intervention is extremely rare, and when follow-up care *is* done, it is typically handled by having the patient revisit the hospital's outpatient clinic. After-care staff are spread too thinly to make more than token home visits to check the progress of discharged persons (table 5.8, item 4). Those who *are* visited are likely to be living in the immediate vicinity, given transportation handicaps. Follow-up rural trips are unthinkable with present staff.

On the other hand, some efforts to assist discharged patients are made. SCP keeps in contact with certain patients through correspondence— mailing them continued supplies of psychotropic medication—and runs a busy walk-in after-care clinic. SH enjoys access to two transitional living units and occasionally uses the Community Mental Health Center in Chai-Nat Province for after-care. PYO keeps in contact with its "gradu-ates" through the Parent's Association and its social workers' efforts to find steady jobs for the trainees. Furthermore, more than any other insti-tution, CGC sends its workers out for school and home visitation and to administer a formal follow-up questionnaire.

In no instance were relatives asked to stay with their hospitalized fam-ily member. Severely disturbed or suicidal patients at PN sometimes had hired watchers observe them for safety reasons, but relatives wishing to stay overnight were required to pay for the bed used. PYO was building a hostel for the parents of retarded children who traveled from the prov-inces for the week-long assessment procedure.

Formal family involvement in terms of training or educating parents and siblings or family therapy was infrequent except at PYO and CGC, as detailed above. The other agencies sought family contact at the point of discharge, informing the family that their after-care responsibilities were to closely observe the released patient, making sure that he con-tinued taking his medication, and to report new symptoms during hospi-tal follow-up visits. Liaison with community agents (priests, police, em-ployers, etc.) for case management was undetected except for the CGC examples cited earlier.

Accessibility

Bangkok accounts for a tremendous proportion of the existent training, research, and therapeutic resources (see table 5.2). The remaining forty million Thai living in seventy-one provinces have access to six provincial mental hospitals (varying in size from 150 to 1,000 beds), three smaller residential clinics, three psychiatric units in general hospitals, and one halfway house. Provincial bedspace is 3,925. Given these figures, it is obvious that individuals who may benefit by admission to the system can only do so by traveling some distance. In fact, at least half of the resi-dents at Bangkok's major centers have journeyed there from the prov-inces. Constricting the availability of sites even more is the fact that three of the nine provincial hospitals and clinics are located in Chiangmai.

Staff perceptions of agency convenience were based on the extent to

TABLE 5.8 Six Alternatives for Providing Continuity with Community Care-giving in Thailand

Alternatives	SCP	SH	PN	PYO	CGC	RH	SP	CU
Active patient follow-up especially by social worker	++	+	+	++	++	+	+	+
Educate or utilize family members as part of treatment plan (especially at discharge)	+	+	++	+++	+++	++	++	++
Relative stays in hospital with patient	−	−	+	++			−	−
Treatment within home or village setting	−	−	−		++	+	+	−
Community agents assist in treatment (teacher, village leader, M.D., police)	+	+	+		++	?	++	−
Participation in community activities during hospitalization encouraged	+	+	−	++			++	++

+++ always
++ sometimes
+ seldom
− never

which they served rural people. SP, SH, and PN personnel handling clients from several parts of the country felt that their agencies were seldom conveniently situated. On the other hand, CGC and CU staff working with those who are drawn from the immediate area believed their locations were often or always conveniently placed.

Additional factors govern the potential use of these sites. These include: cost, hours of operation, availability of empty beds, and policies regulating admissions. On the positive side, there was almost unanimous agreement that persons with little or no money may use the treatment program. Public funds support the basic operations of each agency, although donations are solicited and some charges are made for drug prescriptions. In addition, a $4 nightly fee is assessed for private patients given special rooms at SCP. Money is collected at PN from those who can afford to pay. CU has a flat $15 charge for admission and collects another $10 for drugs and $5 for recreation therapy materials. At PYO parents are expected to contribute clothing and pay for educational materials while RH charges only for psychological testing.

Given these minimal requirements to receive services from public institutions, it is clear that cost is not a restriction to access for most middle-class and some lower-income people living near these resources. However, for poor people living in far-flung provinces to come to Bangkok or Chiangmai for help, the economic hardship and cost in time away from farming or village work—and the expense of travel—is well beyond their means.

Legally there were no strictures governing admission criteria. While this does make it easy for relatives, police officers, or local judges to place a person in the hospital, it also takes away safeguards regarding such commitment. Thailand operates on an informal system (Curran and Harding 1977). The hospital medical officer makes the decision to admit except on those occasions when the patient is sent on a court order. Only one physician is required to do the certification and length of stay is indefinite. Appeals, periodic review, and discharge procedures are neither specified nor required under this informal system. In many cases, however, patients are voluntary or brought in by family members who can be as adamant about release as they were about admission.

Overcrowded facilities can also limit access and, based on staff opinion, every agency except CU experiences user overload as a very serious problem. PYO, for example, has a waiting list of more than 100 retarded children hoping to gain access to its classrooms. The fact that each of these hospitals has between 10,000 and 60,000 outpatient contacts per year takes its toll on the quality of consultation available. Importantly, it forces the patients and their families to endure a great deal of waiting and frustration just to see the physician. An administrator at PN described how families from the provinces began lining up at 4:00 A.M. to talk with the doctor. This condition, therefore, is a major hindrance to accessibility.

Staff Evaluation of Resource Strength

Several interesting discoveries emerge from judgments about twenty-one potential problems hindering agency operations offered by sixteen interviewees at seven sites (table 5.9). First, almost half of the items were endorsed as problematic (60 percent or more rating an item as very serious or moderately serious), while only four items were clearly not viewed as major issues. Second, looking at how staff within individual agencies responded (not shown in table 5.9), workers at SP and CU in Chiangmai had unique answers. Except for five items, they denied experiencing difficulties with these potential deficits. PYO, CGC, and SH were at the opposite extreme. Staff there saw two-thirds or more of the problems as critical. Interestingly, there was general disagreement among SCP professionals on which problems were serious, reflecting acute differences among the disciplines.

The problem groupings in table 5.9 expose the specific deficits felt by respondents. The first group of items shows clear agreement that funding for future programs is highly uncertain. The seriousness of these three items was clearly recognized by SH personnel. The next grouping reveals an unquestionable consensus across all sites that administrators, treatment staff, and follow-up personnel are in critically short supply. This correlates with previous data on the manpower situation and the assertions of WHO consultants.

In contrast, the items dealing with psychiatric workers' sense of alienation from other professionals and social institutions were more positive. Only CGC and PYO reported lack of relationships as a moderate concern. This is peculiar because CGC is especially well-connected in the Bangkok network (see fig. 5.3). It may be that CGC staff, who base their effectiveness on being able to make smooth referrals, are sensitive to this process and expect it to work better. A very slight majority felt unsupported by fellow professionals.

Patient overload—within the "crowdedness" grouping—is a unanimous complaint, except at the twelve-bed Chiangmai unit. Moreover, almost all residential sites find it problematic to separate different kinds of patients. At issue is the need to separate violent patients from the rest of the population and to provide special rooms for children, the elderly, recent intakes, and so forth. The lack of building space to carry on special functions such as occupational therapy is also widespread. In sum,

TABLE 5.9 Staff Perceptions of Resource Deficits in Thailand (N=16)

Potential problem	Problem seriousness			
	Very serious	Moderately serious	Slightly serious	Not a problem
1. Lack of help from government	19%	33%	14%	33%
2. Not enough money for present treatment program	12.5%	31%	12.5%	44%
3. Not enough money for future treatment programs	25%	37%	12.5%	25%
4. Not enough trained administrators	31%	37.5%	31%	
5. Not enough diagnostic staff	19%	31%	31%	19%
6. Not enough treatment staff	56%	12%	31%	
7. Not enough follow-up staff	50%	50%		
8. Lack of relationship with other institutions		31%	19%	50%
9. Other professionals don't support the program	6%	50%	19%	25%
10. Long waiting list	12.5%	12.5%	12.5%	62.5%
11. Not enough rooms to separate different kinds of patients	12.5%	56%	12.5%	19%
12. Lack of building space	12.5%	44%	12.5%	31%
13. Too many patients	69%	19%		12.5%
14. Lack of money for equipment and research	50%	25%	6%	19%
15. Library is not good enough	12.5%	6.3%	19%	63%
16. Little information about new treatments and new research findings	19%	44%	19%	19%
17. Lack of epidemiological data regarding mental health	44%	25%	19%	12.5%
18. Staff relations are not good		12.5%	37.5%	50%
19. Not enough treatment supplies	6%	37.5%	19%	37.5%
20. Lack of transportation services	12.5%	38%	12.5%	38%
21. Low success rate of treatment	6%	50%	19%	25%

the perception of crowdedness is acute, fostered by sheer patient numbers and inadequate architectural spaces.

The last grouping pulls together items focusing on two aspects of research: the materials required to carry it out and its availability to guide program operations. It is clear that grants supporting research are one of the lowest priorities within the mental health system. Nearly all staff were disturbed by the lack of opportunity to conduct research, while CGC and PYO personnel were especially concerned about not having an adequate library. Elsewhere, SCP does have a modern, well-supplied library open to investigators in the Bangkok area.

Furthermore, all but one or two Bangkok professionals expressed distress at the absence of knowledge in regard to new therapies and assessment of disorder in the community. Other items suggest that interviewees overwhelmingly disregard the notion that staff relations were not good. Opinions on availability of treatment supplies and transportation were equivocal, except at SH, PYO, and SCP, where these two problems are regarded as important. Item 21 is included as a general frustration index to determine if the pattern of perceived deficits results in a sense of inability to carry out successful interventions. Although only one practitioner (at SCP) reported that low treatment success was a very serious problem, 50 percent saw their success rate as a moderately serious concern.

Interestingly, only two staff at the recently opened Chiangmai University Clinic plus two others from SCP felt success rate was no problem at all. The remainder saw the issue of treatment outcome as somewhat problematic, suggesting a pervasive dissatisfaction with the programs' ability to have a positive impact. While widely felt, this sense of treatment failure is not expressed as a significant crisis, but rather as a core component of everyday experience for those who choose to work as mental health providers in a system that just barely meets their minimum support requirements.

COMMUNITY INTEGRATION AND ACCEPTANCE OF MENTAL HEALTH SYSTEM

Institutions can reduce their community isolation through active liaison with responsible persons in the patient's natural environment. Assistance from intimates in the patient's social network boosts the chances of continuity of care and breaks down the agency-community barriers detrimental to program acceptance.

Previous discussion of table 5.8 centered on the recognition that persons from the patient's social environment were seldom partners in case management until discharge. The residential programs in particular were not prepared to cooperate with relatives in formulating treatment plans, undertaking family therapy, or having staff train them as collaborators during hospitalization. There is no watcher or amah system as in the Philippines and Taiwan. The treatment plan is the physician's exclusive domain, an international attribute of medical institutions. Of course, visitation is encouraged and relatives are allowed to bring in food and money in some places. But only at discharge is there a widespread effort to communicate expectations regarding the family's role. Namely, to watch the person for new symptoms, make sure that his medication is taken regularly, and return him for appointments.

In sharp contrast, when practitioners carry out consultation work at schools and counseling and health centers, they do not hesitate to use nonprofessional allies. The community mental-health-oriented CGC and the facility for retarded children have the deepest outside penetration in regard to treatment. Both seek to arm parents with new skills for managing their children's behavior problems,. including helping the parents cope with the stress of having impaired children. In short, except for the two cases mentioned, the role given concerned outsiders is restricted to after-care activities. Given the extreme shortage of staff assigned to after-care services and the resulting access barriers, it is hard to visualize how the role could be fulfilled in a meaningful way. Thus, for the most part, it appears that Thailand is without more than superficial community integration through treatment involvement.

A second avenue for fostering intimacy between mental health programs and recipients involves solicitation of community input into institutional policies and objectives. Input formats include community advisory boards and needs-assessment surveys to uncover which users are underserved. Among the Thai sites sampled, no formal community involvement was present either through steering committees or surveys of user-perceived needs. There were, however, studies dealing with drug use among high school and college youth which reported prevalence rates and suggested education and drug counseling. The absence of advisory boards replicates the Taiwanese and Philippine findings. The director of PN did mention the existence of an advisory group made up of interested physicians and lay persons, but it has since disbanded.

Undoubtedly, the desire to allow community input is a policy decision that must be made within the bureaucracy of the Ministry of Public Health and not by the individual institutions. If a single coordinating committee were to be established to guide all services, community integration would be served by having community representation on the central planning board. Provisions should also be made for community input at the local level for individual institutions. However, there appears to be little precedence for this approach and no future discernible plan for it.

A final measure of community integration is derived from practitioner judgments of their clinic's acceptance (table 5.10). One-fourth of the respondents were maximally disturbed that their clinics were unknown or misunderstood by community people. Only 12 percent found this not to be a problem. There is "moderate" concern that the public is reluctant to become involved in the psychiatric system until the last possible moment. Yet, a strong consensus is held that once involved, patients cannot return to their homes without the burden of social stigma. This social tainting of psychiatric contact appears uniform throughout Southeast Asia.

The Hill Tribe people around Chiangmai have an additional fear associated with mental hospitals: the risk of being arrested for growing opium when they come from their mountain villages into the grasp of authorities. Once involvement has been established, however, rejection of the treatment offered and disbelief in its efficacy are not seen as major issues. What may be operating is either a mobilization of hope that comes from making the choice to come in for help or a cultural norm of

TABLE 5.10 Staff Perceptions of Agency Acceptability in Thailand (*N*=16)

| | Seriousness of problem | | | |
Questionnaire item	Very serious	Moder- ately serious	Slightly serious	Not a problem
1. Community people don't know about or understand the treatment program.	25%	37.5%	25%	12.5%
2. Community people have a bad opinion of the treatment program and use it as a last chance.		37.5%	44%	19%
3. Patients and their families don't believe the treatment will help.		19%	37.5%	44%
4. Patients returning home have problems because people know they were in a mental hospital.	6.3%	62.5%	19%	12%
5. People with traditional beliefs about mental problems won't use the treatment program.	12.5%	31%	50%	6%
6. People go to "folk doctors" instead of using the treatment program.		31%	69%	

not expressing negative attitudes toward someone in the position of authority (like a physician).

The issue of program rejection by tradition-minded persons is taken up in the last two items of table 5.10. Here again it appears that respondents were mindful of an incongruity between their service system and beliefs and practices of a segment of the population. Only one practitioner did not feel some level of concern associated with the problem of persons with traditional conceptions of disorder not using agency services. Forty-four percent saw this condition as "moderately serious" or worse.

The use of folk healers in lieu of modern psychiatry was uniformly recognized as problematic. Interviewees did not denote the use of folk doctors as threatening. Yet, the esteemed position of folk doctors in rural Thai society influences the acceptance and use of modern medicine. To the extent that indigenous healers (including Buddhist monks) are easily accessible, attend to patient symptoms in expected ways, and are viewed as effective, such healers perpetuate reluctance to use public services except as a final alternative.

The three sources of evidence regarding community integration of Thailand's mental health programs point unmistakably toward their isolation. Formal intercourse is minimal between institutional handling of patients and important figures in the patient's home environment who could be helpful. CGC was the only consistent exception to this rule. Community liaison with programs to help plan procedures and objectives was conspicuously absent, as were needs assessment approaches to find gaps in the resource system. Finally, staff expressed the opinion that their services were little understood, moderately stigmatizing, and somewhat alien to those who cling to traditional theories of health care. In short, there is good reason to suspect that the Thai mental health system is not well integrated and has little acceptability in the community as a whole.

CULTURAL CONTINUITY AND ACCOMMODATION OF MENTAL HEALTH SERVICES

Available ethnographic accounts and interviews with therapists themselves suggest the presence of several prominent cultural forces guiding client and community commerce with mental health institutions. To the extent that individual facilities are responsive to these forces, it is assumed that their acceptability is enhanced along with their level of community integration and continuity. Examples of cultural accommodation in Thai agencies are reported along the five dimensions contained in the previous case studies.

Thai Family Role in Regulating Commerce with Institutions

As we argued regarding Chinese and Filipino patients, the primary role of the Thai family must be understood by practitioners for its regulation of patient involvement with outside helpers. Regarding matters of mental health, the family inculcates notions of individual identity, decides to tolerate or act on evidence of pathology, serves as the principal referral source, and follows its own set of expectations on what is proper involvement in interaction with health services.

Unquestionably, the immediate family grouping is by far the most powerful affiliation held by any Thai. Its primacy as a social unit cannot be overstated: while loyalty to the nuclear family is enduring, individual identity and cooperation with other social groupings tend to be transitory and pragmatic (Henderson 1971). Resembling a modified Confucian system, the Thai social structure places the father at the head of the household; children are reared by mothers or female members and are taught to give high respect and obedience to parents (Sangsingkeo 1969).

Balanced against this press for conformity to family mores is the fundamental Buddhist value of individualism. Each person must remain responsible first to himself or herself because individual actions are the basis of accumulation of merit or demerit. Thus, we may expect that: (1) deviance is primarily the kinship group's concern and (2) the wider community has little obligation in cases of individual deviance; rather it permits one to follow one's own path or create one's own karma.

Support for these two premises comes from several sources. First, findings presented earlier indicated that family members were the dominant referral source into psychiatric agencies. Visuthikosol and Suwanlert (1977) observed that close to 80 percent of Srithunya's admissions were brought by mothers, fathers, siblings, and children of patients. Readiness to refer and hospitalize appears to be based, as it was in the Philippines, more on the inability to handle violent and abrasive behavior than on distress at the presence of psychological impairment per se.

For example, extremely withdrawn, inhibited, and passive children (prominent in American clinics) are seldom brought to the Child Guidance Clinic. In fact, therapists reported a high percentage of presenting complaints from family members centered on themes of violence and uncontrollability. Assaultiveness against others, burning down the house, and expression of paranoid ideas were mentioned as behaviors especially upsetting of the household and neighbors.

Sangsingkeo (1958) suspects that family overprotectiveness prevents some needy persons from receiving psychiatric care. Impaired women from well-to-do families sometimes pass their entire lives in the care of servants without the outside world being aware of their status. This exact situation was described by Dasnanjali (1971) regarding the responses of families with retarded children. Seen as the results of reincarnation, the retarded child is simply fed, clothed, and cared for as the family's quiet burden.

Traditional theories of illness greatly influence family reaction to patients. When the cause is seen as temporary possession by a spirit or imbalance of body elements, relatives remain genuinely accepting of the person (Ionescu-Tongyonk 1977). Self-treatment and home remedies are the first line of defense and skillfully performed by household heads among the Hill Tribes (Kunstadter 1978). Otherwise, recognition of ill health prompts a consultation with a fortune teller for advice on which of the many folk specialists available is most proper (Suwanlert 1976a). On these occasions, it is not unusual for patients among northern Thai and Hill Tribes people to draw upon the medical system of another nearby ethnic group. Participation in the medical context of another culture is based on such practical considerations as convenience, low cost, high perceived effectiveness, and even social prestige (Kunstadter 1978). It is this exact situation that gives rise to the referral of a patient to a psychiatric hospital, in itself a cross-cultural expedition. When an exorcism ritual fails after forty-eight to seventy-two hours to dislodge the possessing spirit, and the victim's behavior becomes unmanageable in the home environment, the family may resort to a mental institution (Suwanlert 1976b).

Wider community reaction to the illness is also as predicted. Dr. Sangsingkeo (1958) summarizes the attitude held with an old saying: "Don't mind the mad; add no blame to the drunk." The disease is given credit for the person's actions rather than the individual himself. Spirit possession is also a natural part of life and does not by itself become a sign of mental illness. The society allows great latitude for idiosyncracy of expression. While deviancy is not condoned, it is considered the concern of the individual unless it becomes extreme.

Besides deciding which behaviors give cause for referral and where to take the patient, the family also decides the role it will enact vis-à-vis the agency and what to expect from the institution in return. According to treatment personnel, the dominant family expectation is that hospitalization will achieve a complete, almost immediate reversal of symptoms. They expect that it will take only one or two sessions so they don't have to keep returning and miss work or classes. Moreover, the family has its own timetable on hospitalization. In some cases, when improvement is not immediately forthcoming, the patient is brought home. This also occurs when the family detects the slightest sign of improvement.

At other times, the family abandons patients to a lifetime of hospital care. Abandonment happens more often with chronic cases and when

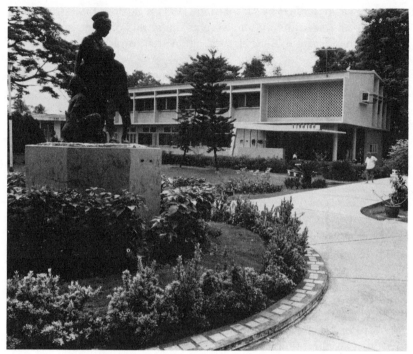

A statue erected by the grateful parents of a patient at Somdej Chaopraya Hospital in Thailand commemorates benevolent nursing care.

relatives cannot afford the burden of patients at home. For the most part, staff perceive families as not preferring to take an active role during hospital care. Some families, staff say, refuse to visit until they are assured the patient is normal. As a general rule, the sites visited reported only rare cooperation with relatives for treatment plans. Most came for visits only occasionally, bringing money or food. Relatives formally spoke with staff only at intake and discharge conferences.

Examples of facility efforts to accommodate to the Thai family system include our earlier descriptions of attempts to involve family members in hospital and postdischarge care (see community continuity of care section). Other examples of accommodation to the family system include the practice at PN, a neurology center, to admit acute psychiatric patients whose families feared that their reputations would be damaged by admission to an acknowledged mental hospital. SP and SH approve family requests for permission to visit native healers where ceremonies are arranged and holy water acquired for purification. Finally, recent community psychiatry experimental wards at SH include group sessions with relatives of patients. Family members of patients on these wards meet to talk with one another on how home care should proceed after discharge, especially how to get the patient to take medication.

In short, agency liaison with patients' families is tenuous up until the point of discharge when efforts are usually made to encourage family participation in an after-care scheme. The lack of involvement prior to that time seems to reflect a mutual agreement. The institution would prefer no interference from the family in its regimen and the family turns over responsibility to the physicians for a cure. If a cure is not forthcoming or it takes too long, families decide either to take their members elsewhere or to abandon them to lifetime custodial care. However, there may be a far larger population of potential cases that families never brought to the attention of these institutions. They take disturbed members to local specialists or simply tolerate them within the home or village.

Accommodation to Popular Indigenous Conceptions of Disorder

Service users carry into treatment a rich array of folk theories regarding the symptoms, causes, treatment options, and probable outcome of their illnesses (Kunstadter 1978). Medical anthropologists have observed that this collection of explanatory notions and nosologies does not form a single, self-contained, or integrated system. Rather, they represent a synthesis of often competing subsystems based on animist traditions, Buddhism, humoral theory from contact with Hinduism and Ayurvedic traditions, plus a dash of Western biomedicine (Hinderling 1973; Kunstadter 1978; Muecke 1979). Major lay explanations are at variance with mental health workers' understanding of psychopathology. Such conceptual discrepancies offer opportunities for cultural sensitivity and accommodation on the part of hospital personnel.

Anthropologists have identified four major indigenous theories of disorder based on ethnographic studies in central and northwestern Thailand (Hanks 1964; Hinderling 1973; Kunstadter 1978; Textor 1960). The two most prominent of these explain illness by the Ayurvedic doctrine of *thaad* (Muecke 1979) and the intrusion of foreign elements, both physical and supernatural. *Thaad* refers to the belief that the human body is composed of various humoral elements in balance with one another. When there is a disturbance in the earth, fire, water, and wind body elements, the person becomes ill (see Muecke 1979). Therapy restores equilibrium, returning the person to health.

The penetration of foreign elements also brings illness. Two sorts of substances may enter an individual—spirits or particles sent by spirits or persons practicing black magic *(khun khon)*. Illnesses caused by witchcraft or the incantation of a magic formula *(khatha)* are thought rare in Thailand. They are difficult to diagnose and only recognizable by social circumstances such as arguments over land rights (Kunstadter 1978; Hinderling 1973). There are many classifications of spirits, though, including the souls and angels of the Hindu pantheon *(thewada)*. Possession by these spirits is generally desirable as it blesses the individual with "higher powers."

However, the intrusion of *phii* spirits is associated with sickness and mental illness. Kunstadter found that among the Hill Tribes of northern Thailand, *phii* spirits were said to cause illness in order to call human attention to their desire to be fed an animal sacrifice (Kunstadter 1978: 191). *Phii* spirits emanate from the dead (especially those who die violently or away from home) and from other living persons, sacred things, or from the village itself. Risk of possession increases when persons violate incest or exogamy taboos, are absent from the village without proper spirit propitiation, and fail to respect other ritual obligations. Possession may also follow family quarrels or wandering near the place where a violent death occurred (Kunstadter 1978; Suwanlert 1976a). Cases of spirit possession were familiar to Thai psychiatrists working with rural populations.

Soul loss and "sin" or karma are two remaining notions of illness etiology. *Khwan* is the Thai concept of body-spirit or life-soul which can reside either inside or outside of the body. *Khwan* bestows life, health, and prosperity when it remains inside. If *khwan* slips away and becomes lost or injured, the person may become ill, chronically weak, or even die (Henderson 1971; Kunstadter 1978).

Buddhist teachings stress that people, through actions, accumulate merit *(bun)* and demerit *(bap)*. The balance of merits and sins determines one's fate or future life form through reincarnation. Kunstadter (1978) notes that "be good, get good" is a Thai prescription for prevention of illness. Disease in general has a "fundamental moral significance, with the severity of illness varying directly with the degree of accumulated demerit" (Muecke 1979: 273). In the instance of congenital birth defects and mental deficiency in children, there is a tendency for parents to view these as reincarnation and not to seek out special services or education for the child (Dasnanjali 1971).

A final folk diagnosis, *lom* (meaning "wind illness"), is worth mentioning because of its focus on mental status. According to Muecke (1979), a chronic episode of this condition may present disorientation and loss of consciousness, grand mal seizures, incoherent speech, and catatonic-like withdrawal. Extreme *lom* is interpreted as direct contact with the spirit world.

Juxtaposed with these ethnomedical accounts are three dominant popular conceptions of psychopathology typically described by hospital staff. The most common understanding relates the problem to a physical anomaly. As in Taiwan and the Philippines, the vast majority of patients complain chiefly of physical discomfort. Frequently mentioned are chest pains, "heart attack," headache, insomnia, weakness, loss of appetite, weight loss, stomachache, etc. At other times, the problem is said to be caused by "bad nerves" *(prasart)* or a neurological disease. It is expected that the physician will check out the brain and nervous system. Loss of physical strength through masturbation and excessive coitus is a reason sometimes cited by parents.

A second lay interpretation mentioned attributes disorder to over-whelming life burdens. Children develop problem behavior before difficult exams or when they haven't studied enough and are failing school. Adults become disturbed when they lose a spouse or parent, when they have to work long hours for little pay, when they feel inferior about their jobs or educational status, and when there is conflict among family members.

Thirdly, moral violations are thought to foster disturbed behavior. Young Chinese men were reported to have strong feelings of guilt regarding masturbation or homosexuality—taboo activities in the eyes of their elders. Guilt associated with sex was even more intensely experienced by Muslim patients from the south. Islamic precepts condemn persons for acts of premarital or extramarital intercourse. Conflicts related to sexual behavior were voiced by women in ward therapy sessions at SH. These women, along with others seen in private practice (Suwana 1969), voiced distress at their spouses' infidelity and the practice of taking a concubine once the wife began rearing the children. It is not surprising that the same women at SH revealed problems with orgasmic dysfunction and impotency on the part of their husbands.

Along similar lines, RH's psychologist had a substantial caseload of men complaining about premature ejaculation. He felt that this problem was endemic in the population due to the fact that Thai men are socialized into an egocentric view of receiving pleasure from their sexual partners. This view hinders their ability to reciprocate in sexual activities and attend to their partners' needs.

Although informally conceived and carried out, institutional accommodation to indigenous theories was noted at several locations. First, doctors seeing patients from northern Thailand had direct experience with spirit possession cases. At the time of this study, Chiangmai psychiatrists had one case of a young girl who had visions of an angel asking her to die and join it in a mountain near the old Thai capital. Another case was a young man who had thought his mother was a *phii* spirit because she would go at night to the water closet, so he attacked her to drive away the *phii.*

Bangkok therapists also reported instances where patients interpreted physical symptoms as spirit-induced. RH staff were treating clients with phobic reactions to the spirit houses kept in the gardens of many Thai homes. Along similar lines, one Bangkok patient explained his disorder as the consequence of urinating too close to a spirit house.

Dr. Sagun Suwanlert at Srithunya Hospital is the recognized expert in diagnosis and treatment of spirit possession. After observing several dozen cases, he concluded that: (1) doctors themselves must bring up the question of possession since clients fear being scolded for prior contact with native healers; (2) "neurotic possession," lasting forty-eight hours or less, is typically in reaction to a seemingly insoluble problem, while "possession psychosis" is the diagnosis of those brought into the hospital after lengthy exorcism has failed to drive out the spirit; (3) the most intense possession period is characterized by numbness of limbs, convulsions, rigid body, and speaking the name of the possessing spirit followed by a period of exhausted sleep and amnesia; (4) possession may be viewed as a socially sanctioned mechanism for handling social conflicts: in trance states, persons can command superior family members to kneel before them or carry out tasks; and (5) therapy with extreme cases may take up to a week; it includes injections of major tranquilizers or antidepressants and supportive talk therapy focused on the problems leading to the possession episode (Suwanlert 1977).

Suwanlert's culture accommodation tactic is to initiate his medical and psychological intervention only after a thorough assessment of how different spirits affect the host patients. A second tactic is simply to maintain a permissive attitude toward patients who pay homage to folk beliefs as long as it doesn't directly conflict with the clinic regimen. At CGC, staff faced with persons insisting that they are possessed simply accept the idea but continue treating what they see as the problem in their own way. Therapists don't attack the belief directly but may offer their own conceptualization during the course of counseling. Neither CGC nor SP staff object to patients visiting folk specialists. In fact, families at SP are allowed to take the patient out to visit priests or herbalists if they ask.

Providing Expected Therapeutics

Logically, the patients anticipate modes of intervention that follow from the perceived roots of their distress. Upon entry to the physician's biomedical territory, patient anomalies are most often communicated through the setting's somatic idiom or at least translated as such. Psychiatrists, interpreting client requests, see themselves as expected to immediately administer medication, or pause long enough to do a brain x-ray or EEG pinpointing what is wrong. Families are particularly keen on the physician using "strong, expensive medicine," perhaps even "medical shock" to modify the mind. They want the same "strong medicine" that is supposedly reserved for private patients because it is deemed most curative.

Drugs administered through intramuscular injection have higher credence than oral medication. Hope is expressed that one or two injections of the right chemicals will bring an immediate reverse and cure. Some families, it was said, simply insist on locking the patient up and the longer the better.

Just as in Taiwan and the Philippines, clients in Thailand enter the medical context for strictly physical as opposed to psychological therapies. Help through a cognitive process mediating psychological conflict is unfathomable except to those urban elite whose educational experiences provide them with a grounding in Western humanism. Recognizing this, CGC staff start counseling with an orientation session to describe their approach.

Older adults ask to see a physician rather than a psychologist or social worker and are less accepting of psychological orientation than younger persons. In any event, therapists seek to be directive and supportive. They give explicit advice on how people should change rather than following a reflective, nondirective model. At one time, CGC tried to initiate group therapy sessions but found a strong opposition which they attributed to a dislike for sharing personal secrets in front of others, especially strangers.

The psychiatrist at CU follows a pills and injections regimen initially to meet patient expectations and build rapport and compliance. Then he shifts to a cognitive-behavior modification strategy based on applying Buddhist meditation. Meditative states are derived through Jacobsonian deep muscle relaxation and breathing exercises. Dr. Chomlong Disayavanish reported employing this integrated behavior therapy/religious meditation technique principally with anxiety-prone patients and those suffering from tension headaches and hypertension.

Possession cases at Srithunya are handled using an accommodation formula worked out by Dr. Suwanlert. First, the patient's beliefs are studied, particularly his schema of the nature of spirits and ghosts. Questioning is then done to learn which symptoms are attributed to possession. It is thought that physician familiarity with the patient's spirit concepts will help explain to the patient the relationship between disturbing states and the personal conflicts causing them. Finally, low dosages of major tranquilizers and supportive psychotherapy taking into account the possession fears are provided.

Suwanlert (1977) adds that the effective psychotherapist, while accepting the patient's schema, must reinterpret it for herself in "modern" concepts of mental illness. Gradually she should educate the patient to a more rational understanding of her particular problem. Other Thai psychiatrists and counselors endorse this reeducative approach for those holding folk conceptions.

In essence, psychiatrists interpret their medically based regimens as closely matching popular conceptions of disorder as a physical/neurological illness. Thai ethnomedicine, on the other hand, points to the wealth of explanatory models of illness that have strictly sacred or social underpinnings and are orthogonal to psychiatry's dynamic/biological nosologies (e.g., Kunstadter 1978; Muecke 1979). Urban as well as rural Thai express a strong preference to consult first nearby folk specialists— of seven generic types—who dispense therapeutics ranging from local pharmacopoeia to holy water, exorcism, and modern drugs as befitting the diagnosis (Kamratana 1973; Suwanlert 1977; Woolley 1974).[3]

Uniquely, the country's greatest supply of indigenous mental health manpower is its 250,000 Buddhist monks and novices (Sangsingkeo 1969). Working from some 22,000 *wats,* the priests act as front-line therapists giving "psychotherapeutic" guidance, instructing troubled individuals to meditate to remove anger and frustration. Buddhist monks have always seemed willing to offer food and shelter to vagrants, the disabled, and those with psychiatric needs but without families' assistance (Henderson 1971). Priests encourage tolerant and understanding attitudes toward social unfortunates using their *wats* as refuges and rehabilitation centers for prepsychotic individuals (Stoller 1959). Monks who have a knowledge of folk medicine frequently gain a reputation as successful healers (Dusit 1972). Priest Phra Charon at Wat Tambrabok, for instance, has reportedly cured 1,000 drug addicts in recent years and was given the Ramon Magsaysay Award for humanitarianism. Possession cases also choose these monks hoping that the spirits will be expelled by the sacredness of the pagoda and rituals using powerful holy water (Suwanlert 1976a).

In a unique opportunity to study reliance on folk therapists for a specific psychological condition, Suwanlert and Coates (1977) interviewed 350 patients in northeastern Thailand during the 1976 *koro* epidemic. *Koro* is a culture-bound syndrome characterized by extreme panic resulting from the impression that the penis is shrinking and retracting into the abdomen and will bring about death. Fostered by ethnic animosity and unstable political conditions, the epidemic affected approximately 2,000 men and women. Among those interviewed—a typical cross-section of young village men—70 percent sought help from native healers, 20 percent made their way to local hospitals, and 5 percent went untreated. Thus, for *koro,* folk treatment was deemed most appropriate. It consisted of ingesting concoctions of watermelon, peppermint, field crabs, and raw eggs or application of a moist local tuber used on other occasions to prevent drunkenness (Suwanlert and Coates 1977).

Accommodation through Staff Qualities and Mannerisms

When asked their understanding of what the therapist's personal manner should be to fulfill the expectations of Thai clients, most respondents reported two prominent qualities: (1) present oneself as a respectable authority figure with expertise and advice which should be followed and (2) temper the authoritarian quality with warmth, friendliness, calmness, and, above all, a helpful and cheerful attitude. Since social norms encourage passivity and deference to those of higher status, therapists wishing open communication with their clients recognized the importance of downplaying their position as authority figures. They did so through a warm and easygoing style of interaction.

Moreover, to establish a good working relationship in counseling, embarrassing topics were not brought up in initial sessions. One psychologist, using deep muscle relaxation, remarked that he avoided having female clients tense and relax their posterior muscles because he believed it would offend them. Apparently, problems related to sexuality are most embarrassing and require an extremely gingerly approach to bring out. The profound shyness of some psychotic patients in the presence of authorities is such that it may take eighty to 100 sessions before patients freely express themselves in therapy interactions (Suwanlert 1970).

Boesch (1972) and Hinderling (1973) bring to light other important attributes of physicians influencing their transactions with clients. First, patients and doctors occupy different strata of the Thai social hierarchy and hence have no basis for a customary relationship founded upon mutual dependency and loyalty. Unless ill, a patient would strongly hesitate to approach a person of the doctor's status (Boesch 1972: 72). He would be more comfortable if introduced by a relative or friend of the doctor, bringing the medical relationship into one of more traditional loyalty.

Status imposes barriers and evokes suspicion in patients because they have no power in the relationship except to reciprocate through money. Differences in education, thinking styles, and basic social values heighten the inability of the two parties to communicate. The physician has another strike against her as a government officer. Historically, rural people associate government agencies with control and taking rather than providing; they lie outside of the bonds of mutual loyalty that bind people in the village (Boesch 1972: 27).

On the other hand, these investigators stress that patients visiting health centers did have expectations that the physicians were competent in diagnosis and therapy, especially when treating serious diseases (Hinderling 1973). Suffering patients were more inclined to travel to a modern physician than to continue nonameliorative treatment with a local, albeit familiar, folk specialist. These same patients were critical of the businesslike, arrogant, often scolding, and inattentive manner of some doctors. Their preference was for someone who consoled them, who explained the illness in a manner that would allow them to have confidence in the healer's knowledge, and who took enough time in the consultation to give the patient a feeling of contact and being looked after. Amazingly, Boesch (1972) found that most office interviews lasted only two minutes. The patients had ten to forty seconds of speaking time to explain their problem. Only a handful of the physicians observed showed sensitivity to these expectations and took the time to console and explain the diagnosis in a friendly, sympathetic manner.

Juxtaposed with clinic culture is that of the local healers. Hinderling (1973) observed that traditional doctors charge very little or even provide financial assistance to patients out of a commitment to the well-being of fellow villagers. They have deep sympathy with the problems others face and are compensated through the confidence people have in them and the making of religious merit (Hinderling 1973: 74). Even if government medical attention were free, the cost of travel, room and board for accompanying family member, and medicine itself are grave burdens for most farming families.

In fact, many of the folk specialists observed by Hinderling practiced as a sideline. They were often retired rice farmers living in houses like those of other villagers. Treating their clients as equals, their payment was usually some small present. Clients were often neighbors who visited before or after work in the fields. However, once a reputation for curing developed, it attracted far-flung patients (Hinderling 1973: 67).

Accommodation in Ward Activities

Ward-level practices reflecting sensitivity to client background were noticed in most institutions. Perhaps the clearest example of this type of accommodation is undertaken at the Buddhist Priest's Hospital in Bangkok. This hospital was set up to serve only priests and novices: it is considered improper for them to mix with laymen in general hospitals. The medical attendants there are all males in line with the taboo against women touching priests. According to the hospital's former chief psychiatrist, Dr. Dusit, psychiatric conditions and pulmonary tuberculosis account for the majority of intakes (Dusit 1972). Psychosomatic and neurotic complaints predominate, and many priests are addicted to bromide drugs taken to relieve psychophysiological symptoms. Since priests are not supposed to have problems and are presumably masters of self-healing, they are reluctant to admit psychological concerns. Physicians must be extremely cautious in their questioning to accord these holy men proper respect. Drug therapy for "diseases of learned men" is deemed most appropriate (Dusit 1972).

Culture accommodation to language was also noted. Most agencies had staff proficient in the various Thai dialects so linguistic matching was common. Hmong and Karen Hill Tribe persons were sometimes brought to SP by missionaries for drug dependence, toxic psychosis, and postpartum psychosis. On these occasions, the language barriers were handled by translators from the nearby Chiangmai Hill Tribe Center.

Moreover, SP made special provisions to ease the admission shock of tribal people. Because it is difficult for them to mix easily with the Thai patients, they are taken off the admission ward as quickly as possible, housed together, and rapidly placed on medication.

These procedures are done so that relatives can take them home as soon as possible. Staff feel that psychotherapy with this population is quite unrealistic because of language and educational differences.

Accommodation was evidenced in other psychiatric wards. Permission is granted at CGC, SH, and SP to attend outside healing rituals although ingestion of medicines from folk doctors is frowned upon. Recreation and occupation therapy at SP and CU focus on familiar and enjoyable activities such as sewing, knitting, flower making, gardening, group singing sessions, and folk dancing.

SH and SCP have pioneered in the design of ward groups as therapeutic communities. Their patients come together to support one another; some assume leadership roles to represent patient viewpoints to the staff. Initially, it was thought contrary to Thai social norms for people to speak in groups. In fact, patients would not speak when their group leaders acted in an authoritarian manner. After ten years of observation of ward groups, it was found that patients are expressive when discussing ward administration, treatment programs, and even their own situations when the therapist creates a permissive and relaxed atmosphere (Visuthikosol and Suwanlert 1976). However, group psychotherapy at SP was discontinued on the male wards when it was found that patient participation was minimal.

Other accommodation practices aimed at "normalizing" the hospital atmosphere. Certain SP staff reside on the hospital grounds and invite patients to visit them in their living quarters. SCP administrators are trying to make the hospital more homey through new dorms without bars and the planned addition of recreation and group activity rooms. SCP prides itself upon its lovely and well-tended gardens. The trees and flowers are being preserved against the press for more space because historically they have been grown as therapeutic instruments to "calm the mind and lift the spirits." Nevertheless, hospitals in general have negative emotional associations for rural Thai; these may prove difficult to over-come. First, they evoke anxiety linked to dying away from home. Thus, the hospital is a dwelling place for malevolent spirits. Secondly, unfamiliar people of higher status and power are encountered there; customary forms of social interaction seem no longer valid. This uncertainty, too, gives rise to user discomfort.

STAFF PERCEPTIONS OF CULTURE ACCOMMODATION

Staff were asked to rate the availability of culture accommodation procedures and to express their personal attitudes on the utility of employing them with traditionally oriented patients. Most respondents perceive their agencies as accommodating in terms of staff adjusting their personal manner to fit patient expectations and inpatient activities being similar to their activities outside the hospital (table 5.11).

A slight majority of interviewees indicated that their programs permitted patients to make choices about their daily activities and encouraged

TABLE 5.11 Perceptions of Institutional Accommodation
Practices in Thailand (*N*=12)

Accommodation practice	Percentage of staff endorsing accommodation item	
	Always/ sometimes	Seldom/ never
1. Native healer involvement in patient care		100
2. Staff seek to reeducate those with traditional beliefs about mental problems	92	8
3. Staff adjust their personal manner to fit patient expectations	83	17
4. A policy exists to find staff whose backgrounds are similar to those of the patients	33	67
5. Inpatient activities are similar to their activities outside the hospital	91	9
6. Patients make choices about their daily activities	65	35
7. Patients are encouraged to participate in community activities outside the hospital— work and recreation	65	35
8. Patient's family helps with hospital care	35	65
9. Problems occur because patients and staff have different social backgrounds	39	61

them to remain involved in work and recreation outside the facility. These two accommodation approaches were in evidence at hospitals with therapeutic community wards, at those offering occupational rehabilitation units, and where families were permitted to take the patient to outside healing rituals.

In marked contrast, staff report shutting out two aspects of patient cultural experience by eschewing native healer involvement and trying to reeducate those with traditional beliefs about mental problems. Even clinicians sensitive to the influence of folk theories on patient experience of psychopathology still work toward the goal of introducing more "modern" concepts into the patients' understanding of their problems. Finally, agencies have yet to introduce policies to involve family members in treatment or hire staff whose backgrounds are congruent with those served even though 40 percent exclaimed that problems do occur because patients and staff have different social backgrounds. This finding fits well with Boesch's (1972) discovery that social distance between physician and patient disrupts efficient delivery of health services in general.

Table 5.12 presents staff evaluation of the utility of sixteen accommodation procedures. The overall endorsement pattern of these professionals mirrors that found for Taiwanese and Filipino respondents: nearly three-fourths of the procedures are overwhelmingly endorsed as useful. For example, those sampled strongly indicated that staff should know the traditional names, beliefs, and healing practices related to mental disorder; community leaders should have a planning role in agency development; and doctors do not have a monopoly on treatment goals and such goals differ between cultures. Moreover, several antiaccommodation items receiving strong support were the same for all three countries: especially, "Staff should try to correct or reeducate patients who maintain their traditional beliefs." Interestingly, although there was absolutely no folk healer involvement within these sites, almost three-fifths were of the opinion that folk healer consultation did have some merit. This may contribute to the willingness of agencies to permit forays to healing temples during hospitalization.

In conclusion, culture accommodation at Thai mental health facilities is most intense at the ward level. This is exemplified by the uniquely designed hospital solely for Buddhist priests, widespread linguistic matching, efforts to release Hill Tribe patients as rapidly as possible, the popularity of therapeutic community wards, an emphasis on recreation and occupation therapy, and the lovely gardens included as important parts of hospital milieu. These efforts fall under the rubric "Making inpatient activities as similar as possible to activities in the community."

Secondly, Suwanlert's transcultural approach to psychiatry is a noteworthy model of accommodation. His efforts are guided by the recogni-

TABLE 5.12 Staff Endorsement of Culture Accommodation Dimensions in Thailand (*N*=23)

Accommodation statement	Percentage of staff endorsing statement
1. Staff should know the traditional names for mental disorder.	100
2. Staff should know the traditional healing practices for mental disorder.	96
3. It is useless for staff to know the traditional beliefs about the causes of mental disorder.	96% disagree
4. Community leaders should help in planning and directing facility activities.	96
5. The doctor alone should decide what the appropriate treatment outcome will be.	96% disagree
6. Staff should adjust their professional manner to fit the expectations of patients from different social backgrounds.	91
7. While in the hospital, patients should remain isolated from community activities.	87% disagree
8. The patient's activities in the hospital should be as similar as possible to activities in the community.	87
9. Patients should go to large central hospitals for their treatment.	87% disagree
10. What is considered the appropriate outcome of treatment should be different for different cultures.	83
11. It is best to hire staff whose social backgrounds are similar to those of the patients.	70
12. The patient and his family should help choose the type of treatment given.	66
13. What is considered "normality" or "good personal adjustment" is the same for all cultures.	65% disagree
14. Only those trained in scientific treatment techniques are qualified to help people with mental problems.	65% disagree
15. It is useless to consult with native healers since most of them cannot really help patients with mental problems.	57% disagree
16. Staff should try to correct or reeducate patients who maintain their traditional beliefs and customs about mental disorder.	13% disagree

tion that if local psychiatrists treating possession cases "have no insight into practices relevant to transcultural psychiatry, they may never find real answers to patient problems" (Suwanlert 1977: 8). This recognition has led him to study regional theories of mental disorder thoroughly and incorporate these cultural insights into assessment of possession cases and clinical responses to them.

Although vitally important, the weakest domain of accommodation is to the cultural pecularities of the Thai family system. The family is central to the person's life, is active in choosing treatment location and time, and expresses ingrained suspicion of government institutions. Only at the point of discharge is there motion towards the family to cooperate in decreasing the likelihood of a readmission. The Child Guidance Center, a program closest to the concept of a community mental health center, does the most to guide complete family involvement in all steps of intervention. This model is unique, however, owing both to traditional hospital regimen and to scarcity of outreach manpower.

NOTES

1. Unstructured interviews were held with Dr. Prasop Ratanakorn, director of the Drug Research and Prevention Center and Special Health Service; Dr. Phon Sangsingkeo, a founder of modern Thai psychiatry; Mr. Kitikorn Meesapya, psychologist within the Division of Mental Health; Dr. Sausuriee Chutikhun, a leading Thai academic psychologist and administrator at the United Nations Asian Development Institute; and Dr. Narongsak Chunnuel, social psychologist at the University of Chiangmai.

2. Prasri Mahaphodi (PM), located in the northeast province of Ubol, replaces RU in this table. This was done because figures on RU were lacking and PM has staffing features characteristic of a large, outlying mental hospital.

3. Hinderling (1973: 64–65) has conveniently summarized the seven categories of healers who function outside the Buddhist *wat*. Fully described are the explanatory systems, education, and methods of healing associated with each type of specialist, including herbalist, midwife, quack, spirit doctor, and so forth.

chapter 6

Modern Psychiatry in Taiwan, the Philippines, and Thailand: Is It Feasible and Culturally Valid?

The preceding chapters set forth comprehensive case studies of psychological service delivery in Taiwan, the Philippines, and Thailand. These accounts detail the status of psychiatric resources within the sociocultural context of developing Asian nations; they form the basis for answering the two central questions of the survey.

First, is it feasible for these countries to embrace the standards of modern psychiatry in the design of mental health systems? Secondly, does an essentially Western model of service delivery manifest cultural sensitivity to these societies as measured by community acceptability and agency accommodations to fit unique cultural patterns? The objective of this chapter is to reiterate the case study findings in light of these two questions.

FEASIBILITY OF DESIGNING MODERN MENTAL HEALTH CARE

Prevailing criteria of "modern psychiatry" were delineated in chapter 1. These criteria were expressed in a seven-variable framework that was then used to analyze the status of mental health services in each country studied.

Having adopted the model of modern psychiatry, are these countries able to allocate resources to achieve comprehensive services; prevention programs; continuity of care within, between, and outside institutions; and accessibility of services? To answer this, a set of general conclusions is drawn from the findings of the three case studies. The conclusions present both the factors mitigating the attainment of modern standards and those instances where successes have been demonstrated.

Conditions Inhibiting Modern Mental Health Delivery

Reviewing the case analyses for Taiwan, the Philippines, and Thailand, it is evident that powerful forces are extant which severely limit the development of viable mental health programs. These forces operate at the national level, involving governmental priorities and economics, and at the level of agency functioning.

Barriers at the National Level

Governmental attention in developing nations is on growth of agricultural and industrial capabilities and on the elaboration of infrastructure supporting them. Social welfare and public health matters are assigned priorities well below these main concerns. Recent figures show Taiwan, the Philippines, and Thailand expending 1.29 percent, 3.05 percent, and 5.1 percent of their respective national budgets on public health.

Mental health services are given low priority within public health administrations. Resource allocations go first toward health infrastructure (building health centers, hospitals, manpower training) and programs for nutrition, environmental sanitation, maternal and child care, infectious disease control, and health education. International agencies extensively fund family planning and population control projects. Only an occasional advisor is made available for program review and consultation on mental health topics.

National executive bodies for planning, policy making, coordinating, and evaluating mental health programs are either weak and ineffective or nonexistent. Without an effective executive committee, proposals for psychiatric service development, implementation, and integration within existing health structures will not be incorporated into national health development plans.

Weak national health leadership and administrative clout also hinder: (1) creation of legislation strengthening and regulating psychiatric services; (2) coordination of university teaching curricula with community needs and governmental demands; (3) recruitment and effective use of qualified mental health manpower; and (4) planning for nationwide coverage and integration of local, regional, and national service units.

Government health insurance covering payments for psychiatric intervention is nonexistent. Without third-party payment, all private and some public psychological services are beyond the economic reach of most citizens. Professionals with an eye to personal income are also discouraged from entering this specialty without insurance schemes.

Independent university psychiatry departments offering comprehensive clinical coursework and practica are quite rare. Standard course-

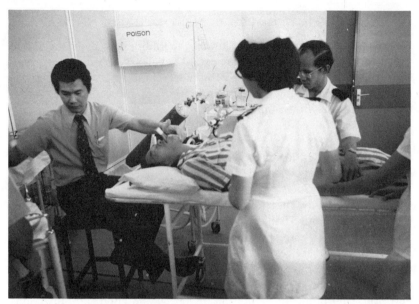

Medical personnel in Singapore administer electroconvulsive shock therapy, a form of treatment used frequently throughout Southeast Asia.

work, internships, and certification for allied professionals such as social workers, are almost completely absent. Throughout these countries and the entire region no more than a tiny handful of master's and doctorate-level clinical psychologists is found.

Qualified professionals exit in disturbing numbers to Western industrial countries. The "brain drain" is prompted by a teaching system that focuses on specialization and disease patterns appropriate to affluent societies, absence of attractive employment, and economic conditions in the home country that cannot support specialized practitioners in the private sector.

Except for Taiwan, there remains an inadequate mapping of the incidence and prevalence of psychological impairment and its link with adverse psychosocial conditions. Empirical documentation of community needs, characteristics of potential service users, and the sociocultural origins of dysfunction is required to focus government attention on these concerns and guide new program creation. Program evaluation to test treatment effectiveness in meeting these needs is the second step which has yet to be taken.

Of singular significance is the extreme maldistribution of mental health resources following the dichotomy between urban and rural living conditions. Hospitals, training institutions, specialty programs of all descriptions, and manpower are concentrated almost exclusively in one or two urban centers in each country. Psychiatry is a Western institution approachable by city-dwelling Westernized elite. It is a cultural island, disconnected from a surrounding sea of rural life and traditions. Rural people are cut off from psychiatry in the same manner they are cut off from each other and their nation's capital: by barriers of geography, transportation, communication, and social distance.

Barriers at the Agency Level

As a rule, individual agencies do not provide a comprehensive array of functions and treatments. *If* the capital cities operate as an integrated referral network, then most specialized services are obtainable to those who can afford them. Psychiatry's core elements—inpatient, outpatient, diagnostics, neurological assessment—are prevalent. But services for special groups and alternatives to inpatient care are rare. Exceedingly scarce are programs for suicide crisis, geriatric patients, substance abuse, transitional living, mental retardation, autism and other childhood disorders, and outreach to discharged patients. Only one or two semicomprehensive community-level centers are available. Most agencies overrely on drug and ECT management, excluding alternative therapeutics. Behavior therapy has just been introduced. It has yet to make an impression.

Preventive mental health functions and indirect services are given low priority. Prevention is difficult to undertake because it demands additional manpower in a system overloaded with existing cases. It is assigned to allied professionals of which there are few and requires a sophisticated understanding of psychosocial stressors in order to conceptualize appropriate interventions. At best, one or two centers in each country exclusively orient their efforts toward public information, education, and consultation. Prevention through ecological change, striving to redirect sociopolitical institutions and ameliorate stress from poverty groups, was not deemed within the purview of any agency visited.

The large residential programs did not maintain sufficient multidisciplinary staffing to allow either meaningful professional/patient contact or fluid transfer from one psychiatric team member to another based on diagnosis or changing needs. There are especially grave shortages of non-medical professionals throughout these systems. Those present perform stereotyped functions. They are denied leadership roles and case responsibility except in a few community-based clinics. Hospital settings are almost totally dominated by nursing and physician personnel. Without the abundance of nurses, the inpatients-to-staff ratios would be astronomically poor. As it is, the small university and private inpatient units are the most adequately staffed, offering the best opportunities for therapeutic contact. Manpower deficiencies are most acute at provincial institutions; treatment is custodial at best. The sheer weight of outpatient contacts reinforces professional inclination towards prescribing and monitoring drug interventions.

Interinstitutional continuity of care, the ability of diverse agencies to function as a unified service system, has two weak points: (1) the inadequate linkage between the mental health and public health systems and (2) the proliferation of "dumping ground" institutions: those with multiple referral sources into them, but few, if any, referral pathways leading back out into the community.

Institutional action aimed at permitting smooth patient transition back into the social environment is another low-priority function. Manpower is deemed too precious for delivering after-care services at the home or village level. Outreach beyond the immediate agency vicinity is unthinkable. Agencies are reluctant to deploy personnel to liaison with relatives in cooperative case management during and after hospitalization. Compounding the problem, there are insufficient alternatives to inpatient care. This hinders the flow of patients from highly restrictive environments to those with minimal supervision. It also forces an overreliance on institutionalization.

Access to psychological care is severely impeded by several conditions: (1) general and specialist services are concentrated almost exclusively in one or two metropolitan districts; (2) those without financial resources can neither afford to travel to these centralized clinics nor pay for private practitioners and the minimal fees for public-funded institutions; and (3) waiting lists and chronic overcrowding of the few respected inpatient units frustrate potential users and are nightmares to outpatients waiting long hours for brief physician consultations. In essence, rural and low-income citizens are disenfranchised from public mental health care.

CONDITIONS FAVORING PROVISION OF MODERN MENTAL HEALTH CARE

Juxtaposed with the limitations, there are also national and agency-level conditions that appear favorable to the provision of modern psychiatry.

Historically, indigenous psychiatrists have created and maintained connections with overseas centers of psychiatric education and research. By necessity, the first group of sojourners received their postgraduate instruction in these centers. As initial couriers of Western mental health technology, they founded the new discipline upon their return. Subsequent generations of students were dispatched along the international pathways forged by their instructors to bring back updated theories and practices. The two-way avenues of interchange between indigenous professionals and overseas colleges have become a fruitful source for alternative conceptions of disorders, treatment strategies, and models of practitioner education.

Consultants and expert advisors from the World Health Organization (WHO) constitute a potent support group for innovation and elaboration of national mental health programs. Except for Taiwan, no longer a member state, these countries may draw upon WHO assistance for several functions: evaluation of existing systems; recommendations for designing new services; guidelines on the creation of national executive structures; input into educational curricula and certification; and research priorities. WHO also provides a framework for regional collaboration on these key functions. More importantly, it seeks to bolster the position of mental health programing within governmental bureaucracies.

Capital cities contain misallocations of hospitals, specialty units, university training centers, and an abundance of multidisciplinary manpower. These resources, concentrated in a relatively small area, offer an essentially modern psychiatric system. This full set of services is more appropriate to the educated upper strata of urban populations whose incomes and medical beliefs render such services accessible to them. In short, a Western standard of psychiatry is feasible within the unique confines of metropolitan capitals. There, economic conditions, "modern" values, and the cosmopolitan life of the nation's elite support and appreciate them.

Institutions within capital cities have created elaborate pathways for mutual consultation and patient referral. This network permits ease of access into the mental health system for referrals from allied agencies and enhances interinstitutional continuity of care when transfer to another facility is appropriate. Taipei has the most formal structure for integration and cooperation of city-wide institutions. Each capital, however, has key agencies whose breadth of ties throughout the network and into the community make them highly influential. This central position is used to transmit information, assist the development of other institutions, introduce innovation, and channel staff and patients among facilities.

The feasibility of achieving a Western standard of service delivery is rendered improbable by the overwhelming impediments arising from both sociopolitical forces and deficits at the level of agency operations. Despite these overpowering restrictions, however, a critical mass of service units and professionals has emerged in the capital cities. Psychiatry is accessible to select urban dwellers and achieves a measure of comprehensiveness when diverse agencies function in a cooperative, integrated manner. Furthermore, historical interchange with foreign training centers and expertise from international consultants have undergirded the creation and expansion of national mental health programs. Despite the continual infusion and updating of mental health technology by international sources, the overall impact is imperceptible. These nations simply cannot allocate sufficient political, economic, educational, and manpower resources to generate a fully functioning delivery system beyond one or two metropolitan enclaves. In brief, the Western model of psychiatry cannot be lauded as even remotely feasible as a standard for nationwide mental health service delivery.

CULTURAL SENSITIVITY OF EXISTING PSYCHIATRIC SYSTEMS

The second issue addressed by the case studies is, succinctly stated, the extent to which programs reflect prevailing community ethos. Culturally accommodating services strive to represent distinct cultural patterns in their policies, plans, and procedures. Cultural sensitivity is also measured by willingness of potential users to draw upon clinic services in times of need and clinic acceptability as a resource option among community members. This section summarizes the case study findings regarding agency acceptability and accommodation—two indices of cultural sensitivity.

COMMUNITY ACCEPTANCE OF EXISTING PSYCHIATRIC SERVICES

The community/agency gap is bridged through active institutional liaison with responsible persons from the patient's natural environment. Yet, there are few formal ways in which community members close to the patient are brought into the procedures for goal setting and therapy administration. Unquestionably, treatment planning and case management are the purview of the medical staff, especially the physician, who remains the final authority.

Acceptability is also strengthened by formal avenues of agency accountability to the opinions of social leaders and service recipients. However, the concept of a community advisory board empowered to assist program specification was alien to every agency except the Philippine Mental Health Association (PMHA). Needs-assessment surveys, a second means of establishing accountability by identifying underserved users, were also absent from program priorities.

In the eyes of service providers, mental institutions are disturbingly alienated and isolated from the ongoing stream of community life. They see their clinics as unknown or mostly misunderstood. Even worse, institutional care stigmatizes those who receive it. Psychiatry is thus reserved as a last resort when all other methods of help have failed. In short, programs are rejected by citizens whose beliefs and health customs are incongruent with what is offered. There are grave doubts about meaningful integration and acceptance of mental health institutions in these communities by the staff who work in them.

Agency penetration by the community was noted at a few key points of contact involving family members. Examples were recorded of family therapy, family education seminars, and spouse counseling. Relatives were sometimes assigned the responsibility of watching for new symptoms, giving medicine, and making sure the patient returned for follow-up visits. Furthermore, institutions encouraged visitation and permitted families to bring in food and money. The most significant correspondence between clinic and patient's social group occurred in Taiwanese and Philippine institutions which allowed relatives to "live in" and take part in the day-to-day management routine.

The PMHA and Taipei's Life-Line Center were the only two programs with administrative accountability to local review boards. Private agencies in general seem to have a better chance of operating under the auspices of review boards whose membership includes wider community interests than just the medical fields.

Agency acceptance was not a problem, according to respondents, after the family made the commitment to bring their distressed member for help. Once this threshold was surpassed, rejection of treatment approaches and disbelief in therapeutic efficacy appear to subside. It may be that agency contact mobilizes hope in a positive outcome. This may be true especially in light of the monumental hardships endured by the family and patient prior to their receiving clinic assistance.

In conclusion, community integration into agency practices chiefly involved family participation in some aspect of in-hospital and discharge care. Still, these gestures cannot begin to offset the profound stigma and alienation experienced by agencies. Stated tersely, psychiatric institutions are unacceptable to most, except when all other avenues have failed and desperation reaches its climax. Small, private outpatient clinics or those educationally oriented and with leadership tied to local interests may be the exception to this strongly negative conclusion.

CULTURE ACCOMMODATION IN AGENCY OPERATIONS

The second index of cultural sensitivity is measurable through efforts to incorporate key customs of community health behavior into institutional environments.

Kinship Role

The preeminent position of Asian kinship groups in controlling the lives of individual family members is generally recognized among mental health workers. The initial point of clinic contact with the family is thought crucial for engendering their cooperation and respect, and halting the widening patient/family chasm which may result in abandonment to institutional care. Preliminary accommodation to gain kinship confidence was undertaken in a variety of ways: entire families were invited in for the intake interview; physicians sought to relieve unspoken fears by fully explaining treatment approaches and asking permission prior to shock therapy; quick, demonstrable improvements via drugs were sought before asking family participation in rehabilitation efforts; and family attendants are allowed to live-in on certain wards. Other examples where the strong emotional attachments between relatives are taken into account include family attendance at ward groups to plan home care, assignment of specific after-care responsibilities to parents and spouses, and permission to bring in food, money, and holy water from sacred healers.

Folk Theories

Sensitivity to popular and folk theories of illness is another requirement of a culturally responsive organization. The most dominant form of accommodation to indigenous conceptions is nonjudgmental acceptance of them. When confronted with such beliefs, it was recognized that attacking them directly would only serve to alienate the patient. One strategy was simply to ignore folk notions or gently point out the difference between traditional and "scientific" concepts. Seasoned therapists recognized that knowledge of folk nosologies and culture-bound syndromes was useful in working effectively with traditional clients. Ethnopsychiatrists, such as Sangun Suwanlert, guide their medical interventions by a thorough understanding of how belief in spirit possession, for example, influences symptom expression and response to treatment. Most workers manifest a permissive attitude toward adherence to folk healing customs as long as it does not interfere with their approach to therapy. A few even permit visitation to priests or herbalists during hospitalization. At minimum, there is a general awareness that patients take a circuitous route to the hospital, arriving only after a variety of local healers and self-cures are exhausted.

Ward Activities

Ward-level activities provide a rich arena for accommodation to family/patient relationship, folk beliefs, and other important aspects of the

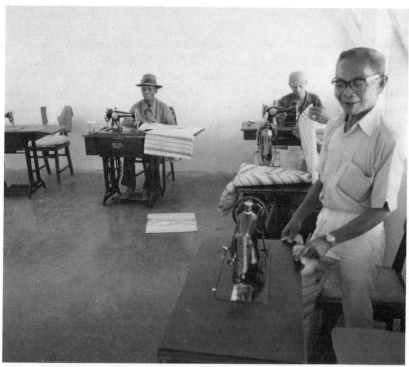

An occupational therapist in Indonesia teaches his patients the tailor's craft.

patient's background. Linguistic matching—the assignment of patients to staff who speak the same dialect—was prevalent throughout these programs. Often, relatives of ill, elderly, suicidal, or unmanageable inpatients were asked to reside on the ward as "watchers" or amahs. The Buddhist Priest's Hospital was set up in harmony with the culture of its residents; all attendants there are male and physicians are careful to accord full respect to the holy men they treat. Recreational and vocational therapies were aimed at familiar pastimes. They also teach skills enabling persons to return to their families capable of making an economic contribution. Ethnic and religious minorities were sometimes permitted to stay together in the hospital and observe their own customs of worship and diet. Practitioners deemed it urgent to stabilize minority patients with drugs and return them quickly to their families because hospitals were even more alien to them than to other groups. At several sites, acreage was devoted to attractive landscaping and flora. Besides giving the residents an opportunity to do their own gardening, these natural scenes were intended to stimulate an aesthetic sense among residents and perhaps induce a relaxed state of mind.

Therapist's Manner

Persons seeking clinic aid appear to hold well-defined expectations of what the therapist's manner should be in order to make them feel secure and confident. The most commonly described attribute was that of an omnipotent authority figure in command of the situation. Yet, equally important, the authoritarian stance should be tempered with a warm, human side. The therapist should allow emotional dependency, be cheerful, friendly, and helpful. It was also best for the therapist to give direct, concrete advice and exude confidence that the intervention will assuredly work. In Taiwan, sensitivity to nonverbal communication was considered a prerequisite as Chinese are reserved in verbal self-expression. In all cases, one should avoid shaming the patient and mentioning embarrassing topics until the relationship is well-established.

Expected Therapeutics

To an overwhelming extent, patients admitted to psychiatric clinics express their presenting problems to staff in somatic terms. Under the influence of the biomedical setting, patients voice expectations that curing measures are physical rather than emotional or religious. Superficially, it appears as if hospital care accommodates to these expectations with its uniform components of psychotropic medication, electroconvulsive shock, bed rest, and vitamin supplements. But ethnomedical data suggest that secular medicine fails to address the body-spirit dualism underpinning folk theories of health and illness. A small number of nonmedically oriented centers do exist and sometimes provide orientation sessions to teach clients what to expect. Therapists interested in applying psychological interventions—talk therapies—first meet their patients' medical expectations in order to build rapport and compliance before shifting to alternative strategies.

INSTANCES OF NONACCOMMODATION

More than 80 percent of those responding to questionnaires endorsed twelve of the sixteen accommodation scale items. Staff unanimously agreed that they should adjust their manner to fit patient expectations, know traditional names for mental disorder, and allow community leader participation in facility development. With such strong, consistent endorsement of these sixteen accommodation statements, it could be concluded that most professionals are favorably disposed to culture accommodation when providing services to traditional client populations. Yet, there are clear discrepancies between these apparent positive attitudes and actual practices found in or missing from clinic procedures. For example, there was a conspicuous lack of involvement of community leaders in planning facility activities. While in the hospital, patients are in fact isolated from community activities, although most staff agree that they should not be. Below are other examples of nonaccommodation to community customs detracting from agency cultural validity.

Patient Reeducation

Many staff consider it proper, even mandatory, to reeducate those patients maintaining traditional conceptions of psychopathology. Personnel strive to teach traditional-minded individuals to view their problems in psychiatric terms. Becoming acquainted with psychiatric methods will presumably make them more psychologically minded. Even those ethnopsychiatrists who have documented the influence of indigenous theories on symptom expression maintain that the effective psychotherapist, while accepting the patient's scheme, must reinterpret it for himself in modern concepts. In brief, the "superstitious" patient must be educated to a more "rational" understanding of his problem. In the expression of this attitude, we recognize how practitioners exposed to the Western medical orientation assimilate values of individual autonomy, psychological mindedness, and secular health. Adopting these values both alienates indigenous professionals from their native cultures and makes them systematically blind to the cultural influences on the illness and care of their patients (Kleinman, personal communication).

Native Healer Rejection

Although there was solid agreement that staff should know the folk healing practices for mental disorder, in no instance was native healer participation sought in management. Most, in fact, eschew folk doctor involvement. They view it as a waste of finances, a delay from proper care, or even harmful. Staff will ask that families stop taking their ailing member to indigenous practitioners while under psychiatric care. When staff feel that such visits interfere with their own therapeutics, they insist on discontinuation of healer contact.

Social Class Differences

Even though it was clearly recognized that social differences between staff and clients was a moderate problem, there was seldom any policy or recommendation that personnel be hired whose backgrounds closely matched those of service users. This problem was most acute in Thailand. Rural Thai are extremely reluctant to approach persons of the physician's status. Communication barriers arise from differences in social status and differences in education, thinking styles, and basic values between the two groups. Patients are put off by the businesslike, arrogant, scolding, and inattentive manner of clinic doctors. They much prefer local healers who spend a lot of time with them, explaining what has caused their illness and expressing genuine concern.

Limited Family Participation

As a rule, institutions prefer minimal interference by family members in the treatment regimen. With pressing shortages of personnel, it is simply too great a luxury in most cases to take the time to permit community members meaningful involvement in the therapeutic routine. Families are invited to visit and staff do encourage their continued contact with the patient to avoid abandonment, but any treatment role relatives do play is generally circumscribed.

Negative Stereotypes

Lastly, mental institutions not only carry the negative connotations of custodial care—confinement places for the "mad" and hospitals from which no one returns—but are also associated with poor souls dying away from home. In Thailand, such places are filled with the wandering spirits of persons who did not have a peaceful death in their homes. These spirits themselves are looking to possess the living and cause illness.

In review, sociocultural elements such as strong kinship ties, indigenous conceptions of illness, expectations of therapist manner and medical applications, are represented in the day-to-day procedures of certain clinics. Such efforts bring a closer correspondence between these Western-derived institutions and the prevailing cultures in which they are embedded. Yet, a careful scrutiny of existing culture accommodation practices shows that many are undertaken at the initial phase of agency-family contact as a method to win confidence, respect, and rapport. Once the initial expectations are met and compliance is established, these same agencies switch into their preferred treatment modalities. With newly won patient cooperation, they coax the uninitiated into accepting established psychiatric procedures.

CONCLUSION

The case study findings are unequivocal on the issue of whether or not the standard of Western psychiatry is feasible as a model for service delivery among Southeast Asian nations. At national or even regional levels, these countries are unable and unwilling to allocate economic, educational, administrative, research, and manpower resources to secure the standards of care prescribed by contemporary criteria of comprehensive service delivery. Extant psychiatric systems, functioning in an integrated fashion, are capable of providing sufficient intervention resources to meet the needs of a circumscribed number of middle- and upper-class residents of these nations' capital cities.

The question of cultural sensitivity of mental hospitals and clinics is less straightforward because community attitudes were not directly assessed. Nevertheless, staff perceive their clinics as alien entities in the ongoing stream of community life. Psychiatric treatment is stigmatizing; it is unacceptable except at the last possible moment as a desperate gesture to relieve suffering. Yet, a tiny scattering of community-based units —staffed mainly by nonmedical personnel—do appear well-connected with diverse community groups. They appear nonthreatening and more acceptable, serving as conduits into the mental health network.

Agency-specific practices of culture accommodation diminish community alienation by strengthening cultural validity. A full range of accommodation tactics was noted, but most tended to be informal and makeshift. Accommodation per se was not elevated to the level of policy or program objective.

Moreover, accommodation undertaken at the initial point of agency contact was intended to win over family confidence and cooperation. Once staff secured the family's commitment to treatment, then clinic-preferred therapy modes were introduced. Tradition-minded patients were reeducated to acquire a more psychological view of their problems and appreciate the advantages of psychiatric methods.

In summary, the sites visited were culturally insensitive and isolated in relation to the healing customs and beliefs of the general population. Their range of appropriateness and accessibility was narrowly restricted to the urban elite. The following chapter considers the implications of culturally unresponsive services and describes two perspectives on designing new programs continuous with the popular health sector.

chapter 7

Culture Accommodation of Mental Health Services and Beyond

(WITH LINDA H. CONNOR)

The foregoing critique of psychiatry in Asia expresses a forceful call for systemic change. It is a daunting challenge to speculate what can be done to reformulate mental health resources to serve the interests of indigenous peoples in the Third World. Our perspective of required change is dualistic. In the immediate future, services should be modified according to guidelines formulated through methods of culture assessment and culture accommodation. In the long term, we must move beyond institutional reform toward strengthening culture-specific alternatives to psychiatric care. Psychiatric resources must be dramatically reshaped to become part and parcel of ongoing, community-controlled helping systems, operating through the myriad social support networks that sustain community health and life satisfaction.

In this chapter, we offer an initial delineation of our dualistic perspective in the hope that it will stimulate reaction among health administrators. We expect further refinement of these preliminary ideas by our colleagues within the disciplines of social science and medicine and would consider the mission a success if the viability of this perspective were tested by Third World workers and those serving diverse groups in industrialized nations.

CULTURE ASSESSMENT IN THE SERVICE OF INSTITUTIONAL REFORM: THE SHORT-TERM PERSPECTIVE

The psychiatric institutions of Asia, alienated and impoverished as we found them, will not be transformed overnight. Even though many are sorely deficient as therapeutic communities and are, at best, custodial warehouses, these institutions still represent the only "home" possible for many of their residents at this time. Hence we would argue for short-term institutional reform based on a unified, culture-specific approach to the provision of helping services. This approach must be capable of coping with the dilemmas outlined in chapter 6 while offering a testable vision of how cultural sensitivity is achievable. The concept of culture accommodation aptly satisfies these demands.

Toward an Integration of Cultural Context with the Design of Services Using Culture Assessment

A working model of culture accommodation specifies the tasks that accommodation must perform. These tasks, viewed as outcome variables or "consequences" of accommodation, are manifested at three levels:

Level One: Structural Qualities

Low resource intensive. Programs created are low budget, nondemanding of professional manpower. They operate without elaborate infrastructure and require minimal administrative functions or institutional facilities.

Enhanced accessibility. The helping service is sited in a natural gathering place easily reached on foot or by bike. System entry procedures that are more attractive to users are followed, especially operating hours, intake questions, cost, time delays, architecture, and child care for waiting parents.

Maximum administrative openness. The program is open to local community review and control of policy formulation, hiring, and finances and therefore generates a sense of community responsibility and "ownership" of services.

Level Two: Social Ecology Qualities

Enhanced acceptability. The helping service is nonstigmatizing and nonalienating and engenders positive attitudes among community members.

Health network inclusive. The program is intimately linked with informal referral pathways used by help-seekers once "illness" management moves beyond the immediate family nexus. It promotes a "psychological sense of community," whereby users perceive themselves as part of a readily available, mutually supportive network of relationships that can be depended upon to ease stress and loneliness (Sarason 1974).

Increased community competency and self-management. The program reinforces existing community skills and coping strategies. Available helpers are supported in case management only when necessary. The overarching aim of this policy is to secure community independence from reliance upon limited institutional resources.

Continuity with prevailing social norms, beliefs, and power relationships. Program practices respect pluralistic life styles and philosophies. No attempt is made to disrupt or modify the unique explanations of disorder, learning styles, standards of community adjustment, or beliefs regarding efficacious curing techniques.

Level Three: Healing and Helping Qualities

Reducing community stressors. The helping service has far-reaching effects when it supports community social action efforts to remove community-identified sources of distress. These may include unemployment, discrimination, unresponsive government bureaucracies, and environmental pollution.

Heightened prognostic expectancies. Service users manifest a strong expectation of treatment success stimulated by the qualities of helpers and the therapeutic procedures undertaken.

User satisfaction. Clients and family members positively evaluate treatment efficacy. Users don't unexpectedly drop out, are willing to reuse the program, and recommend it to kinsmen, friends, and neighbors.

What antecedent conditions help determine these outcomes? Table 7.1 presents a three-phase model of culture accommodation, showing the linkage between antecedent and consequent conditions. Two antecedent phases are necessary. First, culture assessment of the local community is accomplished by constructing an ethnographic description of relevant dimensions. Added to the description are priorities contributed by local decision makers and others, including women in the household, who directly manage illness episodes. Second, accommodation implementation is attempted by translating assessment findings into a plan to modify a helping system or design a new program. Literature in the disciplines of medical anthropology, transcultural psychiatry, and minority mental health converge to suggest important culture assessment dimensions.

FOUNDATIONS OF CULTURE ASSESSMENT

Study of ethnomedicine and social support networks provides departure points for determining attributes of a culture or community group that must be understood prior to implementing an accommodation program (see Draguns 1980; Fabrega 1977; Marsella and White 1982; and Mitchell and Trickett 1980 for reviews). The literature offers three contributions: (a) culture-specific (emic) definitions of abnormality and causal explanations; (b) sociocultural correlates of disorder, including formal models

TABLE 7.1 Culture Accommodation Model

Antecedent Conditions		Consequent Conditions
Phase 1: Culture assessment	*Phase 2: Accommodation implementation*	*Outcome and validating criteria*
Semantic illness network	Translate culture assessment data into helping program in terms of:	Structural qualities:
Analysis of culturally defined problem:	Siting/architecture	Low resource intensive
Explanatory model:	Goals/objectives	Enhanced accessibility
Classification	Policies/procedures	Maximum administrative openness
Labeling	Organizational social climate/manning level	
Etiology	Personnel	Social ecology qualities:
Attitudes and norms vis-a-vis sick role	Therapeutics	Enhanced acceptability
Norms of personal adjustment	Administrative style	Health network inclusive
Expected ways and means of curing:	Community relations	Increased community competency, self-management, and psychological sense of community
Social support networks		Continuity with prevailing social norms, beliefs, power relationships
Healers		
Tactics of social influence		Healing/helping qualities:
Expected community relationship with agency:		Reduced community stressors
Community control		Heightened prognostic expectancies
Structure and social climate		User satisfaction
Folk healer integration		
Personnel characteristics and manners		

relating sociocultural stress, disintegration, immigration, and rapid social change to rates of psychological problems; and (c) sociocultural
responses to disorder such as family involvement and formally prescribed procedures for healing and psychotherapy.

These three domains can be transformed into a set of assessment questions to be answered through an ethnographic study of the recipient community and through political decision making at the local level. Ideally,
the culture assessment exercise should obtain some measure of political
legitimacy prior to its initiation. One strategy is to carry out the exercise
under the auspices of an umbrella organization representing the interests
of local constituencies. Briefly, the design of a culture accommodation
treatment program follows an assessment of: cultural perceptions of
problem behavior; philosophy and norms of individual adjustment; social support networks and folk healing practices; and expected community relationship with the agency.

Analysis of a Culturally Defined Problem

A typology of problem behavior as conceptualized by culture members is
the first assessment component. As in ethnomedical analysis (Kleinman
1980), questions are posed regarding episodes of behavioral disorder and
how such occurrences are classified, labeled, explained, and responded
to by members of the informal support networks and formal care providers. Problem behavior typologies, anchored in cultural belief systems,
are intimately linked with behavioral options for therapy and cannot be
understood separately. The composite network of meanings that the sufferer cognitively experiences as the interrelation of problem conception, life stress, fears about the disorder, social reactions of family and
friends, and therapeutic expectations constitutes the community's "semantic illness network" (Good 1977; Good and Good 1980; Kleinman
1978, 1980) and accounts for the cultural patterning of illness in a setting.

Several interrelated elements compose the problem typology. The first
of these is the indigenous classification scheme used to identify and label
disturbing behaviors (e.g., Jocano 1973; Muecke 1979; Wu 1982). An
important consideration is the process of person/group interaction and
the covert rules governing the assignment of a label (Ullmann and Krasner 1975; Carr 1978). No behavior per se is deviant—the social label is
applied by group members observing violations of social expectations
(Draguns 1980; Frank 1973). Behavior is labeled abnormal following several considerations: the person's role and status; frequency and duration
of the action; the time and setting in which it takes place; and power
inequality between the label recipient and those labeling (Bandura 1977;
Fabrega 1971; Kilbride 1979; Marsella 1979).

Another problem typology element involves mapping the perceived etiology of each disorder type. Some conditions are thought to be caused by such sources as "spoilt brain" (Orley 1970) or "wind" entering the body (Chen 1970). Many world cultures understand sickness as the result of intrusion into the body of some sort of malevolent influence (Moerman 1979). Geoff White (1982) observes that the common mode of reasoning about illness in American culture—interpreting certain somatic complaints as psychological in origin—is in fact a minority interpretation when cast in world perspective. For example, research with Chinese university students discovered that physical complaints are perceived explicitly in somatic physiologic terms or with reference to situational demands rather than being mediated by emotional or personality concepts preferred by their American- and European-ancestry counterparts (Higginbotham 1981; White 1982). Fabrega (1977) adds that sometimes illness episodes provide social diagnoses, reflecting areas of interpersonal weakness, disruptions, predicaments, or vulnerabilities within the immediate group of the sick person. Following determination of the problem's origins, each culture prescribes an appropriate *location* for therapeutic intervention. Depending on the problem, the intervenor directs ministrations toward the person, social group, supernatural world, or physical environment (Higginbotham 1976).

The final problem typology element is the social reaction or attitude toward each "type" of deviant. In fact, the attitude of the family and immediate social group may be the most crucial determinant of the natural course of problem behavior and treatment outcome (Lambo 1962; Sangsingkeo 1958; Waxler 1974, 1979). In some cases, the individual himself is not held responsible and maintains family support (Maguigad 1964). Ordinary role obligations are suspended, the equivalent of a cultural "time out," or task demands are reduced to more manageable levels for the individual without the risk of stigma (Connor 1979; Ritchie 1976). It seems particularly important that the family abstain from messages that alienate or reject the "ill" person to insure an episodic rather than degenerative outcome (Howard 1979; Waxler 1979). Some observers suggest that in belief systems where outside forces such as sorcerers or possessing spirits are blamed, the sick role may be shed rather quickly (Dean and Thong 1972; Kleinman 1977; Suwanlert 1976a). In other cases, particularly when the individual has been violent and embarrassing and repeatedly has brought suffering onto others, this process is reversed (Jackson 1964). The sick role stays with the person along with an attitude of rejection (Sheper-Hughes 1978). The individual is often banished from the village. If institutionalized, he or she is likely to be abandoned by relatives (Colson 1971; Suwanlert 1976a).

Norms of Personal Adjustment

The second component of culture assessment attends to the specific values and expectations of adjustment in the community. An accommodating program sets treatment objectives based on knowledge of socially accepted roles, standards of interpersonal relations, and boundaries of behavior for individuals in specific situations. Value orientations toward core cultural dimensions like time, man-nature relations, personal versus group goals, and human nature itself are also accounted for (Papajohn and Spielgel 1975). The behavioral qualities a person should ideally possess according to community consensus are termed *areté* (Goldschmidt 1971). It is toward the cultural *areté* that therapy attempts to resocialize the nonconformist (Draguns 1975). However, using *areté* as the outcome criterion of resocialization and skills training should be balanced against ethical considerations of individual rights, client consent and choice, and the long-range benefits for the person in a changing environment. The culture assessment consultant should also be aware that within-culture value differences may be as vivid as those compared cross-culturally.

Expected Ways and Means of Curing

A people's explanation of behavioral disorder and what constitutes normal functioning makes it possible for them to organize effective therapeutic strategies (Young 1976). The "action" component of the semantic illness network involves making treatment decisions—such as selecting appropriate care-givers—that follow logically from the illness label, perceived etiology, severity and chronicity, and from reasoning about what must change to permit health restoration. Contrasting semantic illness networks sanction unique patterns of choice among available treatment alternatives and specify whether informal or formal helping sources will be drawn upon and the sequence of their use (Kleinman 1978). However, it is quite important for policy makers to avoid assuming a culture uniformity myth regarding such patterns. Individuals sharing a common ethnicity within particular communities have been found to differ markedly regarding mental health beliefs and preferred treatment strategies (Bestman, Lefley, and Scott 1976; Lo, Fung, Woo-Sam, and Samelu 1980).

Figure 7.1 presents a model summarizing the processes linking culturally derived explanations of disorder and community coping actions. Briefly, it proposes that distinct explanatory models, derived from cultural folk theories about health, are conceptual resources communities employ to effectively meet the disruptive impact of illness and disability. Explanatory models apply labels to specific illness episodes evoking associated beliefs and attitudes regarding etiology and causality, covarying

Figure 7.1

Processes Linking Explanatory Models within the Semantic Illness Networks
and Social Support Networks

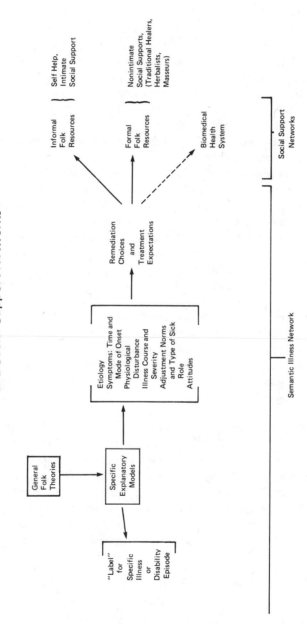

symptoms, illness course, physiological disturbance, and expected social roles related to the particular disorder (Kleinman 1980). Most importantly, these inferences become guides for narrowing the range of treatment alternatives in health care decision making. Explanatory models direct the sufferer and his or her caretakers toward appropriate or sensible remedies expected to produce the most efficacious cure. Figure 7.1 depicts treatment choices as distinct subcomponents within a person's social support resource network. Furthermore, treatment resources are conceptualized along two dimensions—informal versus formal care mode and folk versus biomedical health system.

Specifically, informal resources for curing or coping with disorder involve self-care and help remedies received from one's intimate psychosocial support network—i.e., family, close friends, workmates, and neighbors (Pattison 1977). The family and intimate associates' wider network of social ties may become activated to contact "formal" folk resources, such as traditional healers or herbalists, should intimate sources prove inadequate or be viewed as inappropriate according to the illness explanation. Nevertheless, both of these care-giving modes operate according to folk theory precepts regarding illness remediation shared by culture members.

In marked contrast, the biomedical health system is both formal, in that medical professionals and institutional settings are seldom available to people as well-integrated components of their psychosocial support network, and it promulgates health practices according to a "scientific" knowledge base. This latter ideology may have little in common with the conventional or sacred wisdom of folk theories. The biomedical care system is always the least intimate resource selection and links into the person's explanatory model to a greater or lesser extent depending on his or her socialization into the culture of modern medicine. By implication, satisfaction with the healing process and evaluation of health outcome by the patient and his or her social network depends in part on the overlap in explanatory models held by practitioners and those seeking therapy.

Analysis of folk helping resources—support networks, healers, and their curing methods—is the third culture-assessment component. In this way, we attempt to understand how the *means* of social influence employed by an agent of behavior change (healer) brings about resocialization to community goals and reassigns valued social roles to alienated members.

Informal Helping: The Role of Social Support Networks

Outside the meager services of modern psychiatry, two levels of care management serve distressed individuals: (a) the natural support network of kinfolk and close associates and (b) the formal system of folk doctors

and specialists of indigenous medicine. Complementing medical anthropologists' study of the popular health sector, community psychologists
have recently achieved a greater understanding of the vital role social
support networks play in preventing, shaping, and diminishing psychological stress and disturbance (Gottlieb 1981; Heller 1979; Pilisuk and
Parks 1981). Mitchell, Billings, and Moos (in press) have taken a careful
look at the wealth of studies measuring the health-promotive and health-
protective effects of social support and conclude that support availability directly benefits health and psychological functioning, regardless of
whether the individual is under stress. However, these reviewers found
inconsistent evidence for the stress-buffering effect of social support,
where support is assumed to indirectly affect functioning through reducing the occurrence and intensity of negative life events. Nevertheless,
social support networks typically provide their members with several
important resources. The most prominent among these are material aid,
physical assistance, intimate interactions, guidance, and interpersonal
feedback (Barrera 1981).

In particular, the family's dominant position as a support network
resource deserves careful attention during culture assessment (Fandetti
and Gelfand 1978; Manson 1980). While some kinship networks can be a
potent source of stress—capable of demanding conformity and delivering aversive judgmental feedback (see Higginbotham, in press)—a dense
family network also has the capacity to mobilize around the suffering
member. Nurturance, security, and intense intimacy are provided to
retrieve the individual's sense of self-identity and feelings of belonging to
a caring social group. Usually the kinship cluster is the most suitable
structure to buffer the distressed members against further stressful events
and maintain them outside of institutional care (Pilisuk 1982). Kleinman
(1980) reported Taiwanese data indicating that 93 percent of illnesses
were first treated in the context of the family and 73 percent of these
never left family care. Moreover, should the illness management move
beyond their domain, the family decides which practitioners are consulted, who will accompany the ill person, how long to remain in care,
whether or not to comply with treatment regimen, and how to evaluate
the outcome (Fabrega 1977; Wintrob and Harvey 1981). Among *kinship-
reliant* groups (Graves and Graves 1980), emotionally stressed persons
turn to support from one particular relative with whom they share not
only kinship but a special bond of affection and trust (Keefe, Padilla,
and Carlos 1979; Fandetti and Gelfand 1978). In contrast, ethnic groups
adopting *self-reliant* adaptive strategies may have no difficulty revealing
feelings to and securing emotional support from resource persons outside
the family such as social workers or psychologists (Graves and Graves
1980).

Formal Helping: The Role of Socially Sanctioned Healers

The second resource tier contains the network of formal helpers available in the local community. The folk practitioner system is distinguished by its intimate link with the user's popular health ideology and its ability in many cases to fulfill client expectations of successful treatment. Regarding accessibility, healers are generally enmeshed physically and functionally in local community life. They live nearby, make house calls, are frequently available at a moment's notice regardless of hour, work without fee or extend credit, and allow repayment in kind (Mackenzie 1977). For example, Balinese spirit mediums extend their interventions beyond physical or mental disorders to mediate village political disputes, elect a temple priest, find a lost cow, and resolve other social problems (Connor 1979). Equally important to fostering accessibility is the need for an absence of social class differences between helper and client (Leslie 1976). Sharing culture rules guarantees that the practitioner lives up to his ethical responsibilities, and, on the client's side, there emerges an ability to reciprocate and remove social debt or obligation. Unfortunately, in urban settings with transient populations, healers may be less enmeshed in the local context of social checks and balances. Opportunities for charlatanism and irresponsible practice arise under conditions of too-rapid social change, anonymity, and reliance upon a cash economy.

The second distinct feature of the folk practitioner is her skillful manipulation of client belief in the therapy's curative power. The concept of "treatment expectations" helps explain why culture accommodation is related to user satisfaction and positive evaluation of a program.

Culture members have set expectations about the processes and techniques of healing (Quah 1977). Different predictions of treatment outcome are based on "met" versus "unmet" expectations (Higginbotham 1977). When expectancies are tapped and included in therapy, the client recognizes that he is receiving the necessary and correct help; it is coming from a recognizable expert possessing the required skill to ameliorate suffering. The client has hope, confidence, and faith in improvement—demoralization and helplessness are counteracted.

Oftentimes the individual attributes of the folk practitioner will elicit faith and hopefulness. Her personal manner, style of speech, rituals, omniscient problem explanation, even style of dress and nonverbal messages are all appropriate to the expectations of patient and audience (Draguns 1975; Frank 1973; Lieban 1977). She knows how to inspire group confidence in the cure and mobilize family and friends as resources for the distressed person (Clark 1959; Dean and Thong 1972; Marriott 1955). Of course, in certain intractable cases, the expert mobilization of psychological and social resources by the healer is insufficient to alter the sufferer's condition. This need not be a weakness of folk practitioner systems as long as these systems make provision for identifying failures, and either refer the patients elsewhere or help to maintain them within the home locality.

In contrast, a negative patient reaction is likely when it is found that what is supposed to happen in order to receive help doesn't occur. Unless the client can be taught to appreciate agency methods, a therapeutic relationship will not develop and the patient and family will go elsewhere. Unfulfilled expectations are sparked by a treatment rationale with low credibility, inadequate explanations of the problem, and a therapist style that is unfavorably evaluated. Ignoring the client's learning style—preferences for action or cognitively mediated learning—and pragmatic needs in relation to environmental demands may also trigger treatment rejection (Goldstein 1973). Since these are associated with incompetent help, positive emotions, trust, and expectations of cure are not aroused.

Westernized doctors have been found to be especially flagrant violators of cultural expectations (Nichter 1978). Professional ideology finds morally offensive the patient's failure to comply with "expert" orders and is intolerant of alternative help-seeking activities (Kleinman 1980). Because it focuses exclusively on the disease process rather than the "total" human, villagers view Western treatment as depersonalizing, mechanistic, and fragmented. Scientific doctors spend too little time providing the assurance necessary to relieve fear among family and friends. Nursing staff, on the other hand, have been observed on occasion to fulfill this function and attempt to mediate the family's experience of institutional settings (e.g., Connor 1982a). Failure to comply with a holistic view of resolving human problems—treating simultaneously the person's physical, spiritual, and social needs—is undoubtedly the biomedical model's greatest shortcoming in the eyes of traditional people (Jaspan 1976; Marsella and Higginbotham 1979).

Formal Helping: Tactics of Social Influence

Formal and informal helpers constitute a legitimate delivery system for bringing to bear the influences of specific therapeutic techniques. Social-influence tactics, however, may operate only in and through the medium of the participants' evolving relationship. Assuming a transcultural perspective, some writers postulate a universality of therapists' behavior-influence tactics (Draguns 1975; Frank 1973; Torry 1972). Elements common to all therapeutic experiences are believed to include therapist and patient sharing a world view; therapist manifesting special personal qualities; manipulation of success expectancy; and the "specialness" of the therapist-client relationship—intense trusting and confiding. Authors following a social learning orientation analyze therapy by examining general processes accounting for human behavior in social situations in all cultures (Higginbotham and Tanaka-Matsumi 1981). Reinforcement procedures like shaping, extinction, and stimulus discrimination are assumed to underly customs and practices concerned with evoking, maintaining, and altering the social behavior of culture members. For example, Naikan therapy in Japan prescribes unique role behaviors, such as reverence for one's parents, but uses social techniques common to behavior therapy to influence clients (Tanaka-Matsumi 1979).

A third typology includes such functions as providing expert testimony, placebo manipulations, and use of modeling (Higginbotham 1976). Also involved are physical exercise, herbal medicines, concoctions for driving away or propitiating spirits, or internal self-healing mechanisms—sleep, meditation, and trance (Prince 1980). Although the cross-cultural researcher is keenly interested in developing these universal (etic) dimensions for comparing indigenous therapies, the task of culture assessment is to discover distinct techniques continuous with the style of social control relied upon in everyday life.

Expected Community Relationship with Agency

The third resource tier in the referral network is the professional health agency. The final culture-assessment component requires appraising the community's expected relationship with the treatment program. Acceptability of the program and its integration into local support networks depends upon the extent to which these expectations are met. For example, there is the issue of community control (Angrosino 1978; Panzetta 1971). Have local leaders been called upon to sanction or sponsor the service? Are personnel selection and funding allocation in the hands of the community, client group, or with the service agency? Before administering treatment, is there an effort to get informed consent? Who may give informed consent—the client, relatives, or village authorities? As a rule, the less community participation in a program's development, the more it is viewed as an unwanted intrusion and external to the community's needs and interests (Panzetta 1971). Consumers' struggles to participate in planning and implementation decisions, on the other hand, both strengthen their economic position and engender community cohesiveness, pride, and a sense of group competency (Kelly, Snowden, and Munoz 1977; Hessler 1977).

A second set of questions concerns expectations of organizational structure, social climate, and activities within the facility. Recipients may have definite preferences regarding location, cost, treatment within the home, types of service units, and the facility's community-like atmosphere (Levine 1978). When a person is suffering, program organizational features may become more salient than, for example, whether the therapy is indigenous or foreign, traditional or modern (Leslie 1977). The user may be especially concerned with how much it will cost, when the clinic is open, the treatment's promised effectiveness, and how long before it takes effect. Some users may need to know whether the agency provides a supportive and sympathetic social atmosphere (Bestman, Lefley, and Scott 1976; Leslie 1977; Moos 1974).

A key policy consideration is the family's expected involvement with the patient during agency contact. The family may insist on having one of its members remain with the patient in the hospital (e.g., Tung 1972), ask to play an active role in diagnosis, therapy, and discharge decisions, or refuse to have any contact whatsoever (Kiev 1972; Wintrob and Harvey 1981).

Community members also have definite ideas about agency personnel. The question arises of whether indigenous healers should be allowed to care for certain patients or be employed as consultants? Some psychiatrists suggest there are times when this is useful (Chen 1979; Wittkower and Warnes 1974; WHO 1975a). Kleinman (1980), however, cites several reasons opposing this integration. In particular, he believes that sacred healers may function best if their services are not organized into bureaucratic treatment settings but instead continue to function in the area between orthodox medical care and folk religion.

If folk practitioners are not among the agency staff, what are present workers expected to know about folk theories, indigenous constructions of illness, and traditional healing? Bestman, Lefley, and Scott (1976) are among the first to specify how ethnic data may be systematically used in clinical diagnosis. They recommend that professionals follow seven steps when managing minority clients. For example: if you cannot claim knowledge of culture background, are unsure of diagnosis or treatment, and suspect a culture-bound syndrome like witchcraft, search for precipitating factors. You should ask the client: "Do you think someone may have done something to you?" If you are *sure* you know how to cure the problem, tell the patient this and state approximately how many days it will take to recover. If the patient says it might be witchcraft, assure him that your therapy will help alleviate the symptoms and try to get a competent faith/folk healer or priest for tandem treatment.

Lastly, age, sex, social status, language capabilities, and ethnicity all play a role in the evaluation of helpers. However, the absolute effect of these factors on treatment outcome is a hotly debated issue in cross-cultural counseling (Higginbotham and Tanaka-Matsumi 1981). Some counselors of American minorities rule out helpers who do not share the client's sociocultural/linguistic background and perhaps even gender. Ruiz and Casas (1981) press for counselor bilingualism and biculturalism as requirements for working with American Chicanos. Partially agreeing,

Draguns (1981) warns that even for bilinguals, second-language usage is tricky. Fleeting allusions and nuances of intonation and meaning can be lost upon the recipient unless that individual is attuned to the subtleties of a specific culture's language usage. Sundberg's (1981) review of Black Americans in counseling lends weight to the notion that minority clients readily approach, are more self-disclosing, and in general prefer to talk with counselors with whom they share racial heritage.

While refraining from the conclusion that matching therapist and client on ethnic variables is necessary for positive outcome, we do assert that agencies should try vigorously to employ persons identified with the user's cultural milieu. Indigenous workers have the trust of their clients and need not spend time proving themselves or overcoming suspicions (Moritsugu 1980). Data from recent studies examining the therapeutic potency of paraprofessionals (Durlak 1979) would lead us to predict that carefully selected ethnic mental health workers can achieve clinical results equivalent to or better than those of professional staff for certain problems. Furthermore, Bestman et al. (1976) and Garrison's (1979) pioneering work serves as a model for discovering effective paraprofessionals and establishing them as "culture specialists" and "culture brokers" in the operation of culturally accommodating mental health services. These ethnic specialists evaluate diagnostic procedures, validate therapeutic methods, and use local social support networks in managing clinic cases.

In summary, we advocate culture assessment as a primary tool for renovating current psychiatric systems. Subsequently, the measure of successful institutional reform will be the attainment of culture-accommodation criteria. Clearly this requires equal contributions of ethnographic analysis and political decision making. However, this short-term view of designing programs with a high level of cultural sensitivity must give way at some point to a long-range perspective. The future of psychiatric care we envisage is founded upon the identification and strengthening of setting-specific health networks. Resources are more effectively diffused through existing cultural forms that provide caring ties to those in distress. The end product of both long- and short-term aspects of our perspective is creation of competent communities capable of actualizing values and goals they select for themselves.

REFORMULATION OF PSYCHIATRIC RESOURCES: THE LONG-TERM PERSPECTIVE

In this final section, we speculate on how resource development might be amassed through amplification of extant care-giving within the community nexus. These propositions are tentative, both in the sense that they require further elaboration to be suitable for particular localities and in that their efficacy remains to be demonstrated. Nevertheless, we risk offering these novel solutions, which depart sharply from current modes of reasoning, because we cannot foresee substantial resolution to the problems enumerated in this volume with the strategies and proposals now circulating within the international mental health network. In essence, our argument responds to Professor Tsung-yi Lin's plea, eloquently stated in his Margaret Mead Memorial Address at the World Congress of Mental Health:

> Mental health in the Third World has reached a point where critical reassessment of goals and reformulation of immediate tasks are imperative in the context of rapidly changing realities. Bold new approaches are needed to meet the overwhelming demands. Priorities in each society must be reordered so as to make best use of indigenous resources efficiently and economically (Lin 1981: 19).

ARGUMENTS FOR REFORMULATING RESOURCE ALLOCATION PRIORITIES WITHIN PSYCHIATRY

Psychiatric institutions in Third World countries are culturally, economically, and politically distant from the populations they are supposed to serve. There are many shortcomings of psychiatric therapy as practiced among peasant and urban masses in the countries for which historical and contemporary information is available. This is despite the fact that psychiatric institutions have appropriated all the resources available for mental health care in these settings. Small-scale, community-based support systems and indigenous healers, working with no government fiscal allocation, are able, on the other hand, to respond constructively to the vast majority of problems. The failures of indigenous providers, as evidenced by the minority of patients who reach custodial psychiatric care, may be more spectacular than their successes. Yet, we have only to observe the clinical failures who have experienced the full repertoire of psychiatric interventions (in Western industrialized societies as well as developing world regions) to realize that there are insufficient grounds for asserting that indigenous healing systems are largely responsible for the chronicity of psychiatric cases.

Medical practitioners in the region under study are members of dominant classes that historically have manifested little political commitment to the problems of the rural and urban populace. Contemporary elites are formed out of groups who for many decades mediated colonial rule to the indigenous populations and who were thereby politically, culturally, and economically oriented to the urban centers of colonial administration and to the mother countries beyond (Gruenbaum 1981). Their education and medical practices reflect these circumstances, even now. Only in recent years has health delivery policy in many developing countries moved away from the colonial heritage of urban-based, individualized medical care to the pursuit of rural-based, primary health care programs with a public health emphasis. This is despite the fact that 80 to 90 percent of the citizens of these countries live and always have lived in rural areas. Practice has been slow to follow new policy and program recommendations, with the majority of human service personnel still located in urban communities and deeply involved in providing elite forms of care to paying private patients (cf. Mejia, Pizurki, and Royston 1979). Training programs growing out of the expertise and value orientations of urban-based practitioners, many of whom are Western-educated, often emphasize the resource deficits of health care infrastructure in rural zones of their own countries while remaining insensitive to the indigenous resources that are already there.

What do elite groups, represented in this case by psychiatric professionals, have to offer the majority of patients? In most cases, what is available is less a comprehensive therapeutic program than physical custodianship and psychotropic medication. It is doubtful whether many of the recipients relinquish their indigenous conceptualizations of their plight for less-satisfying medical models. In fact, it is pertinent to acknowledge the complex ways in which disturbed behavior is interpreted and treated in most folk cultural settings, in contrast to the paucity of diagnostic and therapeutic models that clinic staff have to offer patients and families. This contrast is one index of the considerable cultural gap that separates the professionalized practitioner from the communities of potential patients. Often the paramedicals in the mental health delivery system may have the greater capacity and incentive to translate seemingly arcane practices of their institutions into an idiom that patients and families can understand (cf. Connor 1982a: 790; Garrison 1979). While many psychiatrists are aware that the biomedical constructions of "mental illness" are alien to their recipient audiences, attempts to facilitate better communication about psychological problems among practitioner, patient, and patient's relatives have been isolated and ad hoc. Paramedicals, who often have a greater commitment to this endeavor and who are better qualified to attempt it, unfortunately are placed in a position where they have no power to implement change within the health bureaucracy.

This last point raises the question of political control over the allocation of mental health care expenditures. It is apparent that the communities from which most patients are drawn have virtually no control over the implementation of health care policies. This is one manifestation of the way in which centralized bureaucracies in these countries control their massive but politically peripheral populations. In the field of health care, the projected development is one in which complex medical manipulations conveyed by a centralized bureaucracy effect a transfer of care from the family and local community to specialists who have little knowledge of local conditions or accountability to local constituents.

We suggest that any long-term solution to the problems of psychological care should have a political dimension: that is, it should be premised on rural community control of a significant proportion of health care resources. This would mean the creation of a body of professionals and paramedicals who strongly identify their interests with those of the villagers they serve. Given the more global approach of indigenous peoples to their own health problems, we would expect to see the incorporation of hitherto isolated psychiatric units into a community health system with more expertise and resources going into local polyclinics which are already established in many countries. Is it not these institutions that should become the hub of the health delivery system—operating at the direction of their local communities and in consultation with indigenous and modern health care-givers—rather than overcrowded offices in the far-off metropolis?

Toward Strengthening Culture-Specific Alternatives to Psychiatric Intervention

The relationship between the rhetoric of health care policy makers and the reality of current health delivery is not without its contradictions. For example, primary health care policies and programs have been hailed as one way of incorporating local communities into the health delivery process. Many authors have described the promise of primary health care ideology as promoting universal access to low-cost basic health care through the training of locally selected community members to be responsible for their own public health services. In brief, these policies portend the equalization and decentralization of limited medical resources within the context of developing Third World nations (e.g., WHO 1978d; Mahler 1981). In some countries, higher policy seeks to incorporate traditional healers into the national delivery system through primary health care programs (Green 1980; Rappaport and Rappaport 1981.) Such policies are more often than not formulated in the absence of any detailed knowledge of the activities of these practitioners or of their position in rural communities. Development and restructuring of local facilities that seek to attenuate, integrate, or assimilate the functions of traditional practitioners, or indeed of other local influentials, may only be intimidating to folk specialists given the present political climates of the countries concerned (e.g., see Esman et al. 1980).

Furthermore, primary health care policies in general enjoin people to take more responsibility for their own health care without giving them the resources or power to do so; ultimately, these programs are imposed from the center. In some countries, villagers are removed from the area of politics but nevertheless are expected to rally in the cause of primary health care programs over the formulation of which they have had no control (e.g., Parlato and Favin 1982). Primary health care projects may end up at best an exercise in political tokenism, or at worst as just another avenue for the introduction of alien values and administrative structures into rural communities (e.g., Uphoff, Cohen, and Goldsmith 1979). For example, Pounds (1982) found that a primary health project set up in Bali called for an implementation strategy emphasizing strong local leadership, but this in fact clashed with Balinese consensus ideology common in village political life.

What alternatives are there to primary health care policies with the shortcomings described above? Can health care resources be channeled along different paths altogether? Could medical and paramedical practitioners be better oriented to the sorts of support systems and prevention regimes that already exist in many rural communities? While there are weaknesses in the indigenous system, this is not in itself sufficient justification for imposing an alien system on populations or expanding it where it has already proved unworkable.

The suggestions we are making are premised on new research and training priorities among health care professionals and a restructured service delivery network. A source of these priorities is the culture accommodation framework engendering commitment to indigenous modes of conceptualizing stress, illness and health, interpersonal breakdown, and efficacious solutions to psychological disturbance. Eventually psychiatry would cease to exist as a distinct category of ideas and practices for dealing with illness in the context of rural health care. The polyclinics already situated in rural districts would emerge as the hub of the service system and become the focus of activities of specialists as well as less-highly trained health workers. This means some early prolonged exposure to rural conditions during the training phase of health providers. Ideally, personnel would be drawn from or assigned to areas where they know regional languages. Moreover, they should be prepared to adopt the role of participant-facilitator—working whenever feasible under the auspices of community organizations with the aim of identifying and supporting the often subtle forms of community care-giving and stress

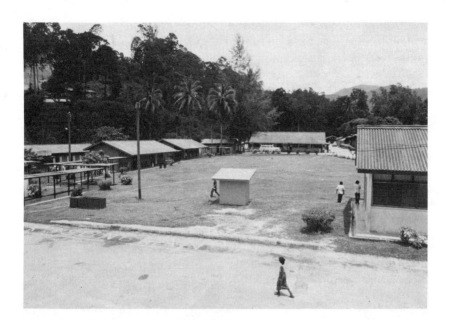

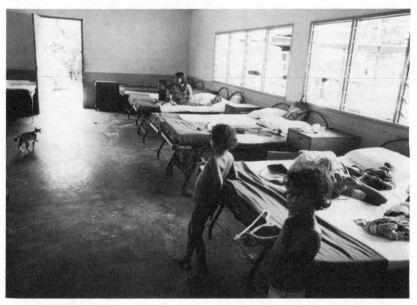

Two views of Gombok hospital, in which Orang Asli families from the jungles of Peninsular Malaysia can receive care in a setting more compatible with their village homes.

mediation embedded in village transactions. Concomitantly the health worker would be encouraged to shed as quickly as possible the "outsider-authority" image that accompanies someone of professional status who is introduced to these settings.

The place of biomedical psychiatry within the newly constituted poly-clinic system would be twofold. First, psychiatrists would become the chief translators of biomedical knowledge and technology to outreach personnel (e.g., nurses). Outreach workers, in the course of their partici-pant-facilitator obligations, would evaluate the advantages of using such knowledge in their negotiations with people in the patient's community. Some psychiatrists, by virtue of language competency or cultural co-membership, may be inclined to serve as a direct translator of the bio-medical model into the popular health idiom for cases referred by the outreach worker (cf. Good and Good 1980). Second, psychiatrists could be called upon for their expertise in neurological evaluation and accurate referral to general medical facilities as well as supervision of prescription medication.

Reformulating Psychiatric Resources: A Balinese Example

A brief example of what we envision as a culture-specific alternative to institutionalized psychiatry can be constructed on the basis of Connor's (1982c) ethnography of Balinese traditional healing. Current expendi-tures to operate the island's mental hospital and sundry outpatient clinics could be reallocated into a two-pronged system for developing multiple care options in lieu of hospitalization. This system would strive both to prevent "failures" from occurring within the indigenous healing nexus, and to bolster village strengths in responding to those "failures" that do emerge.

Indigenous healers (called *balians*) in Bali probably number several thousand. The word *balian* has generally been translated as "traditional healer" in ethnographic literature, but the significance of *balians'* func-tions extends beyond this sphere: they are consecrated practitioners who perform many priestly functions, and they are often highly esteemed people with some influence in the affairs of Balinese rural communities. *Balians* operate in a diverse range of healing capacities, none of which are mutually exclusive. Some specialize in reading, transcribing, and interpreting archaic Javanese-Balinese manuscripts about medicine, magic, and mysticism. Others work as midwives, spirit mediums, mas-seurs, and bonesetters. As well, there are numerous practitioners who traffic in charms and rituals to render the body invulnerable to both physical and magical attack, who peddle love potions, and who sell pro-tective amulets with accompanying ceremonial prescriptions for almost any purpose. Although their skills are diverse, all *balians* struggle with misfortune, disease, and death on behalf of individuals and communities by deploying their spiritual powers as mediators between a domain of supernatural activity of which they have privileged knowledge and their client's immediate concerns.

Preventing "failures" among Balinese healers. Defined simply, a "failure" emerges in the traditional Balinese healing system when, in the judgment of those concerned, a psychological illness episode persists unaccountably in the face of diverse specialist interventions, continues to cause distress to the patient and family, and finally moves into the "official" health sector of district hospitals and local polyclinics. Connor's (1978, 1982a) survey of mental hospital patients and their families showed that in cases of psychological breakdown and interpersonal stress, almost 80 percent of patients visited one or more traditional healers before moving into the official health sector. For reasons indicated above, patients and families are generally extremely reluctant to move outside the traditional health sector for problems of this nature. Help-seeking priorities for other illness categories may differ from this pattern. Yet, in the case of psychological problems, resource reallocation should aim primarily to reduce the number of failures in an indigenous system that is already working efficiently. This would proceed through finding out and remedying what has led to *balian* failure, thereby reducing the number of persons needing to move into alienating institutionalized forms of patient management.

For example, if specific government health and economic policies are undercutting opportunities for the healers to learn and effectively practice their craft, then these policies should be reviewed in light of their adverse health consequences. At minimum, government agencies should acknowledge and support the operation of healers as primary health providers for their spheres of expertise. While doing so health ministries must cautiously avoid measures to license, regulate, or monitor folk specialists or co-opt their allegiance through providing monetary incentives (e.g., Indonesian Ministry of Health 1978). Such measures invariably produce a reduction in maneuverability for sacred practitioners by undercutting their ritual base and distancing them from the influence of local residents and mutual interdependency. However, when discussing the problem of *balian* failure, we cannot discount the fact that one factor may be incompetent and irresponsible healers. But in these cases, there are existing controls: such practices usually experience declining clientele or great pressure to conform to local ethical and procedural standards.

Failures by local healers can also be expected with cases that have identifiable neurological, nutritional, and disease etiologies. There is no reason why *balians* cannot be taught to identify such circumscribed conditions—which many already do anyway—and call in the ambulatory polyclinic nurse for consultation and perhaps shared management of the case. Cultural construction of illness is not violated in this instance since the division between treating causes as opposed to merely reducing symptoms enables the client to accept the expertise contributed by both types of providers.

However, this collaboration requires the utmost sensitivity on the part of the polyclinic nurse. He or she must be trained to approach such situations not as an outside authority figure, but as a colleague assisting the *balian* to manage the difficult cases who are at risk of becoming failures. Nurse sensitivity to this situation could be enhanced through selecting trainees who live in the areas they will serve and developing a training curriculum that emphasizes establishment of positive one-to-one working relationships with district *balians*.

Currently, however, health officials take a diverging perspective regarding *balians*. Administrators presume that the *balians* will fail early or will not be consulted at all by prospective patients. Official presumption of these shortcomings helps build a rationale for expansion of the bureaucratic resource base.

Strengthening the community's capacity to care for therapeutic failures. Invariably, some cases will not be managed successfully by the interlocking resource system of family, healer, and polyclinic nurse. It may be that family networks and resources are too impoverished to offer social and economic support or that the family interaction pattern is itself a dominant source of the patient's distress. Similarly, the condition may be of such severity, duration, or aggressiveness that neither *balian* nor polyclinic nurse is capable of achieving desired changes. How can resource allocation at the community level succeed in obviating the need for a last-resort referral to mental hospital custodianship?

Figure 7.2 presents a multiple-option system in which diverse small-scale settings are strengthened or created to care for the myriad failure types possible. At the hub of our proposed system is the local polyclinic. Under the supervision of community leadership, it will establish and coordinate the activities of a network of social settings aimed at maintaining patients near their homes and kin. At the heart of the polyclinic operations are ambulatory nurses, each of whom has a set of positive ties with the district's *balians* and village leaders and with many patients living at home. When someone can no longer be cared for within the home and healer nexus, the nurse may already know intimately the patient's circumstances or at least be known by the family and some of the healers who have previously been consulted. At this point, the nurse would assess the patient's condition and discuss with those concerned what the best referral option would be.

Four referral options are plausible. First, and most intimate, the pa-

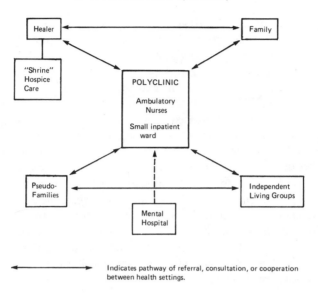

Figure 7.2
System of Culture-Specific Alternatives
to Institutional Psychiatry

Indicates pathway of referral, consultation, or cooperation between health settings.

tient might be encouraged to move into a *balian*'s shrine hospice. Here, he or she could observe ritual healing practices under the guidance of the *balian* and with an occasional visit from the polyclinic nurse. For this purpose, the polyclinic might assist carefully selected *balians* to build and furnish new pavilions in their houseyards. Second, each polyclinic would have a small number of inpatient beds which would handle the immediate needs of certain acute cases—bedrest, nutrition supplements, medicine for physical illnesses, and stabilization through expert application of psychotropic drugs. From the polyclinic, the patients could be referred back to their family or to the *balian*'s hospice. In addition, patients could be boarded with a pseudo-family household in a nearby town or join an independent living group operating their own halfway house and economic enterprise.

These final two options are settings with which the polyclinic would have close and enduring ties. Pseudo-families would be households cultivated by the clinics in town and subsidized to house and befriend patients until they could either return home, join an independent living group, or find more permanent sanctuary elsewhere. In some cases, the pseudo-family would assume long-term care arrangements. The independent living group is an option developed to meet the requirements of those who do not have homes to return to and who could, in a group context with minimal nurse supervision, care for themselves. The living group home would aim to construct a stable, long-term social support network centered on some form of farming or business enterprise that would enable the group to secure a measure of self-sufficiency. Each group home would remain small and intimate, with new ones being formed as numbers require. It might be that some pseudo-family households would serve as initial organizers and long-term stabilizing forces in the development of independent living groups.

Figure 7.2 also suggests that the existing mental hospital in Bali could be depopulated through referral of certain patients back into the community through the polyclinic-based system. Ideally, the hospital as it is currently structured would eventually disappear altogether. The hospital campus might become useful as a site for independent living groups interested in farming or workshop enterprises. Patients who have committed crimes of violence and continue to be a danger to society are a separate group of distressed individuals and are perhaps best treated within the prison system. It is hoped that the combination of supportive settings and carefully monitored medication (if necessary) will insure that this alternative system of community-based and least-restrictive options will serve effectively the mental health needs of all other Balinese patients for whom *balian* treatment was not successful.

DILEMMAS AND BARRIERS HINDERING RESOURCE REALLOCATION

The changes we propose will be profoundly resisted by those whose status has been attained through the current health order. Clearly, a fundamental restructuring of health delivery systems requires a political solution in the first instance (see Smith 1982; Werner 1981; Baer 1982). Turning the primary orientation away from the cities and toward rural areas demands a different ideology of rule among the nation's elite. These changes are a formidable challenge because they run against the interests of those holding bureaucratic authority.

A second dilemma involves the limitations imposed by the biased language we use to couch our images of community health. Even the term "health delivery" is a misnomer in the new conceptualization we wish to construct because it implies a population of passive recipients. Terms of this order, framed to serve the interests of professional guilds, ignore the fact that people do a great deal about their own health already and that specialized practitioners (both indigenous and bureaucratic) see only the tip of the iceberg of actual illness episodes. The challenge is to build a lexicon capable of grounding researchers more fully in a "health" and "prevention" mode, rather than an "illness" mode. The question becomes, "What keeps people well and how do we strengthen those processes?" not "What makes people ill?"

One shortcoming of this approach is that it does not take into account the highly disrupted conditions of many urban poor. The concept of community we employ may be inappropriate when applied to transient populations experiencing the disorganized life settings found in capital cities throughout the Third World. Our ideas are premised on an image of community loosely defined in terms of organizational potential and subjective feelings of identity of interest with regard to critical issues facing a group of people. Through this definition, community is always relative and is molded to meet the specific circumstances of different health organizational contexts. What is considered "the community of interest" will change, for example, depending on the level of health organization and responsibility under consideration—whether it becomes the polyclinic, nursing post, district hospital, or some larger unit. Similarly, we must allow that many rural areas are themselves transformed by the capitalization of agriculture, land shortages, and social relations dependent upon wage labor. In these circumstances, the concept of community as the primary resource for health and human well-being may be idealistic, and it may be that other health care models are more appropriate. Our rationale for concentrating on rural populations is that the majority of people in the countries researched here are living in rural villages.

Despite these obstacles, we remain committed to pursuing culture-specific alternatives to psychiatry as the most promising policy for resolving the issue of community mental health resource development in the Third World. We hope others will join us in transforming this briefly sketched perspective into a set of readily testable empirical questions. The answers, when they emerge, will be found in the experience of researchers and practitioners committed to working with communities in the actualization of their visions of health for all.

Appendix
Field Survey Procedure and Questionnaires

Initial entry into the network of mental health care providers, researchers, and trainers was perhaps the most difficult step during my one-month visits in each country. It required the generous assistance of a host-country sponsor who provided suggestions of where to go and whom to interview and who made the required introductions. The primary task after breaking into the psychiatry network was to learn its critical elements. That is, who are the national leaders of psychiatry? Who are the government decision makers? Who are central figures in mental health administration, in psychiatric research and education, and among those collaborating with WHO personnel? Allied professionals peripheral to this network—clinical psychologists, social workers, etc.—along with ethnopsychiatrists and anthropologists specializing in traditional healing were also sought out.

The task was to develop an exhaustive overview of formal and informal care available to community members seeking help with psychological complaints. In this vein, private, religious, and public sources of services alike were taken into consideration. On several occasions, visits to healing shrines to witness shamanistic healing ceremonies were arranged. I was accompanied to these shrines by ethnopsychiatrists and anthropologists who translated and explained the ceremonies taking place. In addition, I visited university and commercial bookstores to find publications related to psychiatry, ethnopsychology, and traditional medicine in each country.

To make the most of my month-long visits to each nation, I had to move quickly to seek out and interview as many diverse elements in the network as possible. The principle was to interview multiple levels of staff within given institutions. Random selection of subjects was impossible under the constraints of an operating treatment center. Rather, subjects represented the different disciplines found in these institutions: psychiatric supervisor, medical line staff, psychologist, nurse, social worker, occupational therapist.

Numerous and varied sites were sampled as well. Besides the major governmental inpatient facilities, a number of small, primarily private, counseling and social welfare agencies were visited. Also approached were local mental health associations and academicians in national universities who trained mental health personnel.

The purpose of this shotgun approach was to obtain the broadest possible understanding of how the elements of the national delivery system fit together as a functioning whole. Each person had his or her own perception of what the system was and how it worked. It was necessary, therefore, to carry out numerous interviews with informants of varying orientations and levels to gain a balanced picture. This effort was intended to inject some degree of reliability into the data.

Several criteria operated as general guidelines for choosing sites to study once the overall network of facilities was known. These were: (1) position significance in the national delivery system (e.g., the Philippines' major inpatient facility, National Mental Hospital); (2) size and historical value (e.g., Thailand's first mental hospital at Dhonburi; Thailand's largest residential center, Srithunya); (3) innovation (e.g., National Taiwan University Hospital's day care and autistic children center); (4) contact with traditional patients and rural/urban balance (e.g., Chiangmai's Suan Prung Hospital housing patients from nearby Hill Tribes); and (5) accessibility to investigation within the time and economic resources allocated for the survey.

Selecting a site, I would make an appointment with the hospital director. During the initial visit, the administrator would be shown the three interview forms and asked for suggestions on which staff members would be available to complete them. Efforts were always made to interview the administrator himself with Questionnaires 1 and 2. Appointments were usually made through the administrator to interview several of the ward supervisors and at least one each of the psychologists, social workers, and psychiatric nurses.

There were far fewer ancillary psychiatric personnel, so it was often difficult to include them. Their comprehension of the nature of the task and grasp of English were such that sometimes they were a little more reluctant to participate. Conversations with them were slightly more problematic. Many of the physicians had training abroad in English; some attended American universities. This was generally not the case with the other personnel. The investigator made appointments with as many professionals as possible, returning to the agency several times until the interviewing was complete.

The general format for interviewing was for me to sit with each respondent and read each item aloud. It was important to explain questions and terms, rephrasing them as necessary to insure comprehension. Through follow-up questioning on certain items and gentle probing for details, I quickly judged whether the staff member provided answers accurately reflecting the meaning of the interview items. I soon learned which terms were understandable to the personnel in different countries; such terms were substituted to improve rapport and communication.

Questionnaire 1 was given to the director or his assistant along with the other two questionnaires, if the director had time. Questionnaire 2 was administered to the other staff singly and was followed by Questionnaire 3. This last form was sometimes handed out to staff who were not interviewed with the other instruments. It was self-explanatory and simple, requiring only that respondents indicate whether they strongly agree, agree, disagree, or strongly disagree with sixteen culture-accommodation issues (see table 4.11 for a complete list of the items in Questionnaire 3).

All interviews were carried out in English or with another staff member present to translate the items into the native language.

QUESTIONNAIRE 1
Administrator's Overview and Description of Program

Background Data

1.0. Facility Title
      1.1. Country
      1.2. City
      1.3. Address

2.0. Physical Environment of Facility
      2.1. Cottage _____ Hospital _____ Other _____
      2.2. Number of rooms
      2.3. Types of living/working spaces
      2.4. Layout of facility and spatial configuration
      2.5. Condition of buildings: excellent good average poor
      2.6. Density and crowding: extremely crowded
                                     moderately crowded
                                     slightly crowded
                                     uncrowded

3.0. Location
      3.1. Relation to city layout
      3.2. Distance to urban center
      3.3. Ease of access

Interview Questions

4.0. Types of services available
    4.1. What are the objectives of this facility and the types of services offered?
    4.2. Are the following services available?

<table>
<tr><td></td><td></td><td>Yes</td><td>No</td><td>Formerly
or
Planned</td></tr>
<tr><td>4.2.1.</td><td>Emergency services</td><td></td><td></td><td></td></tr>
<tr><td>4.2.2.</td><td>Inpatient services</td><td></td><td></td><td></td></tr>
<tr><td>4.2.3.</td><td>Partial hospitalization</td><td></td><td></td><td></td></tr>
<tr><td>4.2.4.</td><td>Transitional living</td><td></td><td></td><td></td></tr>
<tr><td>4.2.5.</td><td>Follow-up services after discharge</td><td></td><td></td><td></td></tr>
<tr><td>4.2.6.</td><td>Outpatient services</td><td></td><td></td><td></td></tr>
<tr><td>4.2.7.</td><td>Specialized services for children</td><td></td><td></td><td></td></tr>
<tr><td>4.2.8.</td><td>Specialized services for the elderly</td><td></td><td></td><td></td></tr>
<tr><td>4.2.9.</td><td>Programs for alcohol and drug abusers</td><td></td><td></td><td></td></tr>
<tr><td>4.2.10.</td><td>Diagnostic and mental assessment</td><td></td><td></td><td></td></tr>
<tr><td>4.2.11.</td><td>Neurological assessment</td><td></td><td></td><td></td></tr>
<tr><td>4.2.12.</td><td>Suicide prevention program</td><td></td><td></td><td></td></tr>
<tr><td>4.2.13.</td><td>Consultation and education service, including the promotion of preventive mental health program.</td><td></td><td></td><td></td></tr>
</table>

5.0. Funding
    5.1. What is the main source of funding for this facility?
        5.1.1. Public_____ Private grants_____
               Private donations_____ Fee for service_____
               Hospital-generated funds_____ Other_____

6.0. Dimensions of the Program
    6.1. How many full-time staff are there?
        6.1.1. Psychiatrists _____
        6.1.2. Psychologists _____
        6.1.3. Nurses _____
        6.1.4. Social workers _____
        6.1.5. Medical doctors _____
        6.1.6. PMAs _____
        6.1.7. Nurse's aides _____
        6.1.8. Occupational therapy workers _____

6.1.9. Recreation therapy _____
6.1.10. Neurology _____
6.1.11. Surgery _____
6.2. How many part-time staff are there for each of the above?
6.3. What is the facility's capacity with regard to:
    6.3.1. Number of inpatient beds
    6.3.2. Number of outpatients
    6.3.3. Other clients
6.4. What is the facility's present occupancy/use regarding:
    6.4.1. Number of inpatient beds
    6.4.2. Number of outpatients served

7.0. Characteristics of Personnel
    7.1. How would you characterize the background of the professional staff with regard to:
        7.1.1. Type of training and therapy orientation of psychiatrists?
        7.1.2. Place of training of psychiatrists?
        M.D. _____ Residency _____
        7.1.3. Ethnicity, language group, and place of origin of psychiatrist?
        7.1.4. Type of orientation and training of psychologists?
        7.1.5. Place of training of psychologists?
        7.1.6. Ethnicity, language group, and place of origin of psychologists?
    7.2. How would you characterize the backgrounds of other staff with regard to their ethnicity, language groups, and place of origin?

8.0. Client Population
    8.1. What geographical areas are the clients drawn from?
    8.2. What language and cultural groups are served by the program within each area?
    8.3. What is the age range of clients?
    8.4. What are the major diagnostic types treated?
    8.5. How many patients are there within each diagnostic type?
    8.6. How many new patients are admitted each year?
        8.6.1. Total
        8.6.2. For each diagnostic type

9.0.   Referral System and Pathways to the Facility
    9.1.   How are the patients referred to the program?
    9.2.   How frequently are each of the following used as referral sources?

	Often	Some-times	Seldom	Never
9.2.1. Medical doctors in private office				
9.2.2. Mental health professionals in private practice				
9.2.3. Other mental health institutions				
9.2.4. Social welfare agencies				
9.2.5. Schools				
9.2.6. Police and courts				
9.2.7. Priests and clergy				
9.2.8. Traditional healers				
9.2.9. Family and friends				
9.2.10. Employer				

    9.3.   What other institutions or agencies is there a close working relationship with?
    9.4.   What proportion of patients are voluntary vs. involuntary?
    9.5.   Where are the patients referred after contact with the facility?
        9.5.1.   Successfully treated
        9.5.2.   Those needing additional treatment

10.0.   Outcome Measures
    10.1.   What is the turnover rate?
    10.2.   What are the discharge criteria?
    10.3.   How are patient-improvement data gathered?

11.0.   Do you have the following programs in primary prevention?
    11.1.   Community education/workshop?
    11.2.   Training of nonprofessionals in the community?
    11.3.   Crisis intervention?
    11.4.   Consultation with other institutions?
    11.5.   Social action, community organization, political action?
    11.6.   Research (listing of all research)?

12.0. How often are the following therapy techniques used?

	Often	Some-times	Seldom	Never
12.1. Chemotherapy				
12.2. Physical therapy				
12.3. Psychotherapy (types)				
12.4. Behavior therapy				
12.5. Group therapy				
12.6. Electroconvulsive therapy				
12.7. Family therapy				
12.8. Orthomolecular				
12.9. Occupational therapy				
12.10. Work therapy				
12.11. Other				

13.0. Patient's Family Involvement
   13.1. In what ways are the patient's family involved in the treatment?
   13.2. Is there a program to train, educate, or work with the patient's family as part of the treatment plan?
   13.3. Are any other individuals in the patient's immediate social group involved in helping with treatment?

14.0. Community Participation
   14.1. In what ways do community members served by the program participate in planning or directing the activities of the program?
      14.1.1. Does the program have consultants from the community? Yes _____ No _____
         14.1.1.a. Who are they?
         14.1.1.b. What are their responsibilities?
      14.1.2. Is there a community advisory board?
         Yes _____ No _____
         14.1.2.a. How many on the advisory board?
         14.1.2.b. Who are they?
         14.1.2.c. How are they selected?
         14.1.2.d. What are their responsibilities?

15.0. What are the future plans for the facility?

QUESTIONNAIRE 2
Staff Perception of Agency

Data Sources

1. Respondent
   1.1. Name
   1.2. Position
   1.3. Professional training
   1.4. Age
   1.5. Sex
   1.6. Where received training
   1.7. How long at this facility
   1.8. Other current affiliations
   1.9. Language and culture group

2. Conditions of interview
   2.1. Location
   2.2. Others present
   2.3. Quality of communication

3. Confidence and reliability: excellent   good   average   poor

4. Time started _____ Time ended _____

5. Written Materials Utilized
   5.1. Types of materials
   5.2. Titles of materials

Patient and Family Conceptions of Disorder

6. Complaints
   In general, what are types of complaints and symptoms that bring the patient to the treatment program? Have you found "culture-bound" or atypical symptoms among patients?

7. Classification
   What names or labels do patients and their families use to describe mental problems? Do they ever use "folk" names?

8. Causality
   How do patients and their families explain the causes of mental problems?

9. Expectations
   Do patients and their families have definite expectations about the treatment program? What are their expectations? If their expecta-

tions are different from the treatment they actually receive, how is this problem handled?

10. Treatment Goals
    What do patients and their families believe the goals or outcome of treatment should be?

11. Professional Manner
    What should the doctor's personal manner be like when meeting with patients?

12. What would you say are the major problems faced by the treatment program?

13. How serious would you say each of the problems is for this program? very serious   moderately serious   slightly serious   not a problem at all   not applicable

    13.1. Lack of help from the government
    13.2. Not enough money for present treatment programs
    13.3. Not enough money to develop new treatment programs
    13.4. Lack of relationships with other institutions (e.g., hospitals, clinics, welfare agencies)
    13.5. People in the community don't request this kind of treatment program
    13.6. Other professionals don't support the treatment program
    13.7. Not enough trained administrators
    13.8. Staff relations are not good
    13.9. Not enough building space
    13.10. Too many patients
    13.11. Not enough treatment supplies
    13.12. Not enough information about mental problems in the community
    13.13. Not enough trained staff for diagnosis
    13.14. Not enough trained staff for treatment
    13.15. Not enough trained staff for follow-up care
    13.16. Staff receive little information about new treatments and new research findings
    13.17. Low success rate of treatment
    13.18. Patients leave treatment program before treatment is finished
    13.19. Community people don't know about or understand the treatment program
    13.20. Community people have a bad opinion of the treatment program and use it only as a last chance

(Continued)

13.21. The staff and patients are different from each other in their social backgrounds

13.22. People with traditional beliefs about mental problems won't use the treatment program

13.23. People go to "folk doctors" instead of using the treatment program

13.24. Community people have problems using the treatment program because of its location, costs, or hours of working

13.25. Long waiting list

13.26. Patients and their families don't believe the treatment will help

13.27. Patients returning home have problems because people know they were in a mental hospital

13.28. Library is not good enough

13.29. Lack of money for equipment and research

13.30. Not enough rooms to separate different types of patients

13.31. Lack of transportation services

Goal Setting

14.0. How often do each of the following help decide the therapy to be used and the goals of therapy?

	always	some-times	seldom	never
14.1. Psychiatrist or doctor-in-charge				
14.2. Other professional staff (psychologist, social worker, nurse)				
14.3. Patient				
14.4. Family of patient				
14.5. Folk healer (e.g., shaman)				
14.6. Police/courts				
14.7. Clergy/priests				
14.8. Friends/neighbors				

	always	often	some-times	never

Staff Accommodation to Patient's Conceptions of Disorder

15.0. Do staff seek to correct or reeducate those patients who maintain traditional beliefs about mental problems?

15.1. Do staff adjust their personal manner to fit the expectations of different patients?

15.2. Are efforts made to find staff whose social and cultural backgrounds (place of birth, language, income level, etc.) are similar to those of the patients?

Adjusting Inpatient Services to Cultural Patterns

16.0. Are the patients' daily activities in the hospital similar to their activities outside of the hospital?

16.1. Do patients make choices about their daily activities?

16.2. Are patients encouraged to participate in community activities outside of the hospital, both work and recreation

16.3. Does the patient's family help with patient care within the hospital?

	always	often	some-times	never

Accessibility of Services

17.0. Is the program located in a place which is easy to visit and convenient for clients?

17.1. Is it possible for people with little money to use the treatment program?

17.2. Is treatment provided within the patient's own home or village setting?

Involving Community Resources

18.0. Are efforts made to use community people who often handle mental problems? For example, religious leaders, family group, "folk" doctors, public health nurses?

References

Ahern, E. M. 1978. Sacred and secular medicine in a Taiwan village: A study of cosmological disorders. In *Culture and healing in Asian societies,* ed. A. Kleinman, P. Kunstadter, E. R. Alexander, and J. L. Gale. Cambridge, Mass.: Schenkman.

Amor, B. 1975. *Focus on mental health resources.* Quezon City: Philippine Mental Health Association.

Angrosino, M. V. 1978. Applied anthropology and the concept of the underdog: Implications for community mental health planning and evaluation. *Community Mental Health Journal* 14.

Aragon, E. 1977. *Manual of operations on the control of mental disease.* Manila: Republic of the Philippines, Department of Health.

Argandona, M., and A. Kiev. 1972. *Mental health in the developing world.* New York: Free Press.

Asuni, T. 1975. Existing concepts of mental illness in different cultures and different forms of treatment. In *Mental health services in developing countries,* ed. T. A. Baasher, G. M. Carstairs, R. Giel, and F. Hassler. Geneva: World Health Organization.

Australia Development Assistance Bureau. 1977. *International training course in culture and mental health.* Sydney: New South Wales Institute of Psychiatry.

Baasher, T. A. 1975. Principles of psychiatric care. In *Mental health services in developing countries,* ed. T. A. Baasher, G. M. Carstairs, R. Giel, and F. Hassler. Geneva: World Health Organization.

Baer, H. A. 1982. On the political economy of health. *Medical Anthropology Newsletter* 14(1):1–17.

Bandura, A. 1977. *Social learning theory.* Englewood Cliffs, N.J.: Prentice-Hall.

Barrera, M. 1981. Social support in the adjustment of pregnant adolescents: Assessment issues. In *Social networks and social support,* ed. B. H. Gottlieb. Beverly Hills: Sage.

Benyoussef, A., H. Collomb, B. Diop, and H. Zollner. 1975. Demographic and economic aspects of mental health care in developing countries. In *Mental health services in developing countries,* ed. T. A. Baasher, G. M. Carstairs, R. Giel, and F. Hassler. Geneva: World Health Organization.

Berne, E. 1950. Some Oriental mental hospitals. *American Journal of Psychiatry* 106:376–385.

_____. 1960. The cultural problem: Psychopathology in Tahiti. *American Journal of Psychiatry* 116:1076–1081.

Bestman, E. W., H. P. Lefley, and C. S. Scott. 1976. Culturally appropriate interventions: Paradigms and pitfalls. Paper presented at the 53rd annual meeting, American Orthopsychiatric Association, Atlanta.

Bhaskaran, K. 1975. Administration and organization. In *Mental health services in developing countries,* ed. T. A. Baasher, G. M. Carstairs, R. Giel, and F. Hassler. Geneva: World Health Organization.

Boesch, E. E. 1972. *Communication between doctors and patients in Thailand, part I: Survey of the problem and analysis of the consultations.* Saarbrucken, West Germany: Socio-Psychological Research Center on Development Planning.

Bowman, K. M. 1959. Culture and mental disease, with special reference to Thailand. *Archives of General Psychiatry* 1:593–599.

Bulatao, J. 1969. Westernization and the split-level personality of the Filipino. In *Mental health research in Asia and the Pacific,* ed. W. Caudill and T. Y. Lin. Honolulu: East-West Center Press.

Burton-Bradley, B. G. 1973. Kava-kava: Mental health in Papua, New Guinea. *World Medical Journal* 20(6):110–112.

Butwell, R. 1975. *Southeast Asia: A political introduction.* New York: Praeger Publishers.

Carr, J. 1978. Ethno-behaviorism and the culture-bound syndromes: The case of amok. *Culture, Medicine and Psychiatry* 2:269–293.

Carstairs, G. M. 1973. Psychiatric problems in developing countries. *British Journal of Psychiatry* 123:271–277.

_____. 1975. Psychiatry in basic medical education. In *Mental health in developing countries,* ed. T. A. Baasher, G. M. Carstairs, R. Giel, and F. Hassler. Geneva: World Health Organization.

Castaneda, F. C. 1974. Comprehensive community mental health program: Its implications for actualization in the Philippines. In *Proceedings of the first national workshop on community mental health nursing.* Manila: Department of Health.

Castaneda, J. P. 1974. Treatment of the mentally ill. In *Proceedings of the first national workshop on community mental health nursing.* Manila: Department of Health.

Caudill, W., and T. Y. Lin. 1969. *Mental health research in Asia and the Pacific.* Honolulu: East-West Center Press.

Cawte, J. 1972. *Cruel, poor and brutal nations.* Honolulu: University Press of Hawaii.

Chance, N. A., H. Rin, and H. M. Chu. 1966. Modernization, value identification, and mental health: A cross-cultural study. *Anthropologica* 8:197–216.

Chang, Y. H., H. Rin, and C. C. Chen. 1975. Frigophobia: A report of five cases. *Bulletin of Chinese Society of Neurology and Psychiatry* 1(2): 13–16.

Chaudhry, M. R. 1975. Staffing requirements. In *Mental health in developing countries,* ed. T. A. Baasher, G. M. Carstairs, R. Giel, and F. Hassler. Geneva: World Health Organization.

Chen, C. C. 1971. Day hospitalization and its relation to rehabilitation in the community. In *5th World Congress of Psychiatry,* ed. R. de la Fuente and M. N. Weisman. New York: American Elsevier Publishers.

————. 1972. Experiences with group psychotherapy in Taiwan. *International Journal of Group Psychotherapy* 22:210–227.

————. 1974. Group therapy with predelinquent schoolchildren in Taipei. In *Youth, socialization, and mental health,* ed. W. P. Lebra. Honolulu: University Press of Hawaii.

Chen, C. C., C. C. Wu, M. K. Huang, and H. G. Hsu. 1975. Experiences with conjoint couple psychotherapy. *Bulletin of Chinese Society of Neurology and Psychiatry* 1(1):19–20.

Chen, P. Y. C. 1970. Classification and concepts of causation of mental illness in a rural Malay community. *International Journal of Social Psychiatry* 16:205–215.

————. 1975. Medical systems in Malaysia: Cultural bases and differential use. *Social Science and Medicine* 9:171–180.

————. 1979. The Iban *manang* in primary health care. Paper presented at the International Conference on Traditional Asian Medicine, Canberra.

Chu, H. M. 1972. Migration and mental disorders in Taiwan. In *Transcultural research in mental health,* ed. W. P. Lebra. Honolulu: University Press of Hawaii.

Clark, M. 1959. *Health in a Mexican-American community.* Berkeley: University of California Press.

Clement, D. C. 1982. Samoan folk knowledge of mental disorders. In *Cultural conceptions of mental health and therapy,* ed. A. J. Marsella and G. M. White. Boston: Reidel.

Climent, C. E., B. S. M. Diop, T. W. Harding, H. H. A. Ibrahim, L. Ladrido-Ignacio, and N. N. Wig. 1980. Mental health in primary health care. *WHO Chronicle* 34:231–236.

Collomb, H. 1972. *Psychiatries sans psychiatres.* Cairo, Egypt: Ed. Etudes Medicales.

————. 1973. Meeting of two systems of patient care with regard to the treatment of mental illness in Africa. *Social Science and Medicine* 7:623–633.

Colson, A. C. 1971. The perception of abnormality in a Malay village. In *Psychological problems and treatment in Malaysia,* ed. N. N. Wagner and E. S. Tan. Kuala Lumpur: University of Malaya Press.

Connor, L. H. 1978. Laporan singkat tentang hasil penelitian pasien pasien penyakit jiwa di Bali. *Majalah Psykiatri Jiwa* (Journal of the Indonesian Psychiatric Association) 11(4):35–50.

————. 1979. Spirit mediums as therapists in Bali. Paper presented at the International Conference on Traditional Asian Medicine, Canberra.

————. 1982a. Ships of fools and vessels of the divine: Mental hospitals and madness, a case study. *Social Science and Medicine* 16:783–794.

————. 1982b. The unbounded self: Balinese therapy in theory and practice. In

Cultural conceptions of mental health and therapy, ed. A. J. Marsella and G. M. White. Boston: Reidel.

―――. 1982c. In darkness and light: A study of peasant intellectuals in Bali. Ph.D. dissertation, University of Sydney.

Cook, T. D., and D. T. Campbell. 1979. *Quasi-experimentation.* Chicago: Rand McNally.

Cooper, B., and H. G. Morgan. 1973. *Epidemiological psychiatry.* Springfield, Ill.: Charles C. Thomas.

Cooper, J. E., R. E. Kendell, B. J. Gurland, L. Sharpe, J. R. M. Copeland, and R. Simon. 1972. *Psychiatric diagnosis in New York and London.* London: Oxford University Press.

Curran, W. J., and T. W. Harding. 1977. The law and mental health: Harmonizing objectives. *International Digest of Health Legislation* 28:725–885.

Darmabrata, W. H. 1971. Day hospital: The possibility of application in Indonesia. *Djiwa* 4(4):74–84.

Dasnanjali, R. 1971. Special problems in providing mental retardation services in a developing country. In *5th World Congress of Psychiatry,* ed. R. de la Fuente and M. N. Weisman. New York: American Elsevier Publishers.

Dax, E. C. 1962. *Assignment report: Survey of mental services, Federation of Malaysia.* Report no. 303. World Health Organization, Western Pacific Region.

De Guzman, L. T. 1974. Opening remarks. In *Proceedings of the first national workshop on community mental health nursing.* Manila: Department of Health.

Dean, S. R., and D. Thong. 1972. Shamanism versus psychiatry in Bali, "Isle of the Gods": Some modern implications. *American Journal of Psychiatry* 129:91–94.

Del Mundo, F., D. Morisky, and M. Lopez. 1976. *The hilot in transition: Integrating family planning and birth attending.* Quezon City: Institute of Community and Family Health, Ateneo de Manila University Press.

Denner, B., and R. H. Price, ed. 1973. *Community mental health: Social action and reaction.* New York: Holt, Rinehart and Winston.

Department of Health, Philippines. 1971. *Annual report for FY 1970–1971.* Manila: Department of Health.

―――. 1975. *National health plan, 1975–1978,* vol. 2. Manila: Department of Health.

―――. 1977. *Annual report for FY 1976–1977.* Manila: Department of Health.

Department of Health, Taiwan. 1964. *Ten year health plan, Taiwan, Republic of China, 1966–1975.* Taipei: Taiwan Provincial Government.

―――. 1970. *Taiwan's health, 1968–1969.* Taipei: Taiwan Provincial Government.

Diesfeld, J., and E. Kroger, ed. 1974. *Community health and health motivation in South-East Asia.* Wiesbaden, West Germany: Franz Steiner Verlag.

Dohrenwend, B. P., and B. S. Dohrenwend. 1965. The problem of validity in field studies of psychological disorder. *Journal of Abnormal Psychology* 70:50–69.

Draguns, J. G. 1973. Comparisons of psychopathology across cultures: Issues, findings, directions. *Journal of Cross-Cultural Psychology* 4:9–47.

―――. 1975. Resocialization into culture: The complexities of taking a world-wide view of psychotherapy. In *Cross-cultural perspectives on learning,* ed. R. W. Brislin and W. J. Lonner. New York: John Wiley and Sons.

―――. 1980. Psychopathology. In *Handbook of cross-cultural psychology,* vol. 6, ed. H. C. Triandis and J. G. Draguns. Boston: Allyn and Bacon.

―――. 1981. Counseling across cultures: Common themes and distinct approaches. In *Counseling across cultures,* revised and expanded edition, ed. P. Pedersen et al. Honolulu: University Press of Hawaii.

Draguns, J. G., and L. Phillips. 1972. *Culture and psychopathology: The quest for a relationship.* Morristown, N.J.: General Learning Press.

Durlak, J. A. 1979. Comparative effectiveness of paraprofessional and professional helpers. *Psychological Bulletin* 86:80–92.

Dusit, S. 1972. Some psychiatric problems at the Buddhist Priest's Hospital in Thailand. In *Transcultural research in mental health,* ed. W. P. Lebra. Honolulu: University Press of Hawaii.

Errion, G. D. 1979. *Principles for accreditation of community mental health service programs,* 2nd ed. Chicago: Joint Commission on Accreditation of Hospitals.

Errion, G. D., and R. S. Moen. 1976. *Principles for accreditation of community mental health service programs.* Chicago: Joint Commission on Accreditation of Hospitals.

Escudero, M. 1972. Mental disorders in a Philippine community: An epidemiological survey. In *Transcultural research in mental health,* ed. W. P. Lebra. Honolulu: University Press of Hawaii.

Esman, M. J., R. Colle, N. Uphoff, and E. Taylor. 1980. *Paraprofessionals in rural development.* Ithaca, N.Y.: Rural Development Committee, Cornell University.

Europa. 1977. *The Far East and Australasia, 1977–1978.* London: Europa Publishers.

Fabrega, H. J. 1971. Medical anthropology. In *Biennial review of anthropology,* ed. B. J. Siegal. Palo Alto: Stanford University Press.

―――. 1977. The scope of ethnomedical science. *Culture, Medicine and Psychiatry* 1:200–228.

―――. 1982. Culture and psychiatric illness: Biomedical and ethnomedical aspects. In *Cultural conceptions of mental health and therapy,* ed. A. J. Marsella and G. M. White. Boston: Reidel.

Fairweather, G. W. 1972. *Social change: The challenge to survival.* Morristown, N.J.: General Learning Press.

Fandetti, D. V., and D. E. Gelfand. 1978. Attitudes toward symptoms and services in the ethnic family and neighborhood. *American Journal of Orthopsychiatry* 48:477–486.

Faraon, P. 1976. Mental health, socio-economic growth and quality of life. *Philippine Journal of Mental Health* 7(1):15–17.

Foster, G. M. 1977. Medical anthropology and international health planning. *Social Science and Medicine* 11:527–534.

Foucault, M. 1971. *Madness and civilization: A history of insanity in the Age of Reason.* London: Tavistock.

Frank, J. 1973. *Persuasion and healing.* New York: Schocken Books.

Gains, A. D. 1982. Cultural definition, behavior and the person in American psychiatry. In *Cultural conceptions of mental health and therapy,* ed. A. J. Marsella and G. M. White. Boston: Reidel.

Garrison, V. 1979. The inner-city support systems project: Adaptation of the Miami model of culturally-relevant mental health care. Paper presented at the annual meeting of the Society for Applied Anthropology, Philadelphia.

German, A. C. 1972. Aspects of clinical psychiatry in Sub-Saharan Africa. *British Journal of Psychiatry* 121:461–479.

Giel, R. 1975. Problems of assessing the needs of the population. In *Mental health services in developing countries,* ed. T. A. Baasher, G. M. Carstairs, R. Giel, and F. Hassler. Geneva: World Health Organization.

———. 1982. An epidemiological approach to the improvement of mental health services in developing countries. *Acta Psychiatrica Scandinavia Suppliment* 65:56–63.

Giel, R., and T. W. Harding. 1976. Psychiatric priorities in developing countries. *British Journal of Psychiatry* 128:513–522.

Goldschmidt, W. 1971. Areté—motivation and models for behavior. In *The interface between psychiatry and anthropology,* ed. I. Gladston. New York: Brunner/Mazel.

Goldstein, A. P. 1973. *Structured learning theory: Toward a psychotherapy for the poor.* New York: Academic Press.

Good, B. 1977. The heart of what's the matter: The semantics of illness in Iran. *Culture, Medicine and Psychiatry* 1:25–58.

Good, B., and M. J. Good. 1980. The meaning of symptoms: A cultural hermeneutic model for clinical practice. In *The relevance of social science for medicine,* ed. L. Eisenberg and A. Kleinman. Dordecht, Holland: D. Reidel.

Gottlieb, B. H., ed. 1981. *Social networks and social support.* Beverly Hills: Sage.

Graves, T. D., and N. B. Graves. 1980. Kinship ties and the preferred adaptive strategies of urban migrants. In *The versatility of kinship,* ed. S. Bekerman and L. Cordell. New York: Academic Press.

Green, E. C. 1980. Roles for African traditional healers in mental health care. *Medical Anthropology* 4(4):489–522.

Gruenbaum, E. 1981. Medical anthropology, health policy and the state: A case study of Sudan. *Policy Studies Review* 1:47–65.

Gunaratne, V. T. H. 1981. Voyage towards health in South-East Asia. *WHO Chronicle* 35:39–46.

Guthrie, G. M. 1971. *The psychology of modernization in the rural Philippines.* I.P.C. papers, no. 8. Quezon City: Ateneo de Manila University Press.

Hanks, J. R. 1964. *Maternity and its rituals in Bang Chan.* Data paper no. 51, Southeast Asia Program. Ithaca, N.Y.: Department of Asian Studies, Cornell University.

Haq, S. M. 1975. Past and present trends in the development of psychiatric services in peninsular Malaysia. *Family Practitioner* 2(1):4–8.

Harding, T. W. 1975. Mental health services in developing countries: Some issues involved. In *Mental health services in developing countries,* ed. T. A. Baasher, G. M. Carstairs, R. Giel, and F. Hassler. Geneva: World Health Organization.

Harding, T. W., and W. J. Curran. 1978. Promoting mental health through the law. *WHO Chronicle* 32:109–113.

Harper, M. S., R. Shapiro, and J. Zusman. 1975. *Education and training of personnel for mental health work in the community.* Report no. 29. World Health Organization, South-East Asia Region, Mental Health Division.

Hartog, J. 1972a. Some institutions for the mentally and socially deviant in Malaysia: Some ethnic comparisons. *Asian Journal of Medicine* 8:170–177.

_____. 1972b. The intervention system for mental and social deviants in Malaysia. *Social Science and Medicine* 6:211–220.

Hassler, F. R. 1971. Mental health activities of the World Health Organization: An overview. In *5th World Congress of Psychiatry,* ed. R. de la Fuente and M. N. Weisman. New York: American Elsevier Publishers.

_____. 1975. Evaluation of mental health services. In *Mental health services in developing countries,* ed. T. A. Baasher, G. M. Carstairs, R. Giel, and F. Hassler. Geneva: World Health Organization.

Heller, K. 1979. The effects of social support: Prevention and treatment implications. In *Maximizing treatment gains: Transfer enhancement in psychotherapy,* ed. A. P. Goldstein and F. Kanfer. New York: Academic Press.

Henderson, J. W. 1971. *Area handbook for Thailand.* Washington: Government Printing Office.

Hessler, R. M. 1977. Citizen participation, social organization and culture: A neighborhood health center for Chicanos. *Human Organization* 36:124–134.

Higginbotham, H. N. 1976. A conceptual model for the delivery of psychological services in non-western settings. In *Topics in culture learning,* vol. 4, ed. R. Brislin. Honolulu: East-West Center.

_____. 1977. Culture and the role of client expectancy in psychotherapy. In *Topics in culture learning,* vol. 5, ed. R. Brislin and M. Hamnett. Honolulu: East-West Center.

_____. 1981. Cultural explanations of illness and adjustment: A comparative study of New Zealand Europeans and Chinese Malaysian students. Paper presented at the Conference on Cultural Adaptation and Health among International Students, East-West Center, Honolulu.

_____. In press. Generalization of treatment gain: A network analysis. In *Psychotherapy and the psychology of behavior change,* 2nd ed., ed. S. West and H. Higginbotham. New York: Pergamon Press.

Higginbotham, H. N., and J. Tanaka-Matsumi. 1981. Behavioral approaches to counseling across cultures. In *Counseling across cultures,* revised and expanded edition, ed. P. Pedersen et al. Honolulu: University Press of Hawaii.

Hinderling, P. 1973. *Communication between doctors and patients in Thailand, part III: Interviews with traditional doctors.* Saarbrucken, West Germany: Socio-Psychological Research Center on Development Planning, University of Saar.

Howard, A. 1979. Polynesia and Micronesia in psychiatric perspective. *Transcultural Psychiatric Research Review* 16:123–145.

Hsu, C. C. 1972. Fellow's final report to WHO. *25th anniversary memorial report of National Taiwan University Hospital, Department of Psychiatry and Neurology.* Taipei: National Taiwan University.

Hsu, C. C., and T. Y. Lin. 1969. A mental health program at the elementary school level in Taiwan: A six-year review of the East-Gate Project. In *Mental health research in Asia and the Pacific,* ed. W. Caudill and T. Y. Lin. Honolulu: East-West Center Press.

Hsu, J. 1976. Counseling in the Chinese temple: A psychiatric study of divination by chien drawing. In *Culture-bound syndromes, ethnopsychiatry and alternative therapies,* ed. W. P. Lebra. Honolulu: University Press of Hawaii.

Ignacio, L. L. 1976. Effects of urbanization on mental health. *Philippine Journal of Mental Health* 7(1):12–15.

Indonesian Ministry of Health. 1978. Primary health care (village community health development) in Indonesia. Paper prepared for the International Conference on Primary Health Care, Alma Ata, U.S.S.R.

Indries, D. H. 1971. Some socio-cultural aspects of psychiatry in Indonesia. *Jiwa* 4(4):111–122.

Inkeles, A., and D. Smith. 1970. The fate of personal adjustment in the process of modernization. *International Journal of Comparative Sociology* 11: 81–114.

Ionescu-Tongyonk, J. 1977. Transcultural psychiatry in Thailand: A review of the last two decades. *Transcultural Psychiatric Research Review* 14:145–162.

———. 1978. The depressive equivalents of Orientals and Occidentals. *Transcultural Psychiatric Research Review* 15:77–78.

Jackson, J. 1964. Toward the comparative study of mental hospitals: Characteristics of the treatment environment. In *The psychiatric hospital as a social system,* ed. A. F. Wessen. Springfield, Ill.: Charles C. Thomas.

Jaspan, M. A. 1976. The social organization of indigenous and modern medical practices in southwest Sumatra. In *Asian medical systems,* ed. C. Leslie. Los Angeles: University of California Press.

Jayasundera, M. G. 1969. Mental health survey in Ceylon. In *Mental health research in Asia and the Pacific.* ed. W. Caudill and T. Y. Lin. Honolulu: East-West Center Press.

Jocano, F. L. 1971. Varieties of supernatural experience among Filipino peasants: Hallucination or idiom of cultural cognition. *Transcultural Psychiatric Research Review* 8:43–45.

_____. 1973. *Folk medicine in a Philippine municipality.* Manila: National Museum.

Kamal, A. 1975. Principles of preventive action in mental health care. In *Mental health services in developing countries,* ed. T. A. Baasher, G. M. Carstairs, R. Giel, and F. Hassler. Geneva: World Health Organization.

Kamel, M., Z. Bishry, and A. Okasha. 1975. Preliminary psychiatric observations in Libya. *Transcultural Psychiatric Research Review* 12:51–52.

Kamratana, S. 1972. Adolescents' attitudes towards religion in Ubon Ratchathany community. *Journal of the Psychiatric Association of Thailand* 17:364–371.

Kapur, R. L. 1975. An illustrated presentation of a population survey of mental illness in south India. In *Mental health services in developing countries,* ed. T. A. Baasher, G. M. Carstairs, R. Giel, and F. Hassler. Geneva: World Health Organization.

Keefe, S. E., A. M. Padilla, and M. L. Carlos. 1979. The Mexican-American extended family as an emotional support system. *Human Organization* 38:144–152.

Kelly, J. G. 1966. Ecological constraints on mental health services. *American Psychologist* 21:535–539.

Kelly, J. G., L. R. Snowden, and R. F. Munoz. 1977. Social and community intervention. *Annual Review of Psychology* 323–361.

Kennedy, J. G. 1973. Cultural psychiatry. In *Handbook of social and cultural anthropology,* ed. J. Honigmann. Chicago: Rand McNally.

Kiernan, W. E. S. 1976a. *Strengthening of mental health services in Thailand.* Field visit report no. 34. World Health Organization, South-East Asia Region, Mental Health Division.

_____. 1976b. *Field visit report on developments in mental health services in Indonesia.* SEA/Ment./33. Geneva: World Health Organization.

Kiev, A. 1972. *Transcultural psychiatry.* New York: Free Press.

_____. 1976. Psychiatry programs for the developing countries. In *Further explorations in social psychiatry,* ed. B. H. Kaplan and A. H. Leighton. New York: Basic Books.

Kilbride, P. L. 1979. Barmaiding as a deviant occupation among the Baganda of Uganda. *Ethos* 7:232–254.

Kinzie, D., and J. M. Bolton. 1973. Psychiatry with the Aborigines of West Malaysia. *American Journal of Psychiatry* 130:769–773.

Kinzie, J. D., J. I. Teoh, and E. S. Tan. 1974. Community psychiatry in Malaysia. *American Journal of Psychiatry* 131:573–577.

Kleinman, A. 1977. Explaining the efficacy of indigenous therapies: The need for interdisciplinary research. *Culture, Medicine and Psychiatry* 1:133–134.

_____. 1978. International health care planning from an ethnomedical perspective: Critique and recommendations for change. *Medical Anthropology* 2:71–96.

————. 1980. *Patients and healers in the context of culture.* Berkeley: University of California Press.

Kleinman, A., and T. Y. Lin, ed. 1981. *Normal and abnormal behavior in Chinese culture.* Boston: Reidel.

Kleinman, A., and L. H. Sung. 1976. Why do indigenous practitioners successfully heal? A follow-up study of the efficacy of indigenous healing in Taiwan. Paper presented at the Workshop on the Healing Process, Michigan State University.

Kline, N. S. 1963. Psychiatry in Indonesia. *American Journal of Psychiatry* 119:809–815.

Kluckhohn, C., and D. Leighton. 1946. *The Navaho.* Cambridge: Harvard University Press.

Ko, Y. H. 1974. A study of the effects of psychotherapy. *Acta Psychologica Taiwanica* 16:141–154.

————. 1975. Student mental health problems in two differently industrialized cities. *Acta Psychologica Taiwanica* 17:25–38.

Kraph, E. E., and J. M. Moser. 1966. A survey of mental health resources. In *International trends in mental health,* ed. H. P. David. New York: McGraw-Hill.

Kunitz, S. J. 1970. Equilibrium theory in social psychiatry: The work of the Leightons. *Psychiatry* 33:312–328.

Kunstadter, P. 1978. Do cultural differences make any difference? Choice points in medical systems available in northwestern Thailand. In *Culture and healing in Asian societies,* ed. A. Kleinman et al. Cambridge, Mass.: Schenkman.

Laing, R. D. 1967. *The politics of experience.* New York: Pantheon Press.

Lambo, T. A. 1962. The importance of cultural factors in psychiatric treatment. *Acta Psychiatrica Scandinavia* 38:176–179.

————. 1966. Patterns of psychiatric care in developing African countries: The Nigerian village program. In *International trends in mental health,* ed. H. P. David. New York: McGraw-Hill.

————. 1977. Mental health: A challenging new role within WHO. *World Health,* December, 2–5.

————. 1978. Psychotherapy in Africa. *Human Nature* 1:32–39.

Lapuz, L. 1972. A study of psychopathology in a group of Filipino patients. In *Transcultural research in mental health,* ed. W. P. Lebra. Honolulu: University Press of Hawaii.

Lebra, W. P., ed. 1972. *Transcultural research in mental health.* Honolulu: University Press of Hawaii.

————, ed. 1976. *Culture-bound syndromes, ethnopsychiatry, and alternative therapies.* Honolulu: University Press of Hawaii.

————. 1982. Shaman-client interchange in Okinawa: Performative stages in shamanic therapy. In *Cultural conceptions of mental health and therapy,* ed. A. J. Marsella and G. M. White. Boston: Reidel.

Leighton, A. H. 1959. *My name is legion.* New York: Basic Books.

————. 1969. Cultural relativity and the identification of psychiatric disorders.

In *Mental health research in Asia and the Pacific,* ed. W. Caudill and T. Y. Lin. Honolulu: East-West Center Press.

Leighton, A. H., T. A. Lambo, C. C. Hughes, D. C. Leighton, J. M. Murphy, and D. B. Macklin. 1963. *Psychiatric disorder among the Yoruba.* Ithaca, N.Y.: Cornell University Press.

Leighton, D. C. 1971. The empirical status of the integration-disintegration hypothesis. In *Psychiatric disorder and the urban environment,* ed. B. N. Kaplan. New York: Behavioral Publications.

Leighton, D. C., J. S. Harding, D. B. Macklin, A. M. Macmillan, and A. H. Leighton. 1963. *The character of danger: Psychiatric symptoms in selected communities.* New York: Basic Books.

Leon, C. 1972. Psychiatry in Latin America. *British Journal of Psychiatry* 121:121–136.

Leslie, C. 1976. Introduction. In *Asian medical systems,* ed. C. Leslie. Los Angeles: University of California Press.

———. 1977. Pluralism and integration in the Indian and Chinese medical systems. In *Culture, disease and healing: Studies in medical anthropology,* ed. L. Landy. New York: Macmillan.

Levine, E. S. 1978. An overview of pluralistic therapy with application to Hispanics. *International Journal of Intercultural Relations* 2:361–371.

Lewis, O. 1955. Medicine and politics in a Mexican village. In *Health, culture and community,* ed. B. D. Paul. New York: Russell Sage.

Li, Y. U. 1976. Shamanism in Taiwan: An anthropological inquiry. In *Culture-bound syndromes, ethnopsychiatry, and alternative therapies,* ed. W. P. Lebra. Honolulu: University Press of Hawaii.

Lieban, R. W. 1967. *Cebuano sorcery: Malign magic in the Philippines.* Los Angeles: University of California Press.

———. 1977. Symbols, signs, and success: Healers and power in a Philippine city. In *The anthropology of power,* ed. R. Fogelson and R. N. Adams. New York: Academic Press.

Lin, T. Y. 1953. A study of incidence of mental disorder in Chinese and other cultures. *Psychiatry* 16:313–336.

———. 1961. Evolution of a mental health programme in Taiwan. *American Journal of Psychiatry* 117:961–971.

———. 1964a. Mental health programme. In *Ten year health plan, Taiwan, 1966–1975.* Taipei: Department of Health, Taiwan Provincial Government.

———. 1964b. *Assignment report on mental health services in Thailand.* Report no. 14. World Health Organization, South-East Asia Region, Mental Health Division.

———. 1967. The epidemiological study of mental disorders by WHO. *Social Psychiatry* 1:204–206.

———. 1971. Psychiatric training for foreign medical graduates: A symposium. *Psychiatry* 34:233–234.

———. 1981. Mental health in the third world. Address to the World Congress of Mental Health, Manila.

Lin, T. Y., and M. C. Lin. 1981. Love, denial and rejection: Responses of Chinese families to mental illness. In *Normal and abnormal behavior in Chinese culture,* ed. A. Kleinman and T. Y. Lin. Boston: Reidel.

Lin, T. Y., H. Rin, E. K. Yeh, C. C. Hsu, and H. M. Chu. 1969. Mental disorders in Taiwan, fifteen years later: A preliminary report. In *Mental health research in Asia and the Pacific,* ed. W. Caudill and T. Y. Lin. Honolulu: East-West Center Press.

Lindemann, E. 1969. Mental health aspects of rapid social change. In *Mental health research in Asia and the Pacific,* ed. W. Caudill and T. Y. Lin. Honolulu: East-West Center Press.

Lo, S., D. Fung, J. Woo-Sam, and R. Samuelu. 1980. Socio-demographic characteristics of Chinese and other Asian psychiatric outpatients. Paper presented at the Western Psychological Association meeting, Honolulu.

London, P. 1965. *The modes and morals of psychotherapy.* New York: Holt, Rinehart and Winston.

Lubis, D. B. 1975. The prospects for psychotherapy in Southeast Asian countries. *Jiwa* 2(2):65-80.

———. 1977. Dynamic psychotherapy for mental patients. Doctoral dissertation, University of Indonesia, Jakarta.

McDermott, J. F., T. W. Maretzki, M. J. Hansen, D. E. Ponce, W. S. Tseng, and J. D. Kinzie. 1974. American psychiatry for export: Special training for foreign medical graduates. *Journal of Medical Education* 49: 431-437.

MacKay Counseling Center. 1976. *Report of the Taipei Life-Line.* Taipei: MacKay Prevention Center and Life-Line Association.

MacKenzie, M. 1977. Mana in Maori medicine—Rarotonga, Oceania. In *The anthropology of power,* ed. R. Fogelson and R. N. Adams. New York: Academic Press.

MacMurray, V. D. 1976. *Citizen evaluation of mental health services: A guidebook for accountability.* New York: Human Sciences Press.

Maguigad, L. C. 1964. Psychiatry in the Philippines. *American Journal of Psychiatry* 121:21-25.

Mahler, H. 1981. The meaning of "health for all by the year 2000." *World Health Forum* 2(1):5-22.

Malakul, S. 1964. *Mental hygiene clinic's report.* Bangkok, Thailand.

Manapsal, L. E. 1969. Epidemiological survey of mental disorder in a Philippine community. *Philippine Journal of Public Health* 13(3).

———. 1974. Extent of mental health problems in the Philippines. In *Proceedings of the first national workshop on community mental health nursing.* Manila: Department of Health.

Manapsal, L. E., E. M. Aragon, R. M. San Pedro, and M. M. Manuel. 1974. Follow-up study of the 86 active mental cases from the epidemiological survey of mental disorder in a Philippine community. *Philippine Journal of Mental Health* 5(1):30-47.

Mangay-Angara, A. 1977. New status for the hilot. *WHO Chronicle* 31:432.

Manson, S. 1980. Problematic life situations: An inquiry into cross-cultural variation of support mobilization among minority elderly. Paper presented at the Western Psychological Association meeting, Honolulu.

———. 1982. New directions in primary prevention of mental health problems among native American and Alaskan Indians. Washington: National Institute of Mental Health.

Margetts, E. L. 1965. Methods of psychiatric research in Africa. In *CIBA symposium on transcultural psychiatry,* ed. A. V. S. DeReuck and R. Porter. London: Churchill.

Marriott, M. 1955. Western medicine in a village of northern India. In *Health, culture and community,* ed. B. D. Paul. New York: Russell Sage.

Marsella, A. J. 1978. Modernization: Consequences for the individual. In *Overview of intercultural education, training, and research: Special research areas,* vol. 3, ed. D. Hoopes, P. Pedersen, and G. Renwick. La Grange, Ill.: Intercultural Network, Inc.

———. 1979. Cross-cultural studies of mental disorders. In *Perspectives on cross-cultural psychology,* ed. A. J. Marsella, R. Tharp, and T. Ciborowski. New York: Academic Press.

———. 1982. Culture and mental health: An overview. In *Cultural conceptions of mental health and therapy,* ed. A. J. Marsella and G. M. White. Boston: Reidel.

Marsella, A. J., M. Escudero, and P. Gordon. 1972. Stress, resources, and symptom patterns in urban Filipino men. In *Transcultural research in mental health,* ed. W. P. Lebra. Honolulu: University Press of Hawaii.

Marsella, A. J., and H. N. Higginbotham. 1979. Applications of traditional Asian medicine to psychiatric services in developing nations. Paper presented at the International Conference on Traditional Asian Medicine, Canberra.

Marsella, A. J., and G. M. White, ed. 1982. *Cultural conceptions of mental health and therapy.* Boston: Reidel.

Meadow, A. 1964. Client-centered therapy and the American ethos. *International Journal of Social Psychiatry* 10:246–260.

Meesook. A. 1975. Cultures in collision: An experience in Thailand. In *Cultures in collision,* ed. I. Pilowsky. Adelaide: Australian National Association for Mental Health.

Mehryar, A., and F. Khajavi. 1974. Some implications of a community mental health model for developing countries. *International Journal of Social Psychiatry* 21:45–52.

Mejia, A., H. Pizurki, and E. Royston. 1979. *Physician and nurse migration: Analysis and policy implications.* Report of a WHO study. Geneva: World Health Organization.

Ministry of Public Health, Thailand. 1976. *Thailand health profile.* Bangkok: Kingdom of Thailand, Ministry of Public Health.

———. 1977. *Annual report of the Division of Mental Health.* Bangkok: Kingdom of Thailand, Ministry of Public Health.

Mintz, N. L., and D. T. Schwartz. 1964. Urban ecology and psychosis: Community factors in the incidence of schizophrenia and manic-depression among Italians in greater Boston. *International Journal of Social Psychiatry* 10:102–119.

Mitchell, R. E., A. G. Billings, and R. H. Moos. In press. Social support and well-being: Implications for prevention programs. *Journal of Primary Prevention.*

Mitchell, R. E., and E. J. Trickett. 1980. Social networks as mediators of social support: An analysis of the effects and determinants of social networks. *Community Mental Health Journal* 16:27–44.

Moerman, D. E. 1979. Anthropology of symbolic healing. *Current Anthropology* 20:59–80.

Moos, R. H. 1974. *Evaluating treatment environments: A social ecological approach.* New York: John Wiley.

Morely, D. 1973. *Paediatrics priorities in the developing world.* London: Butterworths.

Moritsugu, J. 1980. Issues in minority mental health: Indo-Chinese and Asian warbride projects. Paper presented at the Western Psychological Association meeting, Honolulu.

Muecke, M. A. 1979. An explication of wind illness in northern Thailand. *Culture, Medicine and Psychiatry* 3:267–300.

Murphy, H. B. M., ed. 1955. *Flight and resettlement,* Paris: UNESCO.

———. 1961. Social change and mental health. In *Causes of mental disorders: A review of the epidemiological knowledge.* New York: Milbank Memorial Fund.

———. 1971. The beginnings of psychiatric treatment in the Peninsula. In *Psychological problems and treatment in Malaysia.* ed. N. N. Wagner and E. S. Tan. Kuala Lumpur: University of Malaya Press.

Murphy, H. B. M., E. D. Wittkower, and N. W. Chance. 1963. A cross-cultural survey of schizophrenic symptomatology. *International Journal of Social Psychiatry* 9:237–249.

———. 1970. The symptoms of depression—A cross-cultural survey. In *Cross-cultural studies of behavior,* ed. I. Al-Issa and W. Dennis. New York: Holt, Rinehart and Winston.

Murphy, J. M. 1972. A cross-cultural comparison of psychiatric disorder: Eskimos of Alaska, Yorubas of Nigeria, and Nova Scotians of Canada. In *Transcultural research in mental health,* ed. W. P. Lebra. Honolulu: University Press of Hawaii.

———. 1976. Psychiatric labeling in cross-cultural perspective. *Science* 191:1019–1028.

Murthy, R. S. 1977. Reaching the unreached. *World Health,* December, 22–27.

National Economic and Development Authority (NEDA), Philippines. 1977. *Five year Philippine development plan, 1978–1982.* Manila: NEDA.

National Health Administration, Taiwan. 1976. *Taiwan's health, 1974–1975.* Taipei: National Health Administration.

———. 1977. *Health statistics: General health statistics, 1976.* Taipei: National Health Administration.

Neki, J. S. 1973a. Psychiatry in South-East Asia. *British Journal of Psychiatry* 123:257–269.

_____. 1973b. Psychiatric education and the social role of the psychiatrist in developing South-East Asian countries. *Social Science and Medicine* 7:103–107.

Nichter, M. 1978. Patterns of resort in the use of therapy systems and their significance for health planning in South Asia. *Medical Anthropology* 2:29–49.

Orley, J. H. 1970. *Culture and mental illness: A study from Uganda.* East-African studies, no. 36. Nairobi, Kenya: East-African Publishing House.

Osborne, O. H. 1969. The Yoruba village as a therapeutic community. *Journal of Health and Social Behavior* 10:187–200.

Otrakul, A., S. Suwanlert, J. Vatanasoporn, and S. Satrasingha. 1975. A survey of Thai adolescents' views on drug abuse. Paper presented at the 31st International Congress on Alcoholism and Drug Dependence, Bangkok.

Padilla, A. M., R. A. Ruiz, and R. Alvarez. 1975. Community mental health services for the Spanish-speaking/surnamed population. *American Psychologist* 30:892–905.

Pande, S. K. 1968. The mystique of western psychotherapy: An eastern interpretation. *Journal of Nervous and Mental Disease* 146:425–432.

Panzetta, A. 1971. *Community mental health: Myth or reality?* Philadelphia: Lea and Febinger.

Papajohn, J., and J. Spielgel. 1975. *Transactions in families.* San Francisco: Jossey-Bass.

Parker, S., and R. J. Kleiner. 1966. *Mental illness in the urban Negro community.* New York: Free Press.

Parlato, M. B., and M. N. Favin. 1982. *Primary health care: Progress and problems. An analysis of 52 AID-assisted projects.* Washington: American Public Health Association.

Pattison, E. M. 1977. A theoretical-empirical base for social system therapy. In *Current perspectives in cultural psychiatry,* ed. E. F. Foulks, R. M. Wintrob, J. Westermeyer, and A. R. Favazza. New York: Spectrum.

Philippine Mental Health Association. 1976. *Annual report.* Quezon City: PMHA.

Pilar, N. N., E. G. Boncaras, and G. P. Santos. 1976. *Social development policies and programs in the Philippines: Focus on the delivery of health services.* SPAR series. Manila: College of Public Administration, University of the Philippines.

Pilisuk, M. 1982. Delivery of social support: The social innoculation. *American Journal of Orthopsychiatry* 52:20–31.

Pilisuk, M., and S. H. Parks. 1981. The place of network analysis in the study of supportive social associations. *Basic and Applied Social Psychology* 2:121–135.

_____. In press. *In search of a cure: Social support and illness.*

Pounds, M. 1982. Strategies of negotiation in three realms of Balinese society. Ph.D. dissertation, University of California, Berkeley.

Prasetyo, J. 1977. *Child psychiatry in Indonesia.* Working paper, Subdivision of Child Psychiatry, Department of Psychiatry, University of Indonesia.

Prasetyo, J., W. E. Humris, B. Hardjawana, M. Budhiman, and L. Mangindaan. 1977. *Some thoughts on the psychiatric treatment of children with emotional disorders in Jakarta, Indonesia.* Working paper, Subdivision of Child Psychiatry, Department of Psychiatry, University of Indonesia.

Prince, R. H. 1980. Variations in psychotherapeutic procedures. In *Handbook of cross-cultural psychology,* vol. 4, ed. H. Triandis and J. C. Draguns. Boston: Allyn and Bacon.

Prince, R. H., and E. D. Wittkower. 1964. The care of the mentally ill in a changing culture (Nigeria). *American Journal of Psychotherapy* 18:644–648.

Quah, S. R. 1977a. *The unplanned dimensions of health care in Singapore: Traditional healers and self-medication.* Sociology working paper no. 62, Department of Sociology, University of Singapore.

———. 1977b. Accessibility of modern and traditional health services in Singapore. *Social Science and Medicine* 11:333–340.

Rappaport, H., and M. Rappaport. 1981. The integration of scientific and traditional healing. *American Psychologist* 36(7):774–781.

Rappaport, J. 1977. *Community psychology: Values, research and action.* New York: Holt, Rinehart and Winston.

Rappaport, J., and J. M. Chinsky. 1974. Models for delivery of service from a historical and conceptual perspective. *Professional Psychology* 5:42–50.

Ratanakorn, P. 1975. Asia and problems of alcoholism. Paper presented at the Sixth Medical and Scientific Conference, Milwaukee.

Reyes, S. S. 1970. An analysis of the progress made by mental patient residents in a half-way community program. *Philippine Journal of Mental Health* 1(2):127–160.

Rin, H. 1969. Sibling rank, culture and mental disorders. In *Mental health research in Asia and the Pacific,* ed. W. Caudill and T. Y. Lin. Honolulu: East-West Center Press.

———. 1972. Fellows report for the World Health Organization. *25th anniversary memorial report of the National Taiwan University Hospital, Department of Psychiatry and Neurology.* Taipei: National Taiwan University.

Rin, H., H. M. Chu, and T. Y. Lin. 1966. Psychophysical reactions of rural and suburban populations in Taiwan. *Transcultural Psychiatric Research Review* 3.

Rin, H., C. Schooler, and W. Caudill. 1973. Culture, social structure and psychopathology in Taiwan and Japan. *Journal of Nervous and Mental Disease* 157:296–312.

Ritchie, J. E. 1976. Cultural time out: Generalized therapeutic sociocultural mechanisms among the Maori. In *Culture-bound syndromes, ethnopsychiatry, and alternative therapies,* ed. W. P. Lebra. Honolulu: University Press of Hawaii.

Rosen, R. M., H. F. Goldsmith, and R. W. Redick. 1979. Demographic and social indicators: Uses in mental health planned in small areas. *World Health Statistics Quarterly* 32:11–103.

Rossi, P. H., and E. Freeman. 1982. *Evaluation: A systematic approach.* Beverly Hills: Sage.

Ruiz, R. A., and J. M. Casas. 1981. Culturally relevant and behavioristic counseling for Chicano college students. In *Counseling across cultures,* revised and expanded edition, ed. P. Pedersen et al. Honolulu: University Press of Hawaii.

Salan, R. 1968. *Mental health in Indonesia: A WHO report.* Working paper, Directorate of Mental Health, Ministry of Health, Republic of Indonesia.

———. 1975. Personal characteristics of first admissions in mental hospitals in Indonesia. *Jiwa* 7(3):33–53.

Sampson, E. E. 1977. Psychology and the American ideal. *Journal of Personality and Social Psychology* 35:767–782.

Sangsingkeo, P. 1958. Community attitudes in Thailand toward social treatment. *Journal of Social Therapy* 4:197–200.

———. 1965. Medical history of psychiatry and mental health. Lecture presented at the Scientific Conference of Siriraj Medical College, Bangkok.

———. 1966. Mental health in developing countries. In *International trends in mental health,* ed. H. P. David. New York: McGraw-Hill.

———. 1969. Buddhism and some effects on rearing children in Thailand. In *Mental health research in Asia and the Pacific,* ed. W. Caudill and T. Y. Lin. Honolulu: East-West Center Press.

———. 1975. Thailand. In *World history of psychiatry,* ed. J. G. Howells. New York: Brunner/Mazel.

Sangsingkeo, P., S. Punahitanont, and R. J. Schneider. 1974. *A survey of Thai student drug use.* Bangkok: SEATO Medical Research Laboratory.

Santoso, R. S. I. 1959. The social conditions of psychotherapy in Indonesia. *American Journal of Psychiatry* 115:798–800.

Sanvictores, L. L. 1976. Mental health and economic growth. *Philippine Journal of Mental Health* 7:18–21.

Sarason, S. 1974. *The psychological sense of community.* San Francisco: Jossey-Bass.

Sarason, S., and E. Lorentz. 1979. *The challenge of the resource exchange network.* San Francisco: Jossey-Bass.

Sartorius, N. 1971. The programme of the WHO on the epidemiology of mental disorders. In *5th World Congress of Psychiatry,* ed. R. de la Fuente and M. N. Weisman. New York: American Elsevier Publishers.

———. 1977. Compete or complement? *World Health,* December, 28–33.

———. 1978. WHO's new mental health programme. *WHO Chronicle* 32:60–62.

Sartorius, N., A. Jablensky, and R. Shapiro. 1978. Cross-cultural differences in the short-term prognosis of schizophrenic psychosis. *Schizophrenia Bulletin* 4:102–113.

Schmidt, K. E. 1965. Communication problems with psychiatric patients in a multilingual society of Sarawak. *Psychiatry* 28:229–233.

———. 1967. Mental health services in a developing country of South-East Asia. In *New aspects of the mental health services,* ed. H. Freemand and J. Farndale. Oxford: Pergamon Press.

Schulberg, H. C., and F. Baker. 1979. *Program evaluation in the health fields,* vol. 2. New York: Human Sciences Press.

Sechrest, L. 1967. Conception and management of mental disorder in some Negros Oriental barrios. *Transcultural Psychiatric Research Review* 4:116.

————. 1969. Philippine culture, stress, and psychopathology. In *Mental health research in Asia and the Pacific,* ed. W. Caudill and T. Y. Lin. Honolulu: East-West Center Press.

Sena, C. T. 1974. Common psychiatric disorders among Filipinos. In *Proceedings of the first national workshop on community mental health nursing.* Manila: Department of Health.

Setyonegoro, K. 1976. *Indonesian computerized recording system.* Working paper, Directorate of Mental Health, Ministry of Health, Republic of Indonesia.

Shakman, R. 1969. Indigenous healing of mental illness in the Philippines. *International Journal of Social Psychiatry* 15:279–287.

Sheper-Hughes, N. 1978. Saints, scholars and schizophrenics—madness and badness in western Ireland. *Medical Anthropology* 2:59–93.

Shore, M. F., and F. V. Mannino. 1975. *Mental health and social change: Fifty years of orthopsychiatry.* New York: AMS Press.

Shweder, R. A., and E. J. Bourne. 1982. Does the concept of person vary cross-culturally? In *Cultural conceptions of mental health and therapy,* ed. A. J. Marsella and G. M. White. Boston: Reidel.

Smith, R. 1982. Primary health care—rhetoric or reality? *World Health Forum* 3(1):30–37.

Steinberg, J., ed. 1971. *In search of Southeast Asia.* New York: Praeger.

Stoller, A. 1959. *Assignment report on mental health situation in Thailand.* Report no. 7. World Health Organization, South-East Asia Region, Mental Health Division.

————. 1963. *Assignment report on mental health situation in Indonesia.* Report no. 13. World Health Organization, South-East Asia Region, Mental Health Division.

Sue, S. 1977. Community mental health services to minority groups: Some optimism, some pessimism. *American Psychologist* 32:616–624.

Sundberg, N. 1981. Research and research hypotheses about effectiveness in intercultural counseling. In *Counseling across cultures,* revised and expanded edition, ed. P. Pedersen et al. Honolulu: University Press of Hawaii.

Suwana, A. B. 1969. Effect of culture change on anxiety in women in Thailand. *Australian and New Zealand Journal of Psychiatry* 3(3):267–270.

Suwanlert, Sangun. 1970. Experience with group psychotherapy. *Journal of the Psychiatric Association of Thailand* 15:289.

————. 1972. Psychiatric study of bah tshi (latah). *Journal of the Psychiatric Association of Thailand* 17:380.

————. 1975. A study of kratom eaters in Thailand. *Bulletin on Narcotics* 27(3):21–27.

————. 1976a. Phii pob: Spirit possession in rural Thailand. In *Culture-bound syndromes, ethnopsychiatry, and alternative therapies,* ed. W. P. Lebra. Honolulu: University Press of Hawaii.

_____. 1976b. Neurotic and psychotic states attributed to Thai "phii pob" spirit possession. *Australian and New Zealand Journal of Psychiatry* 10:119–123.

Suwanlert, Sangun, and D. Coates. 1977. Epidemic koro in Thailand: Clinical and social aspects. Unpublished manuscript, Srithunya Hospital, Dhonburi, Thailand.

Szasz, T. 1978. *The myth of psychotherapy: Mental healing as religion, rhetoric, and repression.* Garden City, N.Y.: Doubleday Anchor.

Tan, E. S. 1971. A look to the future—quo vadis? In *Psychological problems and treatment in Malaysia,* ed. N. N. Wagner and E. S. Tan. Kuala Lumpur: University of Malaya Press.

Tan, E. S., and N. N. Wagner. 1971. Psychiatry in Malaysia. In *Psychological problems and treatment in Malaysia,* ed. N. N. Wagner and E. S. Tan. Kuala Lumpur: University of Malaya Press.

Tanaka-Matsumi, J. 1979. Cultural factors and social influence techniques in Naikan therapy: A Japanese self-observation method. *Psychotherapy: Theory, Research and Practice* 16:385–390.

Teoh, J. K., J. D. Kinzie, and E. S. Tan. 1972. Referrals to a psychiatric clinic in West Malaysia. *International Journal of Social Psychiatry* 18:301–307.

Tenny, A. M. 1971. Computers in transcultural psychiatry: Indonesia recording systems projects, phase I. *Transcultural Psychiatric Research Review* 8:201–205.

Textor, R. 1960. An inventory of non-Buddhist supernatural objects in a central Thai village. Ph.D. dissertation, Cornell University.

Thong, D. 1976. Psychiatry in Bali. *Australian and New Zealand Journal of Psychiatry* 10:95–97

Thursz, D., and J. L. Vigilante, ed. 1978. *Reaching people: The structure of neighborhood services.* Beverly Hills: Sage.

Tjahjana, L. 1976. Socio-cultural and socio-economic factors in mental rehabilitation in Indonesia. *Jiwa* 9(1):55–69.

Torrey, E. F. 1972. *The mind game.* New York: Bantam Press.

Tseng, W. S. 1975. The nature of somatic complaints among psychiatric patients: The Chinese case. *Comprehensive Psychiatry* 16(3):237–244.

_____. 1976. Folk psychotherapy in Taiwan. In *Culture-bound syndromes, ethnopsychiatry, and alternative therapies,* ed. W. P. Lebra. Honolulu: University Press of Hawaii.

_____. 1978. Traditional and modern psychiatric care in Taiwan. In *Culture and healing in Asian societies,* ed. A. Kleinman, P. Kunstadter, E. R. Alexander, and J. L. Gale. Boston: G. K. Hall.

Tseng, W. S., and J. Hsu. 1969. Chinese culture, personality formation and mental illness. *International Journal of Social Psychiatry* 16:5–14.

Tsuei, J. 1978. Proposal for development of comprehensive rural care. Unpublished manuscript, University of Hawaii, International Health Program, School of Public Health.

Tung, T. M. 1972. The family and the management of mental health problems in Vietnam. In *Transcultural research in mental health,* ed. W. P. Lebra. Honolulu: University Press of Hawaii.

Ullmann, L. P., and L. Krasner. 1975. *A psychological approach to abnormal behavior.* Englewood Cliffs, N.J.: Prentice-Hall.

United Nations Educational, Scientific, and Cultural Organization (UNESCO). 1975. *Population education in Asia: A source book, no. 4: Population quality of life times.* Bangkok: UNESCO Regional Office for Education in Asia.

Uphoff, N. T., J. M. Cohen, and A. A. Goldsmith. 1979. Feasibility and application of rural development participation: A state-of-the-art paper. Ithaca, N.Y.: Rural Development Committee, Cornell University.

Van der Kraan, A. 1980. *Lombok: Conquest, colonization, and under development, 1870–1940.* Hong Kong: Heinemann Educational Books.

Visuthikosol, Y., and Sangun Suwanlert. 1976. Therapeutic community in the large mental hospital. Paper presented at the 3rd Regional Seminar on Psychotropic Medication, Bangkok.

———. 1977. Community and hospital services for Thai schizophrenics. Paper presented at the VI World Congress of Psychiatry, Honolulu.

Vreeland, N., G. B. Hurwitz, P. Just, P. W. Moeller, and R. S. Shinn. 1976. *Area handbook for the Philippines.* Washington: Government Printing Office.

Wagner, N. N., and E. S. Tan. 1968. Adolescence in Malaysia. *Jiwa* 1(4):24–30.

Waxler, N. E. 1974. Culture and mental illness: A social labeling perspective. *Journal of Nervous and Mental Disease* 159:379–399.

———. 1979. Is outcome for schizophrenia better in nonindustrialized societies? The case of Sri Lanka. *Journal of Nervous and Mental Disease* 167:144–158.

Weinberg, S. K. 1970. Culture and communication in disorder and psychotherapy in Ghana, West Africa. *Transcultural Psychiatric Research Review* 7:37–39.

Werner, D. 1981. The village health worker: Lackey or liberator? *World Health Forum* 2(1):46–68.

Westermeyer, J., and W. Hausman. 1974. Cross-cultural consultation for mental health planning. *International Journal of Social Psychiatry* 20:34–38.

White, G. M. 1982. The role of cultural explanations in 'somatization' and 'psychologization.' *Social Science and Medicine* 16:1519–1530.

Widjono, E. 1975. Drug dependence in Indonesia. *Jiwa* 2(2):57–62.

Wig, N. N. 1975. Training of psychiatrists. In *Mental health services in developing countries,* ed. T. A. Baasher, G. M. Carstairs, R. Giel, and F. Hassler. Geneva: World Health Organization.

Windle, C., R. D. Bass, and C. A. Taube. 1974. PR aside: Initial results from NIMH's service program evaluation studies. *American Journal of Community Psychology* 2:311–327.

Wing, J. K., J. L. T. Birley, J. E. Cooper, P. Graham, and A. P. Isaacs. 1967. The reliability of a procedure for measuring and classifying present psychiatric state. *British Journal of Psychiatry* 113:499.

Wintrob, R. M., and Y. K. Harvey. 1981. The self-awareness factor in intercultural psychotherapy: Some personal reflections. In *Counseling across cultures,* revised and expanded edition, ed. P. Pedersen et al. Honolulu: University Press of Hawaii.

Wittkower, E. D., and G. Dubreuil. 1973. Psychocultural stress in relation to mental illness. *Social Science and Medicine* 7:691–704.

Wittkower, E. D., and P. E. Termansen. 1968. Transcultural psychiatry. In *Modern perspectives in world psychiatry,* ed. J. G. Howells. London: Oliver and Boyd.

Wittkower, E. D., and H. Warnes. 1974. Cultural aspects of psychotherapy. *American Journal of Psychotherapy* 28:566–573.

Wolff, R. J. 1965. Modern medicine and traditional culture: Confrontation on the Malay peninsula. *Human Organization* 24:339–345.

Woolley, P. O. 1974. *Syncrisis: The dynamics of health.* Vol. 12: Thailand. Washington: Department of Health, Education and Welfare.

Woolley, P. O., C. A. Perry, L. J. Gangloff, and D. L. Larson. 1972. *Syncrisis: The dynamics of health.* Vol. 4: The Philippines. Washington: Department of Health, Education and Welfare.

World Bank. 1976. *The Philippines: Priorities and prospects for development.* A World Bank country economic report. Washington: World Bank.

World Federation for Mental Health. 1961. *Mental health in international perspective.* New York: World Federation for Mental Health.

World Health Organization. 1950. *First report.* WHO technical report series, no. 9. Geneva: WHO Expert Committee on Mental Health.

———. 1963. *Training of psychiatrists.* Twelfth report of the Expert Committee on Mental Health. WHO technical report series, no. 252. Geneva: World Health Organization.

———. 1964. Mental health research: A summary report of suggested priorities (mimeo). Geneva: WHO Scientific Group on Mental Health Research.

———. 1971. Mental disorders in old age. *WHO Chronicle* 25(12):558–566.

———. 1973. *Report of the International Pilot Study of Schizophrenia.* Geneva: World Health Organization.

———. 1975a. *Organization of mental health services in developing countries.* Sixteenth report of the WHO Expert Committee on Mental Health. WHO technical report series, no. 564. Geneva: World Health Organization.

———. 1975b. *Mental health services in developing countries.* Papers presented at a WHO seminar on the organization of mental health services, Addis Ababa, November 1973. Geneva: World Health Organization.

———. 1975c. *Seminar on the place of psychiatry in South-East Asia: Report on the Third Seminar.* Report no. 24. World Health Organization, South-East Asia Region, Mental Health Division.

———. 1975d. *Schizophrenia: A multinational study.* Public health papers no. 63. Geneva: World Health Organization Press.

———. 1976. *Report of the first meeting of the coordinating group for the mental health programme.* Geneva: World Health Organization.

———. 1977a. *Report of the second meeting of the coordinating group for the WHO mental health program.* Geneva: World Health Organization.

_____. 1977b. *Inter-country group meeting on mental health.* Group meeting report no. 1/7. World Health Organization, South-East Asia Region.

_____. 1977c. *Annual statistics, 1977,* vol. 3. Geneva: World Health Organization.

_____. 1977d. Mental health services in the countries of the WHO South-East Asia Region. Paper presented at the Inter-country Group Meeting on Mental Health. Group meeting report no. 1/7. World Health Organization, South-East Asia Regional Office.

_____. 1977e. Protecting populations at risk. *World Health,* December.

_____. 1978a. *Mental health in South-East Asia Region.* Report on an inter-country group meeting, 6–10 December, 1977, New Delhi, India. Report no. 38. World Health Organization, South-East Asia Region, Mental Health Division.

_____. 1978b. *The work of WHO, 1976–1977.* Biennial report of the director-general to the World Health Assembly and the United Nations. Geneva: World Health Organization.

_____. 1978c. *Official records.* Geneva: World Health Organization.

_____. 1978d. *Primary health care: Report of the International Conference on Primary Health Care, Alma-Ata, U.S.S.R.* Geneva: World Health Organization.

_____. 1980. *Sixth report of the world situation, 1973–1977.* Part I: Global analysis. Geneva: World Health Organization.

_____. 1981a. *Social dimensions of mental health.* Geneva: World Health Organization.

_____. 1981b. *Handbook of resolutions and decisions of the World Health Assembly and the Executive Board,* vol. 2, 4th ed., 1973–1980. Geneva: World Health Organization.

Wu, D. Y. H. 1982. Psychotherapy and emotion in traditional Chinese culture. In *Cultural conceptions of mental health and therapy,* ed. A. J. Marsella and G. M. White. Boston: Reidel.

Yap, P. M. 1968. Cultural bias in psychiatry and mental health. *New Zealand Journal of Psychiatry* 11:8–16.

Yeh, E. K. 1972. Paranoid manifestations among Chinese students studying abroad. In *Transcultural research in mental health,* ed. W. P. Lebra. Honolulu: University Press of Hawaii.

Young, A. 1976. Internalizing and externalizing medical belief systems: An Ethiopian example. *Social Science and Medicine* 10:147–156.

Author Index

Subject Index